BIOPSY INTERPRETATION SERIES

BIOPSY INTERPRETATION OF THE GASTROINTESTINAL TRACT MUCOSA

Volume 1: Non-neoplastic

Second Edition

BIOPSY INTERPRETATION SERIES

Series Editor: Jonathan I. Epstein, MD

Biopsy Interpretation: Pediatrics
Aliya N. Husain, 2014

Biopsy Interpretation of the Gastrointestinal Tract Mucosa, 2/e, Vol. 2: Neoplastic
Elizabeth A. Montgomery and Lysandra Voltaggio, 2012

Biopsy Interpretation of the Upper Aerodigestive Tract and Ear, 2/e
Edward B. Stelow and Stacey E. Mills, 2012

Biopsy Interpretation of the Breast, 2/e
Stuart J. Schnitt and Laura C. Collins, 2012

Biopsy Interpretation of the Lung
Saul Suster and Cesar Moran, 2012

Biopsy Interpretation of the Gastrointestinal Tract Mucosa, 2/e, Vol. 1: Non-Neoplastic
Elizabeth A. Montgomery and Lysandra Voltaggio, 2011

Biopsy Interpretation of the Central Nervous System
Matthew J. Schniederjan, Daniel J. Brat, 2011

Biopsy Interpretation of the Bladder, 2/e
Jonathan I. Epstein, Mahul B. Amin, and Victor E. Reuter, 2010

Biopsy Interpretation of Soft Tissue Tumors
Cyril Fisher, Elizabeth A. Montgomery, and Khin Thway, 2010

Biopsy Interpretation of the Thyroid
Scott L. Boerner and Sylvia L. Asa, 2009

Biopsy Interpretation of the Skin
A. Neil Crowson, Cynthia M. Magro, and Martin C. Mihm, 2009

Biopsy Interpretation: The Frozen Section
Jerome B. Taxy, Aliya N. Husain, and Anthony G. Montag, 2009

Biopsy Interpretation of the Uterine Cervix and Corpus
Anais Malpica, Michael T. Deavers and Elizabeth D. Euscher, 2009

Biopsy Interpretation of the Liver, 2/e
Stephen A. Geller and Lydia M. Petrovic, 2009

Biopsy Interpretation of the Breast
Stuart J. Schnitt and Laura C. Collins, 2008

Biopsy Interpretation of the Prostate, 4/e
Jonathan I. Epstein and George Netto, 2007

Biopsy Interpretation of the Upper Aerodigestive Tract and Ear
Edward B. Stelow and Stacey E. Mills, 2007

Biopsy Interpretation of the Gastrointestinal Tract Mucosa
Elizabeth A. Montgomery, 2005

BIOPSY INTERPRETATION SERIES

BIOPSY INTERPRETATION OF THE GASTROINTESTINAL TRACT MUCOSA

Volume 1: Non-neoplastic

Second Edition

Elizabeth A. Montgomery, M.D.
Professor of Pathology, Oncology, and Orthopedic Surgery
Department of Pathology
Johns Hopkins Medical Institutions
Baltimore, Maryland

Lysandra Voltaggio, M.D.
Assistant Professor of Pathology
Department of Pathology
George Washington University Hospital
Washington, District of Columbia

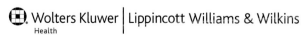
Wolters Kluwer | Lippincott Williams & Wilkins
Health
Philadelphia • Baltimore • New York • London
Buenos Aires • Hong Kong • Sydney • Tokyo

Senior Executive Editor: Jonathan W. Pine, Jr.
Product Manager: Marian A. Bellus
Vendor manager: Alicia Jackson
Senior Marketing Manager: Angela Panetta
Senior Manufacturing Manager: Benjamin Rivera
Creative Director: Doug Smock
Production Service: SPi Global

Printed in the People's Republic of China

Library of Congress Cataloging-in-Publication Data
Montgomery, Elizabeth (Elizabeth A.), 1958-
  Biopsy interpretation of the gastrointestinal tract mucosa. Volume 1, Non-neoplasia / Elizabeth A. Montgomery, Lysandra Voltaggio. – 2nd ed.
    p. ; cm. – (Biopsy interpretation series)
  Non-neoplasia
  Includes bibliographical references and index.
  ISBN 978-1-4511-0960-3 (alk. paper)
  1. Gastrointestinal mucosa–Biopsy. 2. Gastrointestinal system–Biopsy. 3. Gastrointestinal system–Cancer–Diagnosis. 4. Gastrointestinal system–Diseases–Diagnosis. I. Voltaggio, Lysandra. II. Title. III. Title: Non-neoplasia. IV. Series: Biopsy interpretation series.
  [DNLM: 1. Gastric Mucosa–pathology. 2. Gastrointestinal Neoplasms–diagnosis.   WI 301]
  RC804.B5M66   2012
  617.4'30597–dc23

                                                                                2011024590

Care has been taken to confirm the accuracy of the information presented and to describe generally accepted practices. However, the authors, editors, and publisher are not responsible for errors or omissions or for any consequences from application of the information in this book and make no warranty, expressed or implied, with respect to the currency, completeness, or accuracy of the contents of the publication. Application of the information in a particular situation remains the professional responsibility of the practitioner.

The authors, editors, and publisher have exerted every effort to ensure that drug selection and dosage set forth in this text are in accordance with current recommendations and practice at the time of publication. However, in view of ongoing research, changes in government regulations, and the constant flow of information relating to drug therapy and drug reactions, the reader is urged to check the package insert for each drug for any change in indications and dosage and for added warnings and precautions. This is particularly important when the recommended agent is a new or infrequently employed drug.

Some drugs and medical devices presented in the publication have Food and Drug Administration (FDA) clearance for limited use in restricted research settings. It is the responsibility of the health care provider to ascertain the FDA status of each drug or device planned for use in their clinical practice.

To purchase additional copies of this book, call our customer service department at (800) 638-3030 or fax orders to (301) 223-2320. International customers should call (301) 223-2300.

Visit Lippincott Williams & Wilkins on the Internet: at LWW.com. Lippincott Williams & Wilkins customer service representatives are available from 8:30 am to 6 pm, EST.

10 9 8 7 6 5 4 3 2

RRS1206

To my sister, Cassandra
Lysandra Voltaggio

To Sasha, Peter, Sean, and Jonathan
Elizabeth A. Montgomery

ACKNOWLEDGMENTS

We acknowledge our fellow pathologists, residents, and fellows for their help in identifying and collecting cases from their daily sign out, and gastroenterology colleagues for supplying wonderful endoscopic photos. We also want to thank Louise Bierig for her role as development editor, Marian Bellus for her role as a product manager, Anoop Kumar for overseeing production, and Jonathan Pine, Senior Executive Editor, for encouraging us to undertake this project. Finally, writing a book is a time-consuming process that often takes time away from other life duties, and we thank our husbands for their patience during this endeavor.

INTRODUCTION TO BIOPSY INTERPRETATION OF THE GASTROINTESTINAL TRACT MUCOSA

GENERAL FEATURES OF GASTROINTESTINAL BIOPSY INTERPRETATION

Probably the key principle of gastrointestinal (GI) biopsy interpretation is that the GI tract has a limited repertoire of responses to a host of injuries, and diagnosing the type of injury in any given biopsy often requires correlation with clinical and endoscopic information. On the other hand, normal biopsies may be obtained from symptomatic patients, and pathologists should not succumb to the temptation of reporting "inflammation," which serves little purpose since inflammatory cells are a normal constituent of the lamina propria. Other patients may be very ill from diseases that are mural or extraintestinal, and mucosal biopsies offer little information to the treating physician. However, some systemic diseases include GI tract manifestations that can be identified if a consistent, systematic approach is used.

When dealing with mucosal biopsies of the GI tract, it should also be noted that the vast majority of specimens display the mucosa and, rarely, a small amount of submucosa. This is especially significant when dealing with lesions that are usually limited to the submucosa and beyond (e.g., lipomas, inflammatory fibroid polyps). Both pathologists and clinicians should be aware that lack of histologic findings does not preclude underlying pathology. Of course, mucosal biopsies should not include muscularis propria. When they do, it is a good practice to contact the endoscopist and discuss the possibility of endoscopic perforation.

OVERVIEW COMMENTS ON THE GASTROINTESTINAL TRACT

Before a discussion of mucosal biopsies can ensue, it is worthwhile to review the overall microscopic anatomy of the GI tract in general.

The innermost layer of the GI tract is the mucosa, consisting of three components:

1. Epithelium (with protective, secretory, or absorptive properties).
2. Lamina propria. This is a loose connective tissue zone supporting the avascular epithelium. In the esophagus, stomach, and small bowel,

it is rich in lymphatics, whereas it is less so in the lower tract. This is of clinical significance in evaluating carcinomas because they can attain lymphatic access with minimal invasion in the upper tract. In the esophagus and stomach, there are few immune cells (lymphoid and plasma cells) in the lamina propria. Some observers regard the presence of plasma cells, no matter how few, as an abnormal finding in gastric biopsies. It is our practice to report inflammation in this site only when there is obvious expansion of the lamina propria (increased dot density) at low power. In the small bowel and colon, lamina propria lymphocytes and plasma cells are more abundant. Neutrophils do not belong in either the lamina propria or the epithelium. Eosinophils are a normal lamina propria constituent and can be particularly prominent in the right colon in the healthy patient. Mucosal biopsies from all sites must be assessed for prominence in the normal inflammatory components, which is usually identified at low power as an abnormal expansion of the lamina propria.

3. Muscularis mucosae. This is a slim double layer of smooth muscle separating the mucosa from the submucosa. It has an inner circular and outer longitudinal arrangement and, in this respect, it can be regarded as a miniaturized muscularis propria. In the normal state, colonic crypts extend down to the superior aspect of the muscularis mucosae. Crypt shortening (usually with basal plasmacytosis) is an indicator of chronic injury.

The mucosa is wholly distinct in the various regions of the GI tract. Note that the muscularis mucosae is considered a component of the mucosa for the purposes of staging invasive carcinomas.

The submucosa is composed of connective tissue and houses Meissner nerve plexus as well as large caliber vessels. The muscularis propria is the main wall of the GI tract and is composed of an inner circular and outer longitudinal layer of smooth muscle. Between these layers is Auerbach nerve plexus. The outermost component is either adventitia or serosa. The former lacks a mesothelial membrane lining.

Parasympathetic ganglion cells are found in the nerve plexi (both Meissner's and Auerbach's), but the submucosal Meissner plexi contain neuronal cell bodies of the intrinsic sympathetic nerve system that function on the local area of the gut. These are the neurons that have chemoreceptors and mechanoreceptors. They synapse on both other ganglion cells and muscle or secretory cells. Ganglion cells are not a normal component of the mucosa and, when identified, are indicative of chronic injury.

The pathologist should be aware of several points in the GI tract that lack a serosa, which is an issue mostly in staging tumors in resection specimens rather than in interpreting biopsies. Most are aware of the lack of serosal tissue in the esophagus, but several retroperitoneal portions of the colorectum share this feature. The posterior surfaces of the ascending and descending colon lack a peritoneal covering and are in direct contact with the retroperitoneum. In contrast, the anterior and lateral surfaces of the ascending and descending colon are covered by a visceral peritoneum (serosa). The transverse colon is entirely intraperitoneal and is supported on a long mesentery that is attached to the pancreas. The descending colon becomes the sigmoid colon at the origin of the mesosigmoid, and the sigmoid colon becomes the rectum at the termination of the sigmoid mesentery. The upper third of the rectum is covered by peritoneum on the front and both sides. The middle third is covered by peritoneum only on the anterior surface. The lower third (also known as the rectum or rectal ampulla) has no peritoneal covering.

In assessing any biopsy from the GI tract, the pathologist should note the gender, age, race/ethnicity (if known), pertinent endoscopic findings, and the site of the biopsy. These pieces of information are all useful in directing interpretation. For example, celiac disease, found in about 1% of all Americans, is virtually never detected in Southeast Asians (Chinese, Korean, and Japanese persons). Collagenous colitis is typically a disease of middle-aged women with a long-standing history of watery diarrhea and a normal colonoscopy. Biopsies from the left colon in a patient with collagenous colitis may be normal, and the pathologist should recommend sampling of the ascending colon if microscopic colitis is a clinical concern. Assessments of all biopsies from infants should include a systematic review of each compartment of the tissue. For example, the epithelial surface is reviewed with an eye toward malabsorptive diseases (such as microvillus inclusion disease in the small intestine), the lamina propria is scanned for the presence of plasma cells (their lack suggests common variable immunodeficiency), and the muscularis mucosae is assessed for eosinophils (which should be absent in the muscularis mucosae).

The type of mucosa in the biopsy is compared to the recorded biopsy site to address metaplasias (or "switched" specimens). For example, gastric biopsies labeled "body" that look microscopically like inflamed antrum should raise suspicion for autoimmune metaplastic atrophic gastritis (AMAG), a condition usually encountered in elderly women of any race. Also, normal architectural structures are noted, such as villous contours of the small intestine. Before making a diagnosis, the features are compared to the history to assure that the interpretation "makes sense" in light of the clinical information. If the information is scant but required or inconsistent with the microscopic findings, this too must be addressed.

Polyps and neoplasms present their own issues but, as for nonneoplastic samples, correlation with history and endoscopic findings often supplies clues in small samples. For example, when interpreting gastric polyps, attention to the appearance of biopsies from adjoining flat mucosa can offer diagnostic information. Furthermore, when the pathologist encounters neoplasms in the small bowel, it is important to recall that carcinomas from other sites can "colonize" the small mucosa and mimic an *in situ* component.

With a consistent systematic approach, the pathologist interpreting gastrointestinal biopsies can provide important information that can occasionally be lifesaving (in certain instances of ischemic disease) and can often be reassuring to the ever-increasing group of patients undergoing GI tract mucosal biopsies. Although it is impossible to cover every conceivable biopsy finding, it is hoped that these slim manuals will provide useful advice on clues that can be found if they are sought.

Elizabeth A. Montgomery, MD
Lysandra Voltaggio, MD

CONTENTS

BIOPSY INTERPRETATION OF THE GASTROINTESTINAL TRACT MUCOSA

Volume 1: Non-neoplastic

Second Edition

1

ESOPHAGUS

The esophagus is about 25 cm and consists of cervical or upper, mid, and lower thoracic portions. It is physiologically constricted in several spots by the cricoid cartilage, aortic arch, left atrium, and diaphragm. Of course, the esophagus is unique in having skeletal muscle (and thus voluntary muscle) surrounding the upper portions. The vagus provides its parasympathetic innervation, whereas the sympathetic innervation is by the cervical and paravertebral ganglia.

Histologically, the squamous mucosa is heaped up in folds. It has abundant turnover and the mitotically active basal layer matures into a surface containing tonofilaments. The superficial layers contain glycogen, whereas the lower layers (the basal layer and a few layers closer to the surface) do not. Beneath is the lamina propria, which contains vascular access and elastic fibers. The muscularis mucosae is a single slender layer in the esophagus, which easily thickens or even duplicates (1,2) when there has been damage to the epithelium (Fig. 1.1). Because of this feature, it is possible to mistake esophageal lamina propria for submucosa and, in turn, mistake muscularis mucosae for muscularis propria, a pitfall in biopsy and endoscopic mucosal resection (EMR) interpretation. There are mucus-producing glands in the submucosa of the esophagus to lubricate the passage of food (Fig. 1.2). These, too, are sometimes a source of diagnostic errors, particularly when assessing mucin stains. These glands normally display alcianophilia (blue color) on Alcian blue (AB) stains (Fig. 1.3). They can also occasionally undergo oncocytic change similar to that seen in salivary glands (Fig. 1.4, e-Figs. 1.1–1.5).

In our institution, each esophageal biopsy is stained with both hematoxylin and eosin (H&E) and periodic acid-Schiff/Alcian blue (PAS/AB) (at pH = 2.5). However, we regard this staining as optional and believe any given laboratory should perform such staining in an algorithm that best supports local laboratory specimen volume and practice patterns. Large numbers of patients are evaluated for Barrett esophagus at our institution, and, because we have sufficient numbers of immunosuppressed patients, it is best to assess biopsies for fungal organisms at the time of initial slide review. Thus, it is most efficient in our practice to perform "automatic" PAS/AB testing.

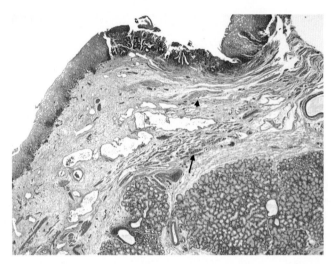

FIGURE 1.1 **Endoscopic mucosal resection showing duplication of the muscularis mucosae.** The original, thicker mucosae is seen below (*arrow*) and a second, more delicate muscle layer is present superficially (*arrowhead*). Mesenchymal tissue between the two layers corresponds to lamina propria, not submucosa. This particular case was an EMR for high-grade dysplasia in Barrett esophagus but any kind of chronic injury can induce these changes.

When scanning squamous mucosa from esophageal biopsies at low magnification, there are a few features to note:

1. Is there parakeratosis? Foci of parakeratosis are likely to harbor Candida sp. and should be examined for this (Figs. 1.5 and 1.6)

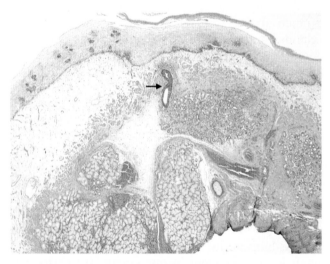

FIGURE 1.2 **Esophageal submucosal glands, endoscopic mucosal resection (EMR).** These mucous-producing glands lubricate the passage of food. An esophageal duct is also present (*arrow*).

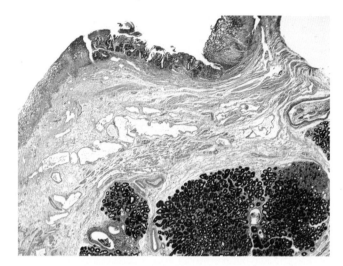

FIGURE 1.3 **Esophageal submucosal glands, Alcian blue/PAS stain, endoscopic mucosal resection (EMR).** Submucosal glands display alcianophilic (blue) staining with this stain.

2. Is the mucosa hyperplastic? If it is hyperplastic with clear cell features, it is worth considering glycogenic acanthosis. If it is hyperplastic and reparative appearing, the lamina propria might occasionally harbor a granular cell tumor.
3. Is there an ulcer? Ulcers are, of course, where infectious agents should be sought.

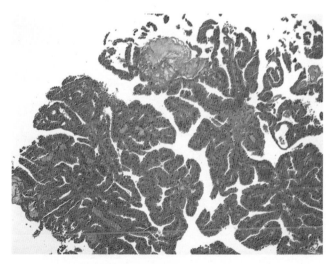

FIGURE 1.4 **Esophageal submucosal glands showing oncocytic change.** The appearance is similar to the oncocytic change seen in salivary glands.

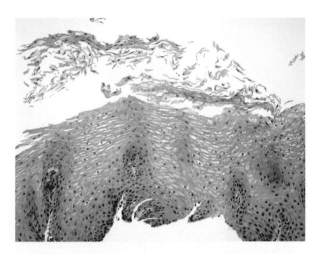

FIGURE 1.5 **Esophageal parakeratosis.** Foci of parakeratosis are likely to harbor *Candida* sp. and should be examined for this even in the absence of inflammation.

Typically, endoscopists record the location of tissue in the esophagus as a measurement (in centimeters) from the incisors. As such, the position of the gastroesophageal (GE) junction is a function of the patient's height: it is often about 35 cm from the incisors in women and 40 cm from the incisors in men. Obviously, these figures differ for tall women or short men, but knowing the location of the biopsy in the esophagus can be helpful when considering interpretations of Barrett esophagus, allergic versus reflux esophagitis, or "inlet patch."

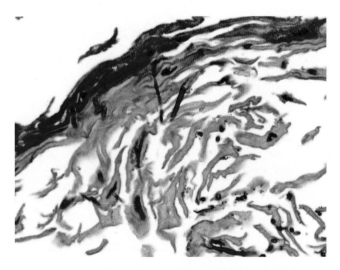

FIGURE 1.6 **Esophageal candidiasis.** Same case as Figure 1.5 stained with a PAS/AB stain showing fungal pseudohyphae within the parakeratotic layer.

INLET PATCH (CERVICAL GASTRIC HETEROTOPIA)

If an esophageal biopsy site is designated as "15 to 20 cm," has a segment of normal squamous esophagus distally, and displays gastric type mucosa, it is probably from an inlet patch. Inlet patches are believed to be embryologic vestiges from early gestation when the esophagus is lined by columnar epithelium. They are found in about 1% of patients undergoing upper endoscopy, when assessed retrospectively through biopsy records. Incidences of up to 10% are recorded (3,4), and they are found in the cervical esophagus and are generally asymptomatic. However, there are occasional complications in the form of local injury (webs, strictures, ulcers, and fistulas) that can result in symptoms (pain and dysphagia). Rarely do carcinomas develop in inlet patches.

Inlet patches may be small, between 0.2 and 0.3 cm and up to about 4 cm. They typically consist of oxyntic type mucosa (containing parietal cells), but a transitional or cardiac pattern (lacking oxyntic glands and negative for gastrin on immunohistochemistry) may also be found (Fig. 1.7, e-Fig. 1.6). Lesions are often inflamed and may occasionally show *Helicobacter pylori*. Intestinal metaplasia in inlet patches is occasionally found. Several studies have explored a link between inlet patches and Barrett esophagus, and indeed these conditions are found together more than coincidence would suggest. Of course, some studies are difficult to interpret since criteria for Barrett esophagus have changed with the recent requirement for intestinal metaplasia to be confirmed before diagnosing lesions as Barrett

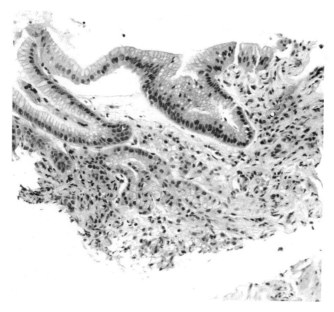

FIGURE 1.7 **Inlet patch.** This biopsy was obtained from 16 cm (from the incisors) and consists of gastric cardiac type mucosa.

esophagus (see Volume 2 for a discussion of Barrett esophagus). Pancreatic tissue may also be a component of "inlet patch."

Gastric heterotopia, of course, is not unique to the esophagus and has been identified in the tongue, duodenum, jejunum, gallbladder, and rectum. However, in some of these sites and in the duodenal bulb in particular, it may be impossible to separate heterotopia from metaplasia. Certainly, it is impossible to do so in the distal esophagus.

PANCREATIC ACINAR CELL METAPLASIA/HETEROTOPIA

Pancreatic acinar cells, or even nodules of pancreatic ductal structures accompanied by a few acinar cells, are often noted on biopsies of the distal esophagus, but typically those from the GE junction. In our institution, these are often found in patients undergoing biopsy evaluation of reflux disease, but are also found commonly in patients who are asymptomatic (80,81). Such foci do not seem to undergo a dysplasia–carcinoma sequence and are probably best regarded as an incidental finding (Fig. 1.8, e-Figs. 1.7

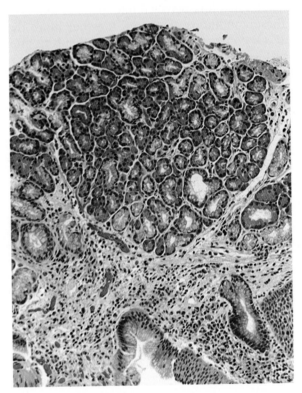

FIGURE 1.8 **Pancreatic acinar cell metaplasia/heterotopia.** Acinar cells or nodules of pancreatic ductal structures with or without acinar cells are not infrequent on biopsies from the distal esophagus.

and 1.8). In our institution, we are in the habit of referring to these foci as "pancreatic acinar cell metaplasia," although they probably are heterotopic.

Foci of pancreatic acinar cell metaplasia/heterotopia superficially resemble foci of gastric oxyntic mucosa, but on closer inspection, cells in the nests contain larger, more fuscinophilic granules than those in parietal cells. On PAS/AB staining, they may display alcianophilia, but, of course, lack goblet cell morphology.

Occasionally, ciliated cell heterotopia (or possibly metaplasia) (e-Fig. 1.9) or oncocytic change of submucosal glands (Fig. 1.4, e-Figs. 1.1–1.5) is found in the esophagus. These are presumably incidental findings.

HETEROTOPIC SEBACEOUS GLANDS

Esophageal sebaceous gland heterotopia is an extremely rare occurrence initially reported as an incidental finding in 4 out of 200 autopsies in 1962 by De La Pava and Pickren (5). Since then, this benign incidental finding has been encountered in the literature predominantly in the form of case reports, many in association with heartburn sensation, abdominal pain, and gastroduodenal peptic ulcer (5–17). Endoscopically these lesions appear as slightly raised, irregular, yellow nodules or plaques that can be solitary or multiple, measuring anywhere from a few millimeters up to 2 cm in greatest dimension. Microscopic exam reveals lobules composed of large, polygonal, clear cells with vacuolated cytoplasm located within the lamina propria surrounded by a chronic inflammatory infiltrate without hair follicles (Fig. 1.9, e-Figs. 1.10 and 1.11). A squamous-lined duct with a granular layer that connects the lobule to the luminal surface may

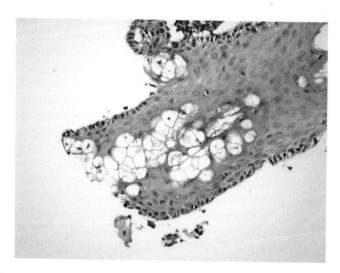

FIGURE 1.9 **Heterotopic sebaceous glands.** Large, polygonal, clear cells with vacuolated cytoplasm are seen here within the squamous epithelium.

or may not be present. Associated hair follicles or other dermal append-
ages have not been observed.

The view that sebaceous heterotopia represents a congenital anomaly
is challenged by the fact that the esophagus is embryologically derived from
the endoderm, while sebaceous glands are ectodermal structures. In addition, to the date of this writing no cases have been reported in pediatric
patients, arguing for a metaplastic process. Nakanishi et al. (12) were able
to identify small areas of sebaceous differentiation arising from globular
nests extending downward from the basal cell layer in an esophagectomy
specimen with concomitant squamous cell carcinoma, Barrett mucosa,
and extensive sebaceous heterotopia. The same authors found that these
foci, along with areas of established sebaceous glands, were immunoreactive only for cytokeratin (14), paralleling the pattern of immunoreactivity
of the normal control epidermis, sebaceous glands, and esophageal basal
layer. Whether congenital or metaplastic, esophageal sebaceous glands are
incidental, benign, inconsequential, and require no patient follow-up.

ESOPHAGEAL MELANOCYTOSIS/MELANOSIS

Esophageal melanocytosis/melanosis is a rare condition of middle aged
adults, with a gender ratio of about 2:1 in favor of men (18). It was first
described in 1963 (19) by De La Pava, who had also noted sebaceous
heterotopia (5). It may be more common in individuals with pigmented
skin than in those with pale skin since the largest series is from India (20)
but, regardless, there are only on the order of 50 reported cases. The terms
"melanocytosis" and "melanosis" are both used in the literature. These
lesions are typically encountered in the lower or middle third of the esophagus where they present as blue to black mucosal macules. In fact, microscopic foci of melanocytosis were detected in about 8% of esophagectomy
samples in one Japanese study (21) whereas only about 2% of esophagi
had macroscopically identifiable melanocytic patches at endoscopy in an
Indian study (20).

When seen on biopsies, esophageal melanocytosis is characterized
by the presence of increased numbers of melanocytes in the basal layer of
esophageal squamous epithelium and an increased quantity of melanin in
esophageal mucosa. On H&E staining the melanocytes are pigment-laden
dendritic cells (Fig. 1.10, e-Figs. 1.12–1.14). Like their cutaneous counterparts, basal melanocytes of the esophagus lack desmosomes and tonofilaments but possess long dendritic cytoplasmic processes that extend between
the keratinocytes, often passing through several layers of cells. The nuclei are
smaller and slightly more hyperchromatic than the nuclei of adjacent keratinocytes. Cells have uniform chromatin and indented nuclear contour. The
nucleoli are inconspicuous. These cells are positive for melanocytic markers,
such as S100 protein, Melan-A, and HMB-45. The underlying lamina propria contains macrophages laden with coarse brownish black pigment on
H&E-stained slides. In most cases, the melanocytes do not exhibit nuclear

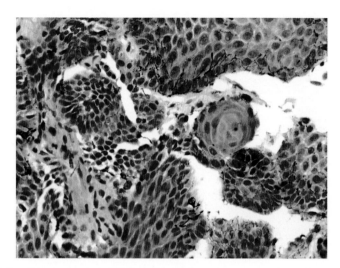

FIGURE 1.10 **Esophageal melanocytosis/melanosis.** Increased numbers of melano-cytes are seen here within the basal layer. Long dendritic cytoplasmic processes extend between the squamous epithelial cells passing through several layers of cells. The nuclei are smaller than the nuclei of adjacent keratinocytes.

or cellular atypia. The overlying squamous epithelium may exhibit reactive basal hyperplasia, acanthosis, and hyperkeratosis but appears mature.

Melanocytosis itself is benign, although there are reports of its associa-tion with melanoma (22–24). However, we are unaware of reports of docu-mented progression from esophageal melanocytosis to esophageal melanoma.

GLYCOGENIC ACANTHOSIS

Glycogenic acanthosis of the esophagus is a common benign entity (25–35) found in up to 15% of esophagi (34), or probably closer to 3% of cases overall (35). It is characterized by single or multifocal plaques of hyperplas-tic squamous epithelium with abundant intracellular glycogen deposits. At esophagoscopy, or on autopsy specimens, these lesions appear as slightly raised, grey–white plaques, which are usually 2 to 10 mm in diameter and may be confluent. They cause a finely nodular or cobblestone mucosal pat-tern, evident on double-contrast views of the well-distended esophagus. The findings are not associated with mucosal ulcerations, luminal narrowing, or mobility disturbance, although some patients may have coexistent hiatal hernia and GE reflux (35). An association with celiac disease has been sug-gested in pediatric patients (36). There is also an association with Cowden disease, especially when diffuse (37–40). In this last setting glycogenic acanthosis can also be seen in the gingival or labial mucosa and similar macroscopic lesions have been reported in the trachea (41,42). However, glycogenic acanthosis does not appear to be linked with diabetes and it does not regress with acid suppression when associated with reflux disease (35).

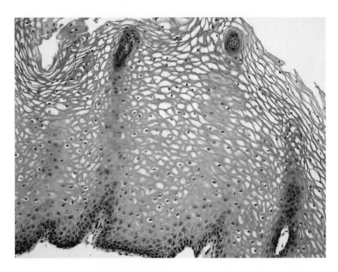

FIGURE 1.11 **Glycogenic acanthosis.** Observe the cleared (glycogen-containing) cells. The endoscopist noted a white thickened area.

In one Japanese study, it was commonly found in adjacent nonneoplastic mucosa in patients with squamous cell carcinoma of the esophagus (43).

In our own material, glycogenic acanthosis has been essentially an incidental finding at routine endoscopy, in which the endoscopist notes a white plaque. A biopsy displays prominent intraepithelial glycogen extending to within one cell layer of the basement membrane, with just a single row (or two) of basal cells between the glycogenized squamous cells and the basement membrane (Fig. 1.11, e-Figs. 1.15 and 1.16). For the endoscopist, the differential diagnosis is with *Candida esophagitis*, whereas pathologists often do not notice glycogenic acanthosis. Probably the most important reason for the pathologist to diagnose patients with glycogenic acanthosis is to provide the endoscopist with an explanation for the abnormal gross appearance of the biopsied focus!

ESOPHAGEAL LEUKOPLAKIA

Leukoplakia refers to a persistent white patch usually encountered in the buccal mucosa that corresponds histologically to areas of hyperkeratosis. Corresponding esophageal lesions are rarely encountered and are sporadically mentioned in the literature (44–46). The endoscopist sees plaques of white, thickened mucosa, or red areas, which are typically more prominent toward the distal third of the esophagus. Biopsies of the affected areas show epithelial hyperplasia and parakeratosis often with an accompanying inflammatory reaction with or without areas of sharp demarcation between a thick basal layer, an acanthotic midzone with vacuolated cells, and a third, superficial, parakeratotic layer (Fig. 1.12, e-Figs. 1.17–1.20) (44). The

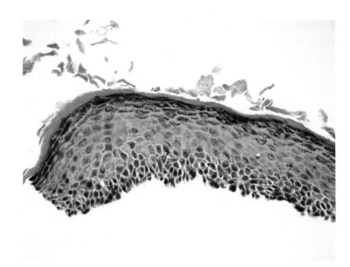

FIGURE 1.12 **Esophageal leukoplakia.** This particular case shows prominent hyperkeratosis and hypergranulosis.

inciting factor for the development of leukoplakia is not clear but chronic irritation seems to play a role as many of the reported cases share esophageal dysmotility with distal constriction and stasis as a common bond (44–46). In fact, extensive areas of leukoplakia have been described in patients with scleroderma and distal esophageal stenosis (45). These patients are known to suffer from dysmotility due to esophageal wall fibrosis.

Whether esophageal leukoplakia represents a preneoplastic lesion is not entirely clear. However, recent work by Taggart et al. (47) suggests an association between esophageal hyperkeratosis and squamous dysplasia/carcinoma in patients without Barrett mucosa. Briefly, this group examined 87 hyperkeratotic esophageal biopsies from 42 patients. Those who underwent endoscopy for reasons other than surveillance for Barrett esophagus had significantly greater history of alcohol consumption, head and neck pathology (squamous carcinoma/dysplasia, leukoplakia, and lichen planus), esophageal squamous dysplasia, and/or squamous carcinoma when compared to those surveyed due to Barrett esophagus (47). Thus it seems that, at least in the non-Barrett setting, esophageal leukoplakia may parallel its oropharyngeal counterpart in terms of risk factors and preneoplastic potential. When we diagnose this condition, we suggest that our gastroenterology colleagues initiate a surveillance program for the patient but this is, unfortunately, not based on high-quality data.

Findings in Mechanical Disorders

WEBS AND RINGS. Endoscopically and radiologically, webs and rings are ledges of mucosa that protrude into the lumen. They are commonly called webs when found in the proximal esophagus and called Schatzki rings when discovered in the distal esophagus or GE junction. Plummer-Vinson syndrome refers to an upper esophageal web, typically in a middle-aged or older woman associated with iron deficiency anemia, glossitis, and cheilosis. The syndrome increases the risk of squamous cell carcinoma in the postcricoid esophagus.

However, when mucosal biopsies are obtained from such structures, there are few pathologic findings. There may be parakeratosis, a response to the process of food passing over the protuberant ring or the constricted segment, and erosions may appear where retained food presses on the static segment proximal to the attenuated lumen. Finding parakeratosis at low magnification is always a signal to check the mucosa for *Candida*, something readily accomplished in our institution since all cases are automatically stained with PAS/AB (Figs. 1.5 and 1.6).

ACHALASIA. Achalasia is a degenerative disorder of the intraesophageal nerves or of the extraesophageal nerves that serve the esophagus, including the vagus nerve. Achalasia is most often primary (idiopathic) but can be secondary to diseases such as Chagas disease (from *Trypanosoma cruzi*), polio, diabetic neuropathy, amyloidosis, etc. Achalasia causes (i) lack of peristalsis, (ii) incomplete relaxation of the lower esophageal sphincter (LES) during swallowing, and (iii) increased resting tone of the LES. There is, therefore, dilatation of the esophagus above the LES. In some, but not all, cases, there are secondary changes to the mucosa including inflammation or even ulcerations, which can become superinfected by *Candida*. Patients classically present with dysphagia. There is a small (5%) risk of esophageal squamous cell carcinoma.

REFLUX DISEASE

In the United States, GE reflux disease (GERD) is the costliest gastrointestinal (GI) disorder and the most common physician diagnosis for GI disorders in outpatient clinic visits (48). A 2002 estimate of the direct cost of GERD was over $9 billion (49). Not surprisingly, many patients undergo endoscopic biopsies in the course of evaluation for reflux symptoms. Findings in these biopsies can range anywhere from "classic" reflux changes (basal cell hyperplasia, elongation of vascular papillae, and intraepithelial eosinophils) to ulcers, intraepithelial lymphocytosis (which correlates poorly with pH studies), or "balloon" cells (which appear distended and have pale abundant pink cytoplasm) (e-Figs. 1.21–1.27).

The classic view on GERD is that it is a reflection of acid reflux. However, we have become increasingly aware that the refluxed material, i.e., the contents of the stomach, consists of duodenal contents mixed with gastric secretions. These stomach contents probably contain a higher percentage of duodenal "juice" than in the past because modern patients often take PPIs and have the benefit of acid suppression (which reduces the volume of gastric secretions and concentrates the secretions refluxed into the stomach from the duodenum). The question in this proton pump era is, "Are the effects of duodenal reflux more severe than those of acid reflux?" Since it is impossible to separate the effects of gastric acid from bile reflux in humans, which can be done in animals (50,51), this question can only be answered indirectly. At the time when Norman Barrett was writing about the condition that now bears his name (52,53), the complications of reflux were severe erosive esophagitis and debilitating stricture formation. But now that ulcers are readily healed by PPIs, the objective is to detect early neoplasia because reflux has been shown as a preneoplastic condition (54).

On epidemiologic grounds, bile is a carcinogen. There are many examples of this phenomenon, but some are especially worth reiterating. For example, patients who have had a cholecystectomy (and who thus secrete constant low levels of bile rather than controlled pulses that accompany boluses of food) have a statistically significant increment in their risk of upper GI (UGI) tract carcinomas (55). Patients who are status post Billroth operations are prone to laryngeal carcinogenesis as well (56). But if the duodenum is diverted in patients who already have had ample injury to the esophagus (e.g., Barrett esophagus with damage to the LES), the risk of progression to dysplasia/carcinoma is reduced (57). In fact, regression of Barrett esophagus in obese patients following Roux-en-Y gastric bypass has been documented (58,59). Similarly, diverting the duodenum in patients who already have low-grade dysplasia may forestall progression to invasive carcinoma (57).

In studying patterns of injury to the esophagus, or any part of the GI tract, it is difficult to separate the cause of the damage when the GI tract has a limited repertoire of responses to a wide variety of insults. For example, we have seen patients with extensive atrophic gastritis (presuming little acid output, if any) whose esophageal biopsies display features identical to those of acid reflux. However, based on the available epidemiologic evidence, it seems likely that the initial injuries may be a result of acid but that carcinogenic bile reflux informs the cycles of repair. Another possibility is that esophageal mucosal injury stems from the combination of bile juices and acidic gastric contents. There is evidence that shows that bile acids combined with an acidic medium (but not either one alone) induces oxidative stress and DNA damage in *ex vivo* Barrett tissue as well as in esophageal cell lines (60). The preneoplastic and neoplastic states that supervene (Barrett esophagus and esophageal carcinoma) are further discussed in Volume 2.

For practical purposes, reflux esophagitis (GERD) is the most common cause of esophagitis. Although most prevalent in adult Caucasian males, reflux esophagitis can occur in both men and women of all races, and even in infants and children.

GERD is caused by reflux of gastric contents into the esophagus, most prominently from reflux of gastric acid and pepsin. However, reflux of alkaline bile and pancreatic secretions (moving from the duodenum into the stomach and then into the esophagus) is increasingly recognized as a contributing factor to esophageal injury in GERD.

Predisposing factors include decreased tone of the LES from alcohol, medications, hypothyroidism, pregnancy, scleroderma, etc.; interference with the function of a normal LES from nasogastric tubes; hiatal hernia; decreased clearance of refluxed material, as in achalasia; and delayed gastric emptying with accumulation of gastric secretions, as in diabetes. Obesity exacerbates all of the aforementioned and is associated with reflux disease. In many patients, no clear predisposing cause is identified.

Reflux esophagitis is an example of an "-itis" that often lacks a prominent component of inflammation. The pathology reflects injury to the squamous epithelium, followed by attempts of the epithelium to regenerate (Figs. 1.13–1.15). Mild features of cellular injury include balloon cells (squamous cells with ballooned cytoplasm from accumulation of plasma proteins) and vascular lakes (dilated small blood vessels in the mucosa, not areas of hemorrhage, which often are seen endoscopically as erythema or redness). Severe injury can result in mucosal sloughing with erosions or ulcers. Regenerative changes include hyperplasia of the basal zone >15% to 20% of the epithelial thickness. The upper limit of the basal cell layer can be defined as the level above which the nuclei are separated by a distance greater than the nuclear diameter (61). There is elongation of the vascular papillae to greater than two-thirds of the epithelial thickness. Inflammation is typically mild and includes scattered eosinophils. Less commonly, scattered neutrophils are present and can be more prominent in cases with more severe injury, including erosions and ulcers. Parakeratosis can be a component as well (but foci of parakeratosis should still be screened for

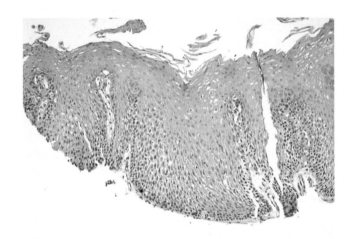

FIGURE 1.13 **Reflux esophagitis.** Basal cell hyperplasia and elongation of the vascular papillae to greater than two-thirds of the epithelial thickness are present. Note scattered eosinophils.

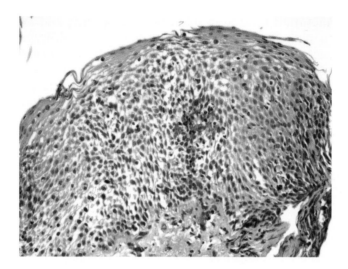

FIGURE 1.14 **Reflux esophagitis.** This higher power image shows basal cell hyperplasia with intercellular edema, scattered eosinophils, and scattered eosinophils.

fungal organisms). Fairly reproducible criteria that have been established by Fiocca et al. (61) as abnormal and associated with clinical reflux include

   a. Thickened basal layer (>15% or 5 to 6 layers)
   b. Increased papillary length (>50% of the squamous thickness)
   c. Intraepithelial eosinophils, neutrophils (>1 to 2 cells/40× field)
   d. Intraepithelial mononuclear cells (>10/40× field)
   e. Dilated/widened intercellular spaces (which may appear as "bubbles" or "ladders")

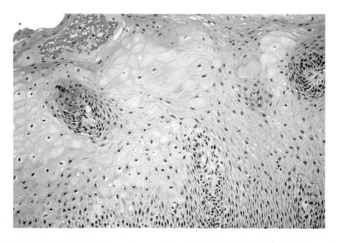

FIGURE 1.15 **Reflux esophagitis.** This particular case shows balloon cells as a result of accumulation of plasma proteins, typically an early change in patients with reflux.

It is important to keep in mind that the severity and extent of the histologic changes that we see on a biopsy do not necessarily correlate well with the severity of the patient's symptoms (heartburn or pyrosis).

Severe complications of GERD are unusual. Complications include development of an ulcer, bleeding from an ulcer, and a stricture formation resulting from scarring, due to deep injury. The complication of Barrett esophagus occurs in approximately 10% of patients with symptomatic reflux.

INJURY DUE TO CHEMICAL OR PHYSICAL AGENTS AND MEDICATIONS

Iron

In our patient population, mucosal iron (ferrous sulfate) is found in about 1% of patients undergoing upper tract endoscopic biopsies. Iron is well recognized for its capacity to cause corrosive injury in the esophagus and, in a hospital population, it is not uncommon to find iron associated with an esophageal ulcer or erosion. While it can be argued that such a phenomenon results from a prior injury in which an iron tablet became embedded, the corrosive and toxic nature of iron itself suggests that just having the pill lodge in the esophagus caused the injury. Either way, it is worth learning to recognize "iron pill esophagitis," and to encourage the patient to ingest the medication in a crushed form with soft food (such as applesauce or yogurt). Using our material at The Johns Hopkins Hospital, where we have a busy endoscopy service, Abraham et al. (62) studied the clinical and histologic features of 36 UGI tract biopsies from 33 patients (24 gastric, 9 esophageal, 1 GE junction, and 2 duodenal) containing characteristic brown crystalline iron material, and evaluated the amount and tissue distribution of the iron. They also investigated the prevalence of iron-associated mucosal injury on the endoscopic examinations. The biopsies typically displayed luminal crystalline iron adjacent to the surface epithelium, or admixed with luminal fibrinoinflammatory exudates (Fig. 1.16, e-Figs. 1.28–1.32). Most biopsies (83%) showed crystalline iron deposition in the lamina propria covered by an intact epithelium, subjacent to small superficial erosions, or admixed with granulation tissue. Three biopsies (8%) demonstrated iron-containing thrombi in mucosal blood vessels. Erosive or ulcerative mucosal injury was present in the majority of biopsies (83%). The amount of iron accumulation in tissue with mucosal injury was greater than in tissue without mucosal injury. Iron medication (usually ferrous sulfate) was confirmed in 25 of 33 patients (76%). However, as an argument for iron-causing injury as a secondary event, half of the patients (17 of 33, 51%) also had underlying infectious, mechanical, toxic, or systemic medical conditions that could have initiated or exacerbated tissue injury.

In order not to miss iron injury in the esophagus (or stomach for that matter), it is worthwhile to pay attention to material in ulcer beds.

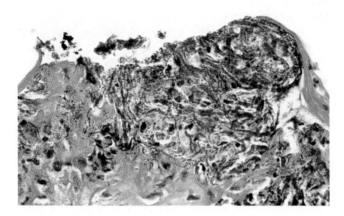

FIGURE 1.16 **Iron pill esophagitis.** Iron appears as crystalline brown-green material on surface epithelium.

On H&E stains, the oxidized iron has a readily recognizable bluish brown color that can be highlighted with iron stain. The same stain can highlight iron embedded in cells deep to the ulcer that is inapparent on H&E stain. Whereas in the stomach iron must be distinguished from mucosal calcinosis, since calcinosis is seldom encountered in the esophagus, esophageal iron-associated injury can be diagnosed without special stains.

Kayexalate

The use of kayexalate (sodium polystyrene sulfonate) for the management of hyperkalemia was approved for use in the United States in 1975. Kayexalate is a cation-exchange resin that can be instilled into the lower GI tract, as an enema preparation, or into the UGI tract, either orally or by nasogastric tube. When administered orally or by nasogastric tube, sodium cations are released from the resin and exchanged for hydrogen ions in the acidic milieu of the stomach. As the resin passes through the intestines, hydrogen is exchanged for potassium, which is then eliminated in the feces along with the remainder of the altered resin, thereby lowering the serum potassium concentration.

In the early use of kayexalate, the resin was typically administered as a suspension in water. Although it was generally well tolerated, some patients were reported to develop gastric and bowel opacifications as a result of concretions of crystalline resin. Therefore, it became increasingly popular to administer kayexalate in a suspension with hypertonic sorbitol. This solution reduces both the frequency of kayexalate bezoar formation and colonic impaction by promoting an osmotic diarrhea. In 1987, Lillemoe et al. (63) reported five uremic patients who developed colonic necrosis temporally associated with the use of kayexalate in sorbitol, which contributed to the death of four of the five patients. That study also provided experimental evidence implicating sorbitol as the agent responsible for colonic necrosis in a rat model.

It has subsequently become apparent that kayexalate also can be associated with severe mucosal injury in the UGI tract, and a series of such cases has been reported by Abraham et al. (64). In most instances, kayexalate is easy to recognize in endoscopic biopsies and the clinician can be alerted if there is associated ischemic GI tract disease or erosive lesions

Kayexalate crystals are lightly basophilic on H&E stain (Figs. 1.17 and 1.18, e-Fig. 1.33), red on PAS/AB and acid-fast stains, and blue on Diff-Quik staining (e-Figs. 1.34–1.36). However, occasionally they seem to absorb bile and can thus be bile pigmented, although this feature is encountered in kayexalate in intestinal biopsies and not in esophageal biopsies. The crystals display a characteristic mosaic pattern that resembles fish scales. The pattern is faintly present in many cases on routine H&E stain, but is better demonstrated on acid-fast, PAS/AB, and Diff-Quik stains. It is this mosaic pattern that distinguishes kayexalate crystals from histologically similar cholestyramine crystals. Kayexalate crystals are refractile but not polarizable.

Taxol Effect, Colchicine Toxicity

Taxol, an antineoplastic agent with a novel mechanism of action, can be associated with striking mitotic arrest associated with epithelial necrosis and ulceration of the esophagus (Figs. 1.19 and 1.20, e-Figs. 1.37–1.39). As a class of drug, taxane chemotherapeutic agents are commonly used to treat malignancies of the esophagus, breast, and lung. Paclitaxel (Taxol) chemotherapy has been associated with dramatic GI mucosal changes, accompanied by an increase in apoptosis (65). Taxol, as reviewed by Rowinsky et al. (66), induces these GI mucosal changes by binding to microtubules, thus promoting polymerization and inhibiting depolymerization. Electron

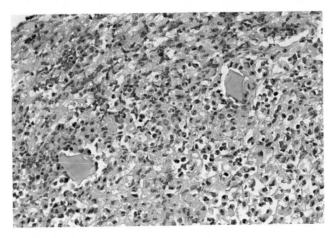

FIGURE 1.17 **Kayexalate injury.** Kayexalate crystals are intimately associated with an ulcer bed.

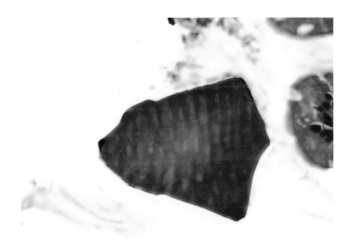

FIGURE 1.18 **Kayexalate crystal.** Sodium polystyrene sulfonate (Kayexalate) crystals display a cracked pattern reminiscent of fish scales.

microscopy has shown this central core of polymerized microtubules surrounded by dispersed chromatin, resulting in a "ring" structure during metaphase (65). Taxanes have been shown to induce unique histologic changes within epithelium of the GI tract associated with cell necrosis in the GI tract (65). As referenced by Hruban et al. (65), in preclinical trials, Taxol had been associated with gastritis and duodenal necrosis in mice and with colonic necrosis in dogs. Reported human drug-related GI effects have included vomiting, diarrhea, mucositis, and neutropenic enterocolitis (66).

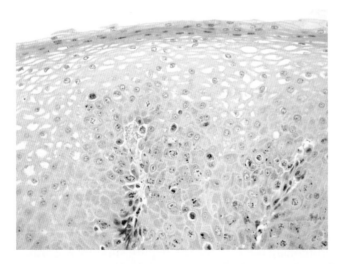

FIGURE 1.19 **Taxol effect.** Esophageal squamous epithelium showing striking mitotic arrest within the proliferative compartment.

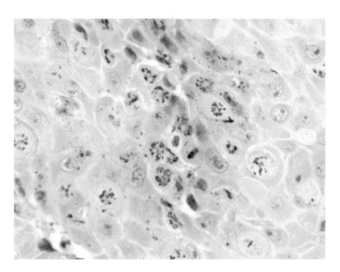

FIGURE 1.20 **Taxol effect.** Higher magnification of Figure 1.19 showing ring mitoses.

Since the mitotic arrest is associated with bundling of intermediate filaments secondary to accumulation of polymerized microtubules (e-Fig. 1.39), the histologic correlate is the presence of arrested mitoses with ring forms. With Taxol, the findings tend to be striking in the esophagus, whereas, in colchicine toxicity, the small bowel is more likely to be severely altered. The ring mitoses are accompanied by prominent apoptosis in all GI tract sites and, regardless of the site, the alterations are found in the proliferative compartment. Thus, in esophageal squamous mucosa, they are encountered in the basal layer, and in the stomach they are seen within the gastric pits. In the small bowel, the epithelial changes are found in the mid crypt but they are in the deep crypts in the colon. The surface cells are uninvolved in all sites. It was initially believed that finding this pattern of injury in a patient taking Taxol indicated clinical toxicity. However, this is not necessarily the case. The medication is administered intravenously on an outpatient basis. If the patient happens to have a GI tract biopsy or resection within 4 days of the administration of the medication, the histologic changes are encountered even in asymptomatic patients (67).

The histologic findings associated with colchicine toxicity are essentially the same as those encountered in patients taking Taxol but are only seen in patients who have clinical toxicity (68). Since it is impossible to separate the effects of the two medications with certainty on histologic examination, it is our practice to contact the submitting clinician caring for the patient to correlate with medication history and determine the need for intervention (colchicine toxicity can require supportive care). That noted, colchicine toxicity is typically encountered in the antrum and small bowel and is described in more detail in Chapter 3.

Mycophenolate

Mycophenolic acid (MPA) is a fermentation product of *Penicillium brevi-compactum* and related fungi. It was isolated in 1898 (69,70). It is an immunosuppressive drug used mainly in patients with solid organ transplants (kidney, liver, heart, lung) to maintain their grafts, but this medication is also administered to patients with a wide range of other conditions including but not limited to nephritis, uveitis, vasculitis, and pemphigus (71–77). In the United States, there are two available preparations for this compound: mycophenolate mofetil (MMF; CellCept; Roche Pharmaceuticals) and mycophenolate sodium (Myfortic, Novartis Inc.). The principal difference between the two preparations is that Myfortic is an enteric coated drug (78) while MMF is not. Thus Myfortic is absorbed in the intestine while MMF is absorbed in the stomach. The efficacy of preventing rejection in transplanted patients and the side effects of the two preparations are similar (70,78).

MPA exerts its immunosuppressive properties by inhibiting the *de novo* pathway of purine synthesis, namely, inhibiting guanosine synthesis for DNA synthesis and cell division (69). Specifically, MPA inhibits inosine monophosphate (IMP) dehydrogenase which is a key enzyme of the *de novo* pathway. In general, almost 100% of B and T lymphocytes depend on the *de novo* pathway for purine synthesis, while this dependency is lower for enterocytes (about 50%). Therefore, by inhibiting guanosine synthesis in lymphocytes, cytotoxic T lymphocytes responsible for cellular rejection and antibody production by B lymphocytes are suppressed in transplanted patients. Although the dependency of enterocytes on the *de novo* pathway for purine genesis is lower than that of lymphocytes, MPA can inhibit the proliferation of enterocytes, leading to epithelial injury.

The side effects of MPA predominantly involve the GI tract and hematopoiesis, and include diarrhea, nausea, vomiting, gastritis, ulcers, opportunistic infections, and anemia (70,79). Since the main side effect of MPA is diarrhea, it is not surprising that colonic injury related to MPA has been documented (80,81). Papadimitriou et al. (80,81) characterized a colonic MPA-induced injury pattern similar to that of graft versus host disease (GVHD), including increased crypt apoptosis, crypt distortion, cellular reparative changes, and increased neuroendocrine cells. The first histologic description of UGI tract MPA-associated damage was documented by Ducloux et al. (82) in 1998 who described villous blunting and crypt hyperplasia in the duodenum of a kidney transplanted patient taking MMF. Parfitt et al. (83) described UGI tract injury caused by MPA and noted the following features: active esophagitis with ulceration or erosion; chemical gastropathy and Crohn-like features in the stomach; and GVHD-like changes and Crohn-like features in the duodenum (83). We have further studied the pathologic features of the UGI tract in patients taking MPA and noted that clinical symptoms tended to correlate with apoptotic counts. In the esophagus, >2 apoptotic bodies per 10 high-power fields

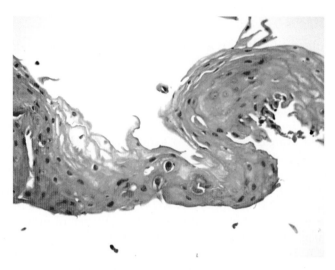

FIGURE 1.21 **Mycophenolate-associated injury.** There is apoptotic damage to squamous epithelial cells. The features are similar to those seen in GVHD. Compare to Figure 1.27.

is in keeping with mycophenolate injury and can be diagnosed as such (Figs. 1.21 and 1.22, e-Figs. 1.40 and 1.41) (84). Of course finding apoptosis is not specific for mycophenolate-associated injury and the findings are essentially identical to those of GVHD such that clinical correlation is always required. Essentially when prominent apoptosis is encountered in mucosal biopsies from patients who have had transplants, those with bone

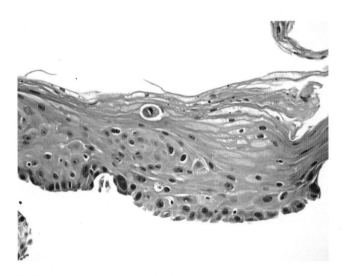

FIGURE 1.22 **Mycophenolate-associated injury.** This example shows prominent apoptosis of the basal layer showing cells with halos that are smaller than lymphocytes. There is a damaged epithelial cell in the superficial portion of the biopsy.

marrow transplants are likely to have GVHD, whereas those who have had solid organ transplants are likely to have mycophenolate-associated mucosal damage. Additionally, cytomegalovirus (CMV) infection (and other viral infections) is also associated with apoptosis.

Fosamax

The bisphosphonates prevent osteoclast-mediated bone reabsorption. Therefore, they have been found to be effective in the treatment of osteoporosis, Paget disease, and the hypercalcemia of malignancy (85). The commercially available bisphosphonates in clinical use include the following:

Alendronate (Fosamax)
Etidronate (Didronel)
Clodronate (Bonefos, Clasteon, Difosfonal)
Pamidronate (Aredia)
Ibandronate (Boniva)
Risedronate (Actonel)
Zolendronate (Zometa, Zomera, Aclasta, Reclast)

Ingestion of alendronate sodium (Fosamax) and related medications by osteoporotic patients has been associated with esophagitis and esophageal ulcer as well as with gastroduodenal ulcers (86–88). Alendronate can damage the esophagus both by toxicity from the medication itself and by nonspecific irritation, secondary to contact between the pill and the esophageal mucosa ("pill esophagitis"). Abraham et al. (89) reported 10 patients who experienced erosive/ulcerative esophagitis while ingesting alendronate. Biopsies from all patients showed inflammatory exudates and inflamed granulation tissue as characteristic of any ulcer site (e-Fig. 1.42). Polarizable crystalline foreign material was present in 6 of 10 biopsies (60%). Multinucleated giant cells, within the inflammatory exudates, were near the crystalline foreign material in 3 of 10 biopsies (30%). Adjacent squamous epithelium typically showed active inflammation and a reactive appearance with enlarged, hyperchromatic nuclei. Multinucleated squamous epithelial giant cells were present in 2 of 10 cases (20%). Microorganisms were unusual; scattered fungi and/or viral inclusions were present in only 2 of 10 biopsies (20%). Although there is no specific histologic finding, it is worthwhile to be aware of this complication with such medicines and relay that concern appropriately to the clinician. There have been reports of esophageal mucosal injury in patients taking all of the bisphosphonates, but it is likely that many of the patients had additional risk factors. In a study that adjusted for the risk of esophagitis, esophageal ulcers, and esophageal perforations before and after initiation of the bisphosphonates, only alendronate, and etidronate were associated with an increased risk of esophageal damage (90).

These agents (i.e., alendronate sodium and related medications) should be avoided in patients with achalasia and other motility disorders of the esophagus, esophageal stricture, or preexisting severe reflux esophagitis. However, patients with reflux disease can probably be treated with a PPI and then safely have bisphosphonate therapy with continued concomitant use of the PPI.

The Food and Drug Administration has also received reports of esophageal cancers developing in patients taking alendronate (91). However, when this issue is studied with proper controls, there seems to be no causal association between bisphosphonate use and esophageal carcinomas (92–97).

Although bisphosphonates are classically associated with esophageal injury, other medications can lodge in this area and induce similar damage. Like with bisphosphonates, pill fragments may be evident microscopically (e-Figs. 1.43 and 1.44).

ESOPHAGITIS DISSECANS SUPERFICIALIS/ "THERMAL INJURY"/ "SLOUGHING ESOPHAGITIS"

These terms have all been used to describe a characteristic pattern of injury consisting of an unaltered basal layer and "mummification" of the superficial squamous epithelium, such that there are "ghost" nuclei (displaying poor uptake of hematoxylin stain) and the mucosa sloughs (Fig. 1.23, e-Fig. 1.45). The condition is uncommon but produces a dramatic endoscopic picture (e-Fig. 1.46) and a blister-like appearance on histologic evaluation (98) that has overlap with skin disorders, especially pemphigus.

The full name for this condition is esophagitis dissecans superficialis. In early reports patients were said to have vomited large esophageal

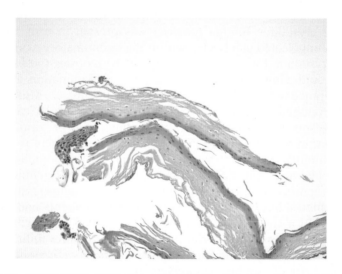

FIGURE 1.23 **Esophagitis dissecans superficialis.** Note the thermal injury pattern, possibly related to ingestion of hot liquids/foods. The upper half of the mucosa has cracked away from the basal layer and has coagulative necrosis. There is little inflammatory response in this field. This may be an early blister.

"casts" with a tubular configuration (99–101) but more typically, the condition is not even suspected until an endoscopist notices whitish strips or streaks ("pseudomembranes") of peeling esophageal mucosa during an endoscopic examination performed for reasons that may be unrelated to the esophagus, although some patients have dysphagia or even strictures (102). The condition is associated with "polypharmacy", skin conditions, heavy smoking, physical trauma (including ingesting hot liquids), immunosuppression, and impaired mobility but the pathogenesis remains unknown. It may be a topical allergic response (similar to the blistering after skin exposure to poison ivy) (98).

At low magnification, unusually long, detached fragments of superficial epithelium can be seen. Most cases have some degree of intraepithelial splitting at varying degrees above the basal layer and in a few cases a distinct bulla is apparent. Most cases show fragments of necrotic epithelium with minimal or no inflammation, in some cases with bacterial colonies. Parakeratosis is common.

CORROSIVE INGESTION

Like the esophageal injury associated with Fosamax, corrosive injury (e.g. lye, bleach) does not result in a specific pattern of injury (although saponification may accompany lye ingestion) and cannot be identified directly (as with iron or kayexalate). However, it can usually be correlated with an ingestion history in a pediatric patient or in a psychiatric setting. Endoscopically, severe ulceration is seen and endoscopists (Fig. 1.24, e-Figs. 1.47–1.50) have described a strong bleach-like odor, even when

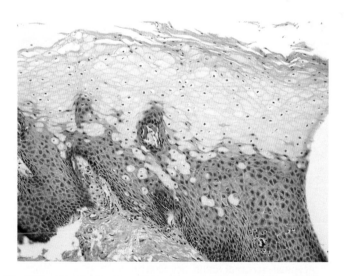

FIGURE 1.24 **Injury due to lye ingestion.** The basal layer is viable while the more superficial aspect of the epithelium appears paler with loss of some nuclei.

the patient has ingested lye. Microscopically, extensive necrosis is found. Those who survive are likely to have severe stricturing disease with all its complications. As a result, such patients require lifetime follow-up as they are prone to develop squamous cell carcinoma (103).

ATYPICAL STROMAL CELLS IN ULCERS/POLYPS

In any biopsy in which there has been injury to the mucosa, reactive fibroblasts can be a component. At times, the reactive fibroblasts can proliferate exuberantly and have atypical (probably hypoxic) features (Fig. 1.25, e-Fig. 1.51). Pseudoepitheliomatous epithelium may also appear in the area of the repairing mucosa (e-Figs. 1.52–1.55). These atypical stromal fibroblasts have been termed "deceptive bizarre stromal cells" (104) and "pseudosarcomatous changes" (105) and can be encountered throughout the GI tract in association with ulcers and polyps (104). If immunolabeling is performed, they are "vimentin-only" proliferations, lacking keratins, S100 protein, muscle markers, and endothelial cell markers. These atypical stromal cells tend to be found at the hypoxic interface between necroinflammatory ulcer debris and the viable granulation tissue layer. This pattern of distribution is obvious on resections, but may be inapparent on superficial biopsies that only include the necroinflammatory exudates and a small portion of hypoxic tissue beneath it. Like atypical fibroblasts associated with radiation, such cells tend to have a low nucleus to cytoplasmic ratio even though they are enlarged and, also like so-called radiation fibroblasts, they often display smudged chromatin. In doubtful cases, rebiopsies can be requested. It is worthwhile to remember that sarcomas invading the esophagus are vanishingly rare and if atypical spindle cells are encountered, the differential diagnosis is generally between sarcomatoid squamous cell carcinoma and reactive fibroblasts.

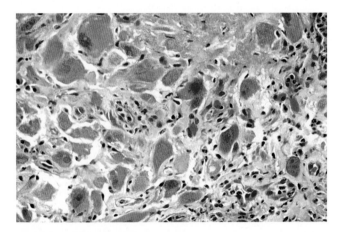

FIGURE 1.25 **Atypical stromal cells associated with ulcers.** Reactive fibroblasts showing low nuclear to cytoplasmic ratio and smudged chromatin pattern are seen. They are typically immunoreactive only with vimentin.

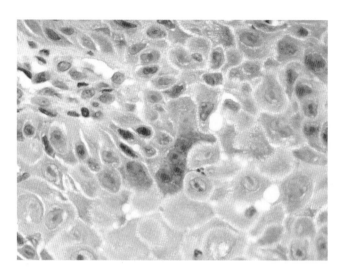

FIGURE 1.26 **Multinucleated epithelial giant cell change.** These are typically confined to the basal zone and display a single or multiple eosinophilic nucleoli with a perinucleolar halo.

MULTINUCLEATED EPITHELIAL GIANT CELL CHANGE

Multinucleated epithelial giant cells are sometimes encountered in squamous mucosa as a reparative change (106) associated with reflux, radiation injury, drug-induced injury, or infection. Microscopically, these cases show multiple multinucleated squamous epithelial cells, usually confined to the basal zone (Fig. 1.26). The nuclei contain a single or multiple eosinophilic nucleoli with a perinucleolar halo, but no inclusions, hyperchromaticity, or atypical mitoses. There are typically associated nonspecific features of active esophagitis such as ulceration, neutrophilic and eosinophilic inflammation, basal cell hyperplasia, and elongation of the lamina propria papillae (e-Figs. 1.56 and 1.57).

GRAFT VERSUS HOST DISEASE

The features of GVHD in the esophagus are similar to those elsewhere; biopsies show intraepithelial lymphocytosis, basilar vacuolization, epithelial apoptosis, and necrosis in severe disease (Fig. 1.27, e-Figs. 1.58–1.60). Some patients manifest characteristic radiologic and endoscopic appearances (49–53,107,108) especially in chronic GVHD, namely, bullous disease, desquamative esophagitis, webs, and strictures. Furthermore, there is literature stating that endoscopic evidence of esophageal webs or strictures in the upper or mid third of the esophagus is sufficient to establish a diagnosis of chronic GVHD (109). This latter setting is histologically characterized by submucosal fibrosis but this layer is seldom present on routine biopsies (107).

On a practical note, we attempt to grade the findings, using mild, moderate, and severe (where severe disease encompasses ulcerations/ erosions).

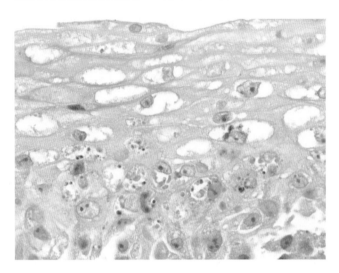

FIGURE 1.27 **Graft vs. host disease.** A case of GVHD showing basilar vacuolization and prominent apoptosis.

We also compare the features in interval biopsies to help monitor the effects of treatment, but we do not perform lymphocyte or apoptotic body counts. When evaluating biopsies from patients for whom GVHD is a clinical consideration, our most important goal is to exclude infectious etiologies, since generally such patients are empirically treated with steroids as well as to learn if the patient is taking medications known to result in prominent apoptosis (e.g., mycophenolate administered for solid organ transplantation) (84).

DERMATOLOGIC DISEASE AFFECTING THE ESOPHAGUS

Dermatologic conditions that are well known to involve the esophagus include pemphigus vulgaris (PV), paraneoplastic pemphigus, mucous membrane pemphigoid, epidermolysis bullosa, lichen sclerosus, lichen planus, pityriasis lichenoides chronica, and toxic epidermal necrolysis. Esophageal involvement by cutaneous diseases is not well recognized by pathologists or clinicians, which delays diagnosis and allows continued esophageal inflammation. In the case of lichen planus, e.g., dysphagia and esophageal strictures are often initially misinterpreted as secondary to the more common GERD.

Lichen planus (110), a subacute to chronic mucocutaneous disorder of unknown etiology, can involve the skin, nails, and mucosal surfaces. Lichen planus of the skin affects both genders with equal frequency at any age, although most patients are middle-aged adults. Cutaneous lichen planus is characterized by eruptions of violaceous, scaling papules, and plaques. These plaques typically are intensely pruritic and are most commonly localized to the extensor surfaces of the forearms and legs. Lichen planus of the mucosal surfaces may include lesions of the perineum, oral mucosa, and pharynx. Unlike cutaneous disease, mucosal lichen planus is predominantly a disease of middle-aged women. Oral involvement, in particular, coexists with skin lesions in approximately 30% to 50% of patients, but it can be the sole disease manifestation.

Even though esophageal involvement by lichen planus is a rarely described manifestation, a prevalence of 26% to 50% has been reported in patients with cutaneous and/or oral disease. The latter figure was reported by Quispel et al. in a study using magnification chromoendoscopy and including detailed histopathologic correlation (111,112). Mucosal stripping, hyperemia, and submucosal plaques are endoscopic features, which are typically limited to the upper and mid esophagus (111–113). In contrast to its oral counterpart, a risk of malignancy is not well established but cases with associated esophageal squamous cell (114,115) and verrucous carcinoma (113) are documented and argue for endoscopic surveillance of these patients. Esophageal lichen planus is an important diagnosis because of its tendency to cause persistent dysphagia, which results from esophagitis and stricture formation. Further trauma from therapeutic dilation can lead to exacerbation of oral lichen planus in a Koebner-like phenomenon.

The pathologic features of esophageal lichen planus differ from those on the skin. The epidermal reaction in cutaneous lichen planus typically includes hypergranulosis, hyperorthokeratosis, acanthosis, and "saw-tooth" elongation of the rete pegs. In contrast, the esophageal epithelium, which does not normally contain orthokeratin or a granular layer, frequently shows parakeratosis, rather than orthohyperkeratosis. Also, esophageal epithelium frequently fails to show hypergranulosis. In addition, the epithelium may be atrophic, rather than acanthotic, or may show variable thinning and acanthosis. The histologic features, therefore, more closely resemble those seen in oral, rather than cutaneous, lichen planus. All sites of involvement reveal the typical band-like inflammatory infiltrate, with a predominance of mature T cells and basal layer degeneration, including characteristic Civatte bodies (Figs. 1.28 and 1.29, e-Figs. 1.61–1.63).

Lymphocytic infiltration alone is not diagnostic of esophageal lichen planus. Medications such as gold, thiazides, and antimalarials can induce lichen planus-like lesions and need to be excluded by clinical history. Nonspecific lymphocytic infiltrates can be seen adjacent to esophageal ulcer sites secondary to infectious or pill-induced esophagitis. Although infectious agents are often easily excluded on biopsy material, exclusion of esophagitis resulting from pill ingestion or caustic substances requires clinical correlation. In addition, lymphocytic infiltrates are occasionally prominent, although often focal, in patients with GE reflux. Reflux can usually be excluded because of the lack of clinical symptoms, the results of pH probe studies, and the failure of the inflammatory condition to respond to intensive antireflux therapy. Other histologic criteria for GE reflux,

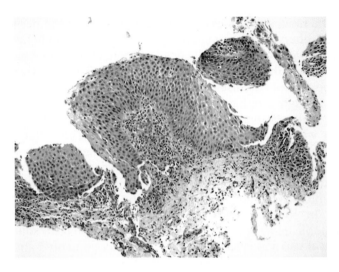

FIGURE 1.28 **Esophageal lichen planus.** A lichenoid infiltrate is seen here underneath an epithelium of variable thickness.

including intraepithelial eosinophils, are usually absent. Furthermore, the typically upper- or mid-esophageal locations of the pathologic findings and stricture sites would be unusual in GERD. However, it is difficult to positively diagnose lichen planus; it can only be suggested and correlated with other features. Systemic treatment is usually required to forestall stricturing disease, whereas topical treatment is often adequate for oral

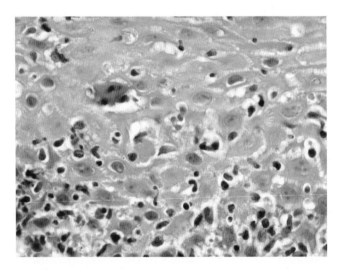

FIGURE 1.29 **Esophageal lichen planus.** Necrotic squamous epithelial cells (Civatte bodies) display brightly eosinophilic cytoplasm.

lesions. Intralesional esophageal steroid injections have been used with some success (116,117).

Pityriasis lichenoides is a group of inflammatory skin disorders that encompasses three entities, namely, pityriasis lichenoides chronica, pityriasis lichenoides et varioliformis acuta, and febrile ulceronecrotic Mucha-Habermann disease. The three are believed to be part of a continuum and the etiology is uncertain. Though not reported in the esophagus as of this writing, one of the authors has encountered such a case (Figs. 1.30 and 1.31, e-Figs. 1.64 and 1.65) in practice. The diagnosis would be next to impossible in the absence of the clinical history.

The bullous diseases are similarly difficult to diagnose in the esophagus, and also must be correlated with clinical findings. When we receive esophageal biopsies showing bullae without an infectious explanation, we typically request that additional biopsies be submitted fresh for immunofluorescence studies.

PV, the most common form of pemphigus, affects men and women equally, especially those in their 4th and 5th decades. Skin and mucous membrane involvement is typical. Although any mucosal surface can be involved, oral lesions are the hallmark of PV; they occur in almost every case and are the presenting sign in half of the affected patients.

Few reports of esophageal involvement in PV exist in early literature because it was thought to be rare; but it is found in most patients when sought (118,119). Because patients with esophageal involvement may be asymptomatic, such involvement has been underrecognized. Although esophageal involvement may be a frequent occurrence in active

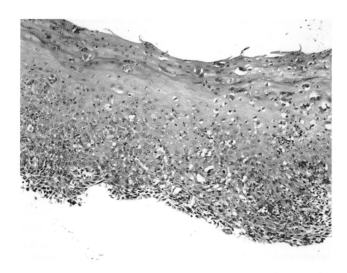

FIGURE 1.30 **Pityriasis lichenoides chronica.** This image shows an esophageal biopsy from a patient suffering from pityriasis lichenoides chronica with intraepithelial lymphocytosis and prominent squamous epithelial cell apoptosis.

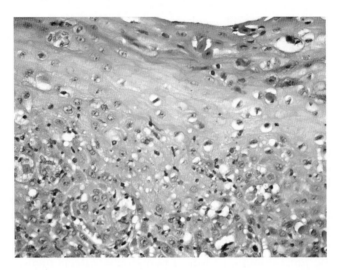

FIGURE 1.31 **Pityriasis lichenoides chronica.** Higher magnification of Figure 1.30 showing intercellular edema, vacuolar degeneration of the basal layer, and necrotic keratinocytes.

mucocutaneous PV, it rarely occurs in the absence of other manifestations of the disease (120).

Odynophagia and dysphagia are the usual symptoms of esophageal PV, as with other mucosal blistering diseases, including herpetic or esophageal candidiasis. Endoscopy is required for diagnosis; it allows evaluation of both the appearance of the lesions and tissue sampling. Essentially normal esophageal mucosa may be seen on initial passage of the endoscope, followed by the appearance of erosions and sheets of sloughed mucosa on withdrawal of the instrument. Erythematous, longitudinal lines can be seen involving the entire organ (119) and Nikolsky sign may observed if elicited (121). Histopathologic findings of suprabasal clefting (cells with a "tombstone" appearance) and acantholysis are features of PV (Figs. 1.32 and 1.33, e-Figs. 1.66 and 1.67); immunofluorescence shows intercellular deposition of IgG and C3. Indirect immunofluorescence detects pemphigus antibodies in about 75% of cases; a negative result can occur if the disease is in remission or in an early localized stage.

Corticosteroids and immunosuppressive agents are considered the first-line treatment in PV. For patients who present with mucosal PV, the disease may remain localized to the mucous membranes or it may progress to skin involvement.

Bullous pemphigoid (BP) affects the esophagus more rarely than the other skin diseases discussed above (122–124). It is a chronic, autoimmune, subepidermal, blistering skin disease that rarely involves mucous membranes. BP primarily affects individuals in the 5th through 7th decades of life, with 65 being the average age at onset.

BP is characterized by the presence of immunoglobulin G (IgG) autoantibodies specific for the hemidesmosomal BP antigens BP230 (BPAg1)

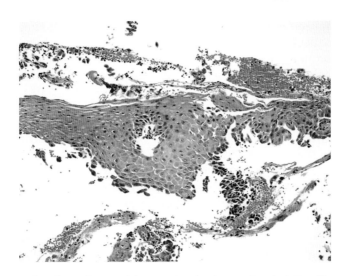

FIGURE 1.32 **Esophageal pemphigus vulgaris.** A suprabasal cleft with acantholytic squamous epithelial cells is present.

and BP180 (BPAg2). IgG autoantibodies bind to the skin basement membrane and activate complement and inflammatory mediators. Eosinophils are characteristically present in bullae, although their presence is not an absolute diagnostic criterion. Serum levels of autoantibodies against BPAg2 correlate with disease activity in some studies.

In France and Germany, the reported incidence is 6.6 cases per million people per year. In Europe, BP was identified as the most common

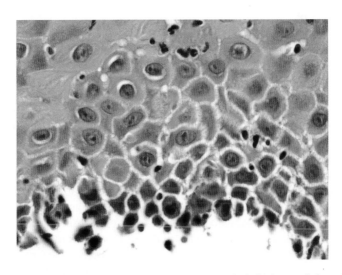

FIGURE 1.33 **Esophageal pemphigus vulgaris.** Acantholysis, intercellular edema, and bullet-shaped nucleoli are seen here.

subepidermal autoimmune blistering disease. The mucosa is affected in 10% to 25% of patients. Limited oral intake may occur secondary to dysphagia. Erosions secondary to rupture of the blisters, which may be found on the palms and soles, may be sufficiently painful to limit patients' daily functions.

Epidermolysis bullosa encompasses a diverse group of rare, potentially devastating hereditary skin disorders characterized by the formation of cutaneous and mucosal blisters at sites of minor trauma. Several mutations involving multiple genes that code for various structural proteins (cytokeratins 5, 14, laminin, type VII collagen, $\alpha6\beta$integrin) within the epidermis and basement membrane give rise to the more commonly observed variants, namely, epidermolysis bullosa simplex (EBS), junctional epidermolysis bullosa (JEB), and dystrophic epidermolysis bullosa (DEB) (125). Clinical phenotypes range from mild to severe with diffuse blister formation, ulceration, scarring, and contractures. The esophagus is amongst the most common sites of GI involvement with dysphagia, odynophagia, blistering, and web formation (45,125–127). Subsequent stricturing disease is common, occurring in the majority of patients with DEB and less frequently in other variants (126,128). Although these patients are at increased risk of skin cancer, esophageal carcinoma is rarely encountered (128,129). Skin lesions show sites of cleavage within the epidermis (simplex form), the dermoepidermal junction (junctional form), or dermis (dystrophic form). While it seems reasonable to assume that histologic features in esophageal tissue would be similar, as of this writing a PubMed search retrieves no studies addressing this specific matter.

ESOPHAGITIS FROM INFECTIOUS AGENTS

Agents affecting the esophagus display the same features as those found elsewhere, but there are some clues based on the background in which they are found. For example, when an infectious etiology is suspected in erosive esophagitis, the endoscopist should biopsy the base of the erosion/ulcer to detect CMV (Figs. 1.34 and 1.35, e-Fig. 1.68); whereas, the epithelium is more likely to demonstrate herpes simplex virus (HSV) (Figs. 1.36 and 1.37, e-Figs. 1.69–1.71). Clues at low magnification show precisely where a search at high magnification in the biopsies is warranted. For example, Greenson (130) has demonstrated that a prominent mononuclear infiltrate adjacent to the infected epithelium often accompanies HSV esophagitis, which is a clue to search for the organism. Likewise, macrophages tend to be present in a perivascular distribution in granulation tissue, which is a clue to search for CMV esophagitis (131). In the case of HSV, the background infiltrate may suggest the need to perform immunohistochemistry for HSV, as viral cytopathic changes may not be apparent on routine H&E stains (e-Fig. 1.68). Generally, it is no problem to recognize *Candida esophagitis* as the epithelium appears sloughed, incrusted with inflammation, and embedded with many yeast and pseudohyphal forms but some cases

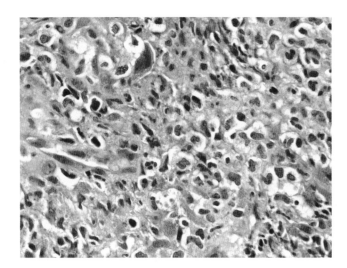

FIGURE 1.34   **Cytomegalovirus (CMV) esophagitis.** The viral cytopathic effect is present in stromal cells (upper left) within an ulcer.

are more subtle and unaccompanied by inflammation. Zones of parakeratosis, however small, are worth studying at high magnification to exclude *Candida* (Figs. 1.5, 1.6, 1.38, e-Figs. 1.72–1.77). Pseudohyphal forms must be sought since budding yeast, alone, might be a reflection of oral contamination or colonization. In our practice, we specify that budding yeast is present (if they are) in a descriptive fashion, but we do not diagnose lesions as *Candida esophagitis* in the absence of pseudohyphal forms.

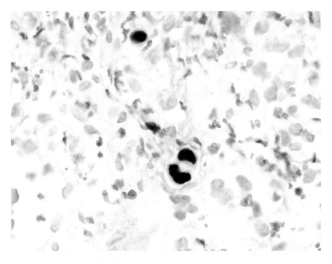

FIGURE 1.35   **Cytomegalovirus (CMV) esophagitis, immunohistochemical stain.** A prominent mononuclear infiltrate adjacent to the infected epithelium often accompanies both CMV and HSV esophagitis.

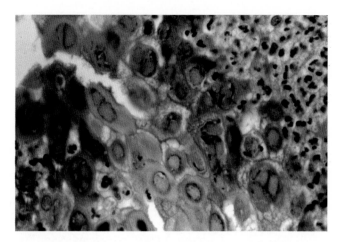

FIGURE 1.36 **Herpes simplex virus (HSV) esophagitis.** Note how the epithelial cells are affected. In this field, there are multinucleated cells with smudged (Cowdry B) inclusions.

Bacterial esophagitis is poorly understood. Of course, esophagitis from various unusual organisms, such as *Actinomyces*, is the grist for case reports, but "garden variety" bacterial esophagitis is a somewhat anecdotal entity. Walsh et al. (132) proposed a definition of bacterial esophagitis as "histopathologically demonstrable bacterial invasion of esophageal mucosa or deeper layers with no concomitant fungal, viral, or neoplastic involvement or previous surgery of the esophagus." Bacterial esophagitis should be considered in immunocompromised patients presenting with odynophagia. Bacterial esophagitis may not be accompanied by an inflammatory response, but by numerous bacterial forms seen "embedded" in the squamous mucosa (e-Figs. 1.78–1.80). Apparently, bacterial esophagitis can be a source of occult sepsis (133).

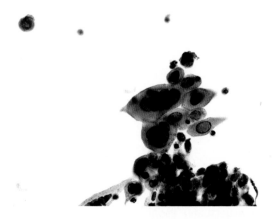

FIGURE 1.37 **Herpes simplex virus (HSV) esophagitis, esophageal brushing.** These cells show the classic viral cytopathic effects (multinucleation, chromatin margination, and molding) of HSV.

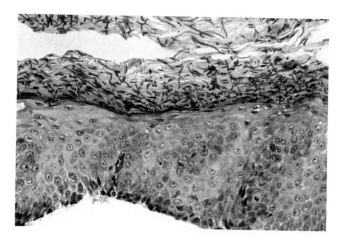

FIGURE 1.38 **Candida esophagitis.** Numerous pseudohyphae are embedded in a parakeratotic layer (PAS/AB stain). Notice there is negligible accompanying inflammation.

As a final note, patients with HIV often have esophageal ulcers attributable to *Candida* sp. or viral agents, but some ulcers in these patients do not seem to have an associated etiologic agent that is readily identifiable. These are often termed "HIV ulcers." Proving whether they are attributable to the HIV virus itself is impossible because the patients have protean infection. But, it is the duty of the pathologist who is evaluating the ulcer to assure that none of the aforementioned organisms is present. This is important because some clinicians inject such ulcers with steroids to provide symptomatic relief to the patient.

ALLERGIC/EOSINOPHILIC ESOPHAGITIS

Overall, eosinophilic esophagogastroenteritis (EG) is an uncommon benign inflammatory condition characterized by eosinophilic infiltration of the GI tract. The diagnostic criteria are

- GI symptoms
- Eosinophilic infiltration of the GI tract, usually with intraepithelial eosinophils
- No evidence of parasitic infestation

Most patients (in addition to their GI involvement) also have a history of allergy, asthma, drug sensitivities, peripheral eosinophilia, and increased IgE levels. Food and inhalant intolerance have been postulated as etiologic factors and some argue for allergy evaluation with skin prick testing in patients with eosinophilic esophagitis (EE). For example, Penfield et al. (134) identified one or more food or inhalant allergens in 21 of 26 (81%) patients with EE who underwent skin testing. The value of such investigations in adults remains uncertain as there is no evidence to support a role for an elimination diet based on their results. In addition, a seasonal variation has been demonstrated with a predominance of newly diagnosed cases during the spring and summer months (135–137). EG predominantly affects patients in their 3rd to 6th decades. However, 15% to 20% of cases are seen in the pediatric age group and, in some cases, milk allergy may be demonstrated.

Any part of the GI tract (from the esophagus to the rectum) can be affected–the stomach and small bowel are commonly involved. Eosinophilic EG can show preferential involvement of the mucosa, muscularis propria, or serosa. Symptoms depend on the site and extent of eosinophilic infiltration. Mucosal disease can present as diarrhea, malabsorption, and protein-losing enteropathy. Submucosal disease presents as obstruction and abdominal pain, and patients can develop eosinophilic ascites with serosal involvement. Rarely do patients present with an acute abdominal emergency necessitating immediate laparotomy.

Patients with EE (limited to esophagus) present with dysphagia, food impaction, and strictures. This finding is encountered in about 6% of adult patients undergoing upper endoscopy and there seems to be a male predominance (138). In children, there is a similar male predominance and probably whites are overrepresented (139). Some of our gastroenterology colleagues provide useful information regarding the endoscopic appearance of the esophagus and pathologists should be familiar with the terminology in order to address the clinical concern. Linear furrows, esophageal rings, esophageal trachealization, and feline esophagus are some of the possible endoscopic scenarios. White mucosal specks, corresponding to foci of eosinophilic microabscesses, may also be seen. In some cases the mucosa appears grossly normal. The differential diagnosis is with reflux esophagitis. However, unlike in reflux esophagitis, the upper and mid esophagus are commonly affected with relative distal sparing. On histologic examination, superficial epithelial clusters of eosinophils that slough into the lumen are more common in EE (Fig. 1.39, e-Figs. 1.81–1.83). Basal cell hyperplasia can be striking (Fig. 1.40), even more so than in cases of GERD, as shown by Steiner et al. (140) in a study where they found a more severe degree of basal cell hyperplasia in pediatric patients with EE than in those with GERD. Besides mucosal involvement, there may be eosinophilic infiltration present deep in the submucosa and muscularis propria, which could explain the fragility of the esophageal wall in these patients. Indeed, they are prone to endoscopic complications, namely, esophageal tears or rupture, in some cases associated with full-thickness esophageal inflammation and high eosinophil density (141–144). Spontaneous esophageal rupture has been reported in some cases (145,146). The eosinophilic infiltrate in EG can be patchy and multiple, localized, or diffuse. In 10% of cases, mucosal biopsies can be nondiagnostic, due to the patchy nature of the disease or mucosal sparing. Multiple and full-thickness biopsies may be necessary to establish the diagnosis. For example, Figure 1.41 illustrates features of EE while Figure 1.42 from the same patient at the same endoscopic examination just shows reflux-associated changes.

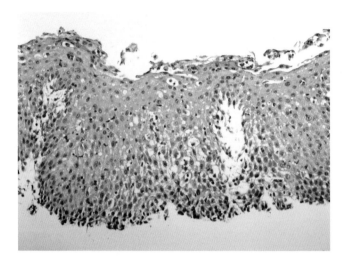

FIGURE 1.39 **Eosinophilic esophagitis.** Note eosinophil clustering along the surface with formation of eosinophilic microabscesses.

Some have proposed that an estimate of the number of eosinophils is a helpful feature to establish the diagnosis. In fact, a consensus agreement sponsored in part by the American Gastroenterological Association (AGA) recommends a minimum of 15 eosinophils/hpf to make a diagnosis of EE (147) although Dellon et al. (148) noted the poor reproducibility of such eosinophil counts. Because some clinicians feel it is necessary to provide concrete numbers, some pathologists are in the habit of counting and

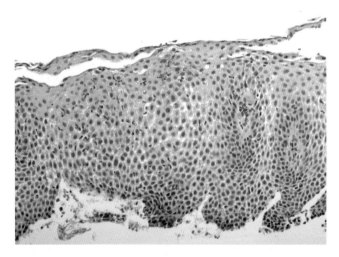

FIGURE 1.40 **Eosinophilic esophagitis (EE).** Numerous eosinophils with superficial clustering in association with a thick basal cell layer.

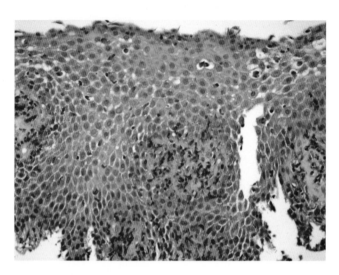

FIGURE 1.41 **Eosinophilic esophagitis (EE).** This biopsy shows features associated with EE. Same patient as depicted in Figure 42.

reporting eosinophils/hpf in biopsies from patients suspected of having EE. Taking this recommendation to heart, especially in isolation, can lead to misdiagnoses as it is well-known that significantly increased intraepithelial eosinophils can be seen in other settings such as severe GERD (149). On the other hand, work by Kephart et al. (150) demonstrates significant extracellular deposition of eosinophil-derived neurotoxin (identified via immunofluorescence) in adult patients with EE, even in the face

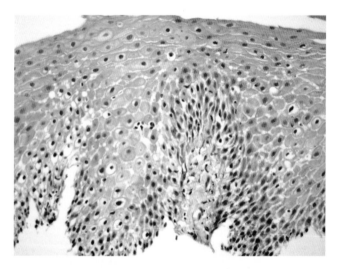

FIGURE 1.42 **Eosinophilic esophagitis.** Only scattered eosinophils with a prominent basal cell layer are seen in a biopsy from the same patient as Figure 1.41. In isolation, these may be interpreted as reflux-associated changes, hence the importance of obtaining multiple biopsies at the time of endoscopy.

of relatively few intact eosinophils in some cases. This finding raises the possibility that, at least in some situations, counting may actually underestimate the degree of tissue involvement in EE. Our approach is as follows: if there are fewer than eight eosinophils per 40× field, reflux esophagitis is favored. Likewise, a count of >24 eosinophils per 40× field better supports EE, especially when seen in a biopsy from the mid or proximal esophagus. Clinicopathologic correlation should be attempted for all cases, especially for those with intermediate "counts" (e.g., pH monitoring studies, stigmata of allergic disease, endoscopic impression). Since reporting number of eosinophils can be misleading, we would prefer not to report counts in our practice but we do offer estimates and we attempt to compare biopsies to prior ones, and estimate whether more or fewer eosinophils are present to help assess response to treatment. While we believe that distinguishing between reflux and EE is a worthwhile endeavor (as patients with EE can show dramatic response to steroids), we also believe that making this diagnosis in a vacuum can result in erroneous diagnoses. A conversation with the gastroenterologist might be of benefit when the clinical and/or endoscopic settings are uncertain.

CROHN DISEASE AFFECTING THE ESOPHAGUS

Reports on the prevalence of esophageal Crohn disease (ECD) vary widely in both adults and children. Decker et al. (151) reported that only 20 of 9,900 (0.2%) adults with Crohn disease (CD), seen over a period of 22 years, had esophageal involvement. A higher prevalence was reported by D'Haens et al. (152), who demonstrated ECD in 14 of 124 (11%) adults. Both of these studies were retrospective and used macroscopic endoscopic evidence as the only criteria for diagnosis, which likely resulted in an underestimation of the prevalence. In contrast, a prospective study of ECD in adults, by Alcantara et al. (153), yielded a prevalence of 5.1%. In the pediatric age group, there have been few prospective and retrospective studies that provide estimates of the prevalence of ECD. In one prospective study, endoscopy identified ECD in 2 of 40 (5%) children with CD, and a total of 17 of 40 (42.5%) had histologic evidence of ECD (154). When only endoscopic criteria were used, Ramaswamy (155) found that about 7% of pediatric patients had ECD but this increased to 17% when biopsy results were incorporated. These findings suggest that the prevalence of ECD in adults and children with CD may be similar, and is at least 5%. Low estimates in some of the retrospective adult studies may be a reflection of patient selection for UGI endoscopy. There is wide variability in the clinical manifestations of ECD, and many patients do not have specific esophageal symptoms. Isolated ECD is uncommon.

ECD is usually associated with advanced ileo-colonic disease, but UGI tract symptoms do not always correlate well with endoscopic and biopsy findings. Cameron (67) reported that UGI symptoms were present in only 15% of children with CD, but found that 42% had endoscopic lesions. Alcantara et al. (153) found that 17% of 41 adults had UGI symptoms, but only 5% had endoscopic ECD. Ramaswamy et al. (155) found that 33% of the children with ECD had specific UGI symptoms, and that there was no difference in the endoscopic findings for children with ECD, whether or not they had UGI tract symptoms. Lenaerts et al. (156) reported dysphagia and/or epigastric pain, nausea, and vomiting more frequently in children with UGI CD, but these symptoms were also seen in children without UGI disease, suggesting that they are not specific to the UGI tract disease. In the pediatric age group, there is often an overlap of symptoms (such as nausea, anorexia, and abdominal pain) between esophageal and small bowel CD. It is, therefore, difficult to identify an UGI site of disease based on clinical evaluation alone. Thus, upper endoscopy and biopsies are important in the evaluation of pediatric inflammatory bowel disease, even in the asymptomatic child.

The presence of histologic abnormalities in radiologically and endo-scopically normal mucosa is not unusual. Hence, endoscopy with biopsy is generally considered the gold standard for diagnosis of early lesions that may be asymptomatic. The spectrum of esophageal injury in CD varies from mild esophagitis with small erosions to transmural involvement with esophageal perforation and fistulization to adjacent organs. In addition to aphthous ulcers, other findings well described in ECD are the presence of erythema, ulceration, erythematous nodules, and polypoid lesions. Pseudomembrane formations, progressive esophageal strictures, and formation of multiple mucosal bridges have been described in advanced stages.

Epithelioid granulomas in the correct clinical setting are considered diagnostic for CD (Figs. 1.43 and 1.44, e-Fig. 1.84). Ramaswamy et al. (155) reported granulomas in 25% of esophageal biopsy specimens in pediatric

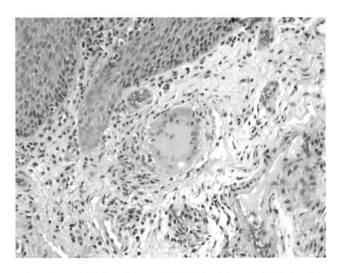

FIGURE 1.43 **Esophageal Crohn disease (CD).** A lamina propria giant cell is seen here.

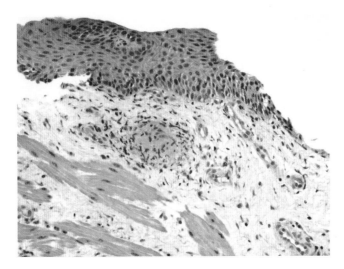

FIGURE 1.44 **Esophageal Crohn disease (CD).** Epithelioid granulomata in the correct clinical setting are considered diagnostic.

CD with ileocolic involvement. In a review of the literature, granulomas were documented in 39% of patients with ECD that was detected at endoscopy with biopsy, and on some surgically resected specimens (157). Focal infiltration with mononuclear cells and histiocytes into the lamina propria, which extends to the muscular layer, is consistent with Crohn esophagitis. Unfortunately, nonspecific upper tract lesions can also be found in pediatric patients with classic ulcerative colitis (158). Additionally, many patients with established CD have slight nonspecific esophageal alterations. For example, some only have prominence in intraepithelial lymphocytes ("lymphocytic eosphagitis") (159) [typically 20 lymphocytes per 40× field in interpapillary areas and 50–55 lymphocytes per 40× field in papillary areas as compared to the figure of >10/hpf considered to associate with reflux disease (61)].

The clinical course of ECD, described by D'Haens et al. (152), was that 8 of 14 patients (57%) had no recurrence of esophageal lesions or symptoms during subsequent disease exacerbations. None of the children in the study by Ramaswamy et al. (155) had repeat endoscopy for recurrence of UGI symptoms. Considering the high prevalence of histologic ECD in children and the low rates of endoscopic ECD in adults, it seems reasonable to suggest that esophageal involvement is unlikely to progress to a more overt disease over time.

"LYMPHOCYTIC ESOPHAGITIS"

As alluded to above, the term "lymphocytic esophagitis" describes a pattern of injury rather than a diagnosis. In one study, this pattern was associated with GERD, gastroduodenitis, celiac disease, carcinoma of the esophagus

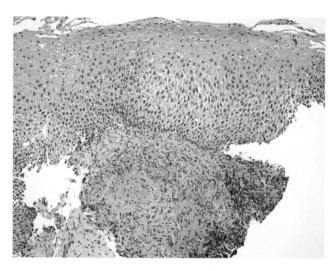

FIGURE 1.45 **Esophageal Crohn disease (CD).** Note the lymphocytic esophagitis pattern and lamina propria granulomata.

or elsewhere, hiatal hernia, gastric ulcer/asthma/hypertension, Hashimoto thyroiditis, cirrhosis/diabetes, and CD (159). Patients typically had 20 lymphocytes per 40× field in interpapillary areas and 50–55 lymphocytes per 40× field in papillary areas. The authors found a striking association between lymphocytic esophagitis and CD, a pattern that we, too, have more anecdotally observed (Figs. 1.45 and 1.46, e-Figs. 1.85 and 1.86). However, other authors found no association between lymphocytic esophagitis and CD compared to

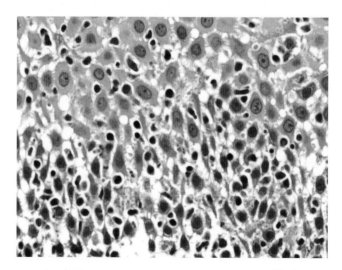

FIGURE 1.46 **Esophageal Crohn disease (CD).** This higher magnification of Figure 1.45 shows intraepithelial lymphocytosis and intercellular edema.

controls (160) and suggested that this pattern is a form of contact mucositis. The findings tended to persist on follow-up sampling. Intraepithelial lymphocytosis is also encountered in patients with esophageal lichen planus.

COMMON VARIABLE IMMUNODEFICIENCY

Common variable immunodeficiency (CVID) is a disease characterized by repeated bouts of infection in association with hypogammaglobulinemia as a result of defective B-cell differentiation and, in some patients, T-cell dysfunction (161,162). Average age at initial diagnosis is series dependent and ranges from 28 to 41.9 years (162–164). Survival 20 years after diagnosis for males and females is 64% and 67%, respectively, compared with 92% and 94% for the general population (162). Besides recurrent infections, patients suffer from a number of associated immune disorders, namely, idiopathic thrombocytopenic purpura, autoimmune hemolytic anemia, rheumatoid arthritis, granulomatous disease, and diabetes mellitus, to name a few (162,163). Some eventually develop chronic lung disease and malignancies, particularly lymphoma (Hodgkin and non-Hodgkin). GI complaints are common and CVID can mimic a host of conditions, both clinically and histologically. Not uncommonly patients carry diagnoses of inflammatory bowel disease (Crohn or ulcerative colitis) and celiac disease (163,165). Small and large bowel changes associated with CVID are further discussed in Chapters 3 and 4. Though nonspecific, esophageal biopsies may present a variety of intraepithelial changes, namely, neutrophils (associated with *Candida* in most cases), lymphocytosis, and apoptosis (Figs. 1.47 and 1.48) (163). Although the latter

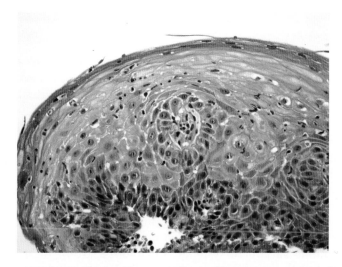

FIGURE 1.47 **Esophageal biopsy from a patient with common variable immunodeficiency (CVID).** CVID is another condition where one can find intraepithelial lymphocytosis (see Fig. 1.45).

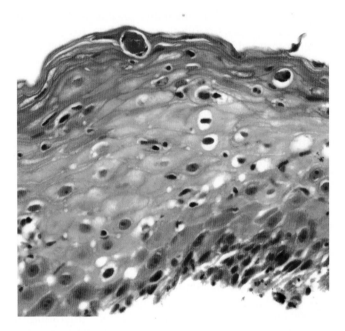

FIGURE 1.48 **Esophageal biopsy from a patient with common variable immunodeficiency (CVID).** Squamous epithelial cell apoptosis is evident in this field.

two features are seen in cases of GVHD and mycophenolate-associated injury, a lack of transplantation history would persuade against such possibility. Acquaintance with histologic patterns in the setting of CVID serves to raise this diagnostic possibility in an undiagnosed patient, provided a suitable clinical scenario.

Systemic Amyloidosis

Both primary (AL type) and secondary (AA type) systemic amyloidosis are well known to affect the GI tract and the esophagus is no exception. Patients may be asymptomatic or may come to clinical attention due to progressive or intermittent dysphagia to solids and liquids, weight loss, and/or regurgitation (166–169). Pseudoachalasia and esophageal dysmotility are common (166,167,170). Manometric studies may reveal anomalies including low or borderline LES pressure, lack of LES relaxation on deglutition, and/or loss of peristalsis in the body of the esophagus; findings that may be explained by amyloid deposition within nerves and/or the esophageal muscle wall (168,170). Endoscopically the mucosa may appear normal or may reveal granularity, erosions, ulcerations, or friability (171,172). Esophageal bullae may be seen in the rare mucocutaneous bullous variant of systemic amyloidosis (169). Biopsies present amorphous, acellular, pink material deposited extracellularly within vascular walls, lamina propria, and muscularis mucosa with the characteristic pink coloration on Congo Red stain and apple green birefringence under polarized light. The frequency of amyloid detection in esophageal biopsies of patients with systemic amyloidosis is the lowest among UGI sites at 72%, compared with 100%, 91%, and 95% for the duodenum, colorectum, and stomach, respectively (172).

REFERENCES

1. Abraham SC, Krasinskas AM, Correa AM, et al. Duplication of the muscularis mucosae in Barrett esophagus: an underrecognized feature and its implication for staging of adenocarcinoma. *Am J Surg Pathol.* 2007;31:1719–1725.

2. Lewis JT, Wang KK, Abraham SC. Muscularis mucosae duplication and the musculofibrous anomaly in endoscopic mucosal resections for barrett esophagus: implications for staging of adenocarcinoma. *Am J Surg Pathol.* 2008;32:566–571.

3. Tang P, McKinley MJ, Sporrer M, et al. Inlet patch: prevalence, histologic type, and association with esophagitis, Barrett esophagus, and antritis. *Arch Pathol Lab Med.* 2004;128:444–447.

4. von Rahden BH, Stein HJ, Becker K, et al. Heterotopic gastric mucosa of the esophagus: literature-review and proposal of a clinicopathologic classification. *Am J Gastroenterol.* 2004;99:543–551.

5. De La Pava S, Pickren JW. Ectopic sebaceous glands in the esophagus. *Arch Pathol.* 1962;73:397–399.

6. Auld RM, Lukash WM, Bordin GM. Heterotopic sebaceous glands in the esophagus. *Gastrointest Endosc.* 1987;33:332–333.

7. Bae JY, Chon CY, Kim H. Sebaceous glands in the esophagus. *J Korean Med Sci.* 1996;11:271–274.

8. Bambirra EA, de Souza Andrade J, Hooper de Souza LA, et al. Sebaceous glands in the esophagus. *Gastrointest Endosc.* 1983;29:251–252.

9. Bertoni G, Sassatelli R, Nigrisoli E, et al. Ectopic sebaceous glands in the esophagus: report of three new cases and review of the literature. *Am J Gastroenterol.* 1994;89:1884–1887.

10. Merino MJ, Brand M, LiVolsi VA, et al. Sebaceous glands in the esophagus diagnosed in a clinical setting. *Arch Pathol Lab Med.* 1982;106:47–48.

11. Nakada T, Inoue F, Iwasaki M, et al. Ectopic sebaceous glands in the esophagus. *Am J Gastroenterol.* 1995;90:501–503.

12. Nakanishi Y, Ochiai A, Shimoda T, et al. Heterotopic sebaceous glands in the esophagus: histopathological and immunohistochemical study of a resected esophagus. *Pathol Int.* 1999;49:364–368.

13. Ramakrishnan T, Brinker JE. Ectopic sebaceous glands in the esophagus. *Gastrointest Endosc.* 1978;24:293–294.

14. Salgado JA, Andrade Filho Jde S, Lima GF Jr, et al. Sebaceous glands in the esophagus. *Gastrointest Endosc.* 1980;26:150.

15. Tak AM, Scott RD, Khan NA. Sebaceous glands in esophagus in gastroesophageal reflux disease. *Indian J Gastroenterol.* 2007;26:36.

16. Thalheimer U, Wright JL, Maxwell P, et al. Sebaceous glands in the esophagus. *Endoscopy.* 2008;40(Suppl 2):E57.

17. Wei IF, Chang CC, Fang CL, et al. Education and imaging. Gastrointestinal: ectopic sebaceous glands in the esophagus. *J Gastroenterol Hepatol.* 2008;23:338.

18. Chang F, Deere H. Esophageal melanocytosis morphologic features and review of the literature. *Arch Pathol Lab Med.* 2006;130:552–557.

19. De La Pava S, Nigogosyan G, Pickren JW, et al. Melanosis of the esophagus. *Cancer.* 1963;16:48–50.

20. Sharma SS, Venkateswaran S, Chacko A, et al. Melanosis of the esophagus. An endoscopic, histochemical, and ultrastructural study. *Gastroenterology*. 1991;100:13–16.

21. Ohashi K, Kato Y, Kanno J, et al. Melanocytes and melanosis of the oesophagus in Japanese subjects—analysis of factors effecting their increase. *Virchows Arch*. 1990;417:137–143.

22. Takubo K, Kanda Y, Ishii M, et al. Primary malignant melanoma of the esophagus. *Hum Pathol*. 1983;14:727–730.

23. Kreuser ED. Primary malignant melanoma of the esophagus. *Virchows Arch*. 1979;385:49–59.

24. Piccone VA, Klopstock R, LeVeen HH, et al. Primary malignant melanoma of the esophagus associated with melanosis of the entire esophagus. First case report. *J Thorac Cardiovasc Surg*. 1970;59:864–870.

25. Bender MD, Allison J, Cuartas F, et al. Glycogenic acanthosis of the esophagus: a form of benign epithelial hyperplasia. *Gastroenterology*. 1973;65:373–380.

26. Berliner L, Redmond P, Horowitz L, et al. Glycogen plaques (glycogenic acanthosis) of the esophagus. *Radiology*. 1981;141:607–610.

27. Ghahremani GG, Rushovich AM. Glycogenic acanthosis of the esophagus: radiographic and pathologic features. *Gastrointest Radiol*. 1984;9:93–98.

28. Glick SN, Teplick SK, Goldstein J, et al. Glycogenic acanthosis of the esophagus. *AJR Am J Roentgenol*. 1982;139:683–688.

29. Jaskiewicz K, Banach L, Mafungo V, et al. Oesophageal mucosa in a population at risk of oesophageal cancer: post-mortem studies. *Int J Cancer*. 1992;50:32–35.

30. Jaskiewicz K, Louwrens HD, Van Wyk MJ, et al. Oesophageal mucosal pathology in a population at risk for gastric and oesophageal carcinoma. *Anticancer Res*. 1989;9:1191–1195.

31. Levine MS. Benign tumors of the esophagus: radiologic evaluation. *Semin Thorac Cardiovasc Surg*. 2003;15:9–19.

32. Rose D, Furth EE, Rubesin SE. Glycogenic acanthosis. *AJR Am J Roentgenol*. 1995;164:96.

33. Rywlin AM, Ortega R. Glycogenic acanthosis of the esophagus. *Arch Pathol*. 1970;90:439–443.

34. Stern Z, Sharon P, Ligumsky M, et al. Glycogenic acanthosis of the esophagus. A benign but confusing endoscopic lesion. *Am J Gastroenterol*. 1980;74:261–263.

35. Vadva MD, Triadafilopoulos G. Glycogenic acanthosis of the esophagus and gastroesophageal reflux. *J Clin Gastroenterol*. 1993;17:79–83.

36. Suoglu OD, Emiroglu HH, Sokucu S, et al. Celiac disease and glycogenic acanthosis: a new association? *Acta Paediatr*. 2004;93:568–570.

37. Eng C. Constipation, polyps, or cancer? Let PTEN predict your future. *Am J Med Genet*. 2003;122A:315–322.

38. Hizawa K, Iida M, Matsumoto T, et al. Gastrointestinal manifestations of Cowden's disease. Report of four cases. *J Clin Gastroenterol*. 1994;18:13–18.

39. Lashner BA, Riddell RH, Winans CS. Ganglioneuromatosis of the colon and extensive glycogenic acanthosis in Cowden's disease. *Dig Dis Sci*. 1986;31:213–216.

40. McGarrity TJ, Wagner Baker MJ, Ruggiero FM, et al. GI polyposis and glycogenic acanthosis of the esophagus associated with PTEN mutation positive Cowden syndrome in the absence of cutaneous manifestations. *Am J Gastroenterol*. 2003;98:1429–1434.

41. Vasovcak P, Krepelova A, Puchmajerova A, et al. A novel mutation of PTEN gene in a patient with Cowden syndrome with excessive papillomatosis of the lips, discrete cutaneous lesions, and gastrointestinal polyposis. *Eur J Gastroenterol Hepatol*. 2007;19:513–517.

42. Nishizawa A, Satoh T, Watanabe R, et al. Cowden syndrome: a novel mutation and overlooked glycogenic acanthosis in gingiva. *Br J Dermatol*. 2009;160:1116–1118.

43. Katagiri A, Kaneko K, Konishi K, et al. Lugol staining pattern in background epithelium of patients with esophageal squamous cell carcinoma. *Hepatogastroenterology*. 2004;51:713–717.

44. Kaye MD. Esophageal leukoplakia. *Gastrointest Endosc*. 1987;33:254–259.

45. Lindsay JR. Esophageal lesions in diffuse scleroderma. *Laryngoscope*. 1949;59:83–112.

46. Watson-Williams E. Fusiform dilatation of oesophagus with spasm; leukoplakia of walls. Specimen and sections of wall. *Proc R Soc Med*. 1929;22:787.

47. Taggart M, Rashid A, Abraham S. Esophageal leukoplakia: risk factors and relationship to squamous neoplasia. *Mod Pathol*. 2010;23:170A (Abstract 749).

48. Shaheen NJ, Hansen RA, Morgan DR, et al. The burden of gastrointestinal and liver diseases, 2006. *Am J Gastroenterol*. 2006;101:2128–2138.

49. Sandler RS, Everhart JE, Donowitz M, et al. The burden of selected digestive diseases in the United States. *Gastroenterology*. 2002;122:1500–1511.

50. Buttar NS, Wang KK, Leontovich O, et al. Chemoprevention of esophageal adenocarcinoma by COX-2 inhibitors in an animal model of Barrett's esophagus. *Gastroenterology*. 2002;122:1101–1112.

51. Byrnes CK, Bahadursingh A, Akhter N, et al. Duodenal reflux produces hyperproliferative epithelial esophagitis—a possible precursor to esophageal adenocarcinoma in the rat. *J Gastrointest Surg*. 2003;7:172–180.

52. Barrett N. Chronic peptic ulcer of the oesophagus and 'oesophagitis'. *Br J Surg*. 1950;38:175–182.

53. Barrett N. The lower esophagus lined by columnar epithelium. *Surgery*. 1957;41:881–894.

54. Lagergren J, Bergstrom R, Lindgren A, et al. Symptomatic gastroesophageal reflux as a risk factor for esophageal adenocarcinoma [see comments]. *N Engl J Med*. 1999;340:825–831.

55. Freedman J, Ye W, Naslund E, et al. Association between cholecystectomy and adenocarcinoma of the esophagus. *Gastroenterology*. 2001;121:548–553.

56. Galli J, Cammarota G, Calo L, et al. The role of acid and alkaline reflux in laryngeal squamous cell carcinoma. *Laryngoscope*. 2002;112:1861–1865.

57. Csendes A, Smok G, Burdiles P, et al. Effect of duodenal diversion on low-grade dysplasia in patients with Barrett's esophagus: analysis of 37 patients. *J Gastrointest Surg*. 2002;6:645–652.

58. Csendes A, Burgos AM, Smok G, et al. Effect of gastric bypass on Barrett's esophagus and intestinal metaplasia of the cardia in patients with morbid obesity. *J Gastrointest Surg*. 2006;10:259–264.

59. Houghton SG, Romero Y, Sarr MG. Effect of Roux-en-Y gastric bypass in obese patients with Barrett's esophagus: attempts to eliminate duodenogastric reflux. *Surg Obes Relat Dis*. 2008;4:1–4; discussion 4–5.

60. Dvorak K, Payne CM, Chavarria M, et al. Bile acids in combination with low pH induce oxidative stress and oxidative DNA damage: relevance to the pathogenesis of Barrett's oesophagus. *Gut*. 2007;56:763–771.

61. Fiocca R, Mastracci L, Riddell R, et al. Development of consensus guidelines for the histologic recognition of microscopic esophagitis in patients with gastroesophageal reflux disease: the Esohisto project. *Hum Pathol*. 2010;41:223–231.

62. Abraham SC, Yardley JH, Wu TT. Erosive injury to the upper gastrointestinal tract in patients receiving iron medication: an underrecognized entity. *Am J Surg Pathol*. 1999;23:1241–1247.

63. Lillemoe KD, Romolo JL, Hamilton SR, et al. Intestinal necrosis due to sodium polystyrene (Kayexalate) in sorbitol enemas: clinical and experimental support for the hypothesis. *Surgery*. 1987;101:267–272.

64. Abraham SC, Bhagavan BS, Lee LA, et al. Upper gastrointestinal tract injury in patients receiving Kayexalate (sodium polystyrene sulfonate) in sorbitol: clinical, endoscopic, and histopathologic findings. *Am J Surg Pathol*. 2001;25:637–644.

65. Hruban RH, Yardley JH, Donehower RC, et al. Taxol toxicity. Epithelial necrosis in the gastrointestinal tract associated with polymerized microtubule accumulation and mitotic arrest. *Cancer.* 1989;63:1944–1950.

66. Rowinsky EK, Donehower RC. Paclitaxel (Taxol). *N Engl J Med.* 1995;332:1004–1014.

67. Daniels JA, Gibson MK, Xu L, et al. Gastrointestinal tract epithelial changes associated with taxanes: marker of drug toxicity versus effect. *Am J Surg Pathol.* 2008;32:473–477.

68. Iacobuzio-Donahue CA, Lee EL, Abraham SC, et al. Colchicine toxicity: distinct morphologic findings in gastrointestinal biopsies. *Am J Surg Pathol.* 2001;25:1067–1073.

69. Allison AC, Eugui EM. Mechanisms of action of mycophenolate mofetil in preventing acute and chronic allograft rejection. *Transplantation.* 2005;80:S181–190.

70. Zolezzi M. Mycophenolate sodium versus mycophenolate mofetil: a review of their comparative features. *Saudi J Kidney Dis Transpl.* 2005;16:140–145.

71. Chan TM. Mycophenolate mofetil in the treatment of lupus nephritis–7 years on. *Lupus.* 2008;17:617–621.

72. Dede F, Onec B, Ayli D, et al. Mycophenolate mofetil treatment of crescentic Henoch-Schonlein nephritis with IgA depositions. *Scand J Urol Nephrol.* 2008;42:178–180.

73. Esmaili N, Chams-Davatchi C, Valikhani M, et al. Treatment of pemphigus vulgaris with mycophenolate mofetil as a steroid-sparing agent. *Eur J Dermatol.* 2008;18:159–164.

74. Lu F, Tu Y, Peng X, et al. A prospective multicentre study of mycophenolate mofetil combined with prednisolone as induction therapy in 213 patients with active lupus nephritis. *Lupus.* 2008;17:622–629.

75. Teoh SC, Hogan AC, Dick AD, et al. Mycophenolate mofetil for the treatment of uveitis. *Am J Ophthalmol.* 2008;146:752–760, 760 e751–753.

76. Wilkins MR, Dart JK. Mycophenolate mofetil for the treatment of severe inflammatory external eye diseases. *Br J Ophthalmol.* 2008;92:578–579.

77. Yalcindag FN, Amer R, Forrester JV. Mycophenolate mofetil in the treatment of ocular inflammation in ANCA-associated vasculitis. *J Ocul Pharmacol Ther.* 2008;24:249–254.

78. Behrend M, Braun F. Enteric-coated mycophenolate sodium: tolerability profile compared with mycophenolate mofetil. *Drugs.* 2005;65:1037–1050.

79. Behrend M. Adverse gastrointestinal effects of mycophenolate mofetil: aetiology, incidence and management. *Drug Saf.* 2001;24:645–663.

80. Papadimitriou JC, Cangro CB, Lustberg A, et al. Histologic features of mycophenolate mofetil-related colitis: a graft-versus-host disease-like pattern. *Int J Surg Pathol.* 2003;11:295–302.

81. Papadimitriou JC, Drachenberg CB, Beskow CO, et al. Graft-versus-host disease-like features in mycophenolate mofetil-related colitis. *Transplant Proc.* 2001;33:2237–2238.

82. Ducloux D, Ottignon Y, Semhoun-Ducloux S, et al. Mycophenolate mofetil-induced villous atrophy. *Transplantation.* 1998;66:1115–1116.

83. Parfitt JR, Jayakumar S, Driman DK. Mycophenolate mofetil-related gastrointestinal mucosal injury: variable injury patterns, including graft-versus-host disease-like changes. *Am J Surg Pathol.* 2008;32:1367–1372.

84. Nguyen T, Park JY, Scudiere JR, et al. Mycophenolic acid (CellCept and Myofortic) induced injury of the upper GI tract. *Am J Surg Pathol.* 2009;33:1355–1363.

85. Lanza F. Bisphosphonate mucosal injury–the end of the story? *Dig Liver Dis.* 2003;35:67–70.

86. Dobrucali A, Tobey NA, Awayda MS, et al. Physiological and morphological effects of alendronate on rabbit esophageal epithelium. *Am J Physiol Gastrointest Liver Physiol.* 2002;283:G576–586.

87. Wallace JL. Upper gastrointestinal ulceration with alendronate. *Dig Dis Sci.* 1999;44:311–313.

88. Peter CP, Handt LK, Smith SM. Esophageal irritation due to alendronate sodium tablets: possible mechanisms. *Dig Dis Sci.* 1998;43:1998–2002.

89. Abraham SC, Cruz-Correa M, Lee LA, et al. Alendronate-associated esophageal injury: pathologic and endoscopic features. *Mod Pathol.* 1999;12:1152–1157.

90. Vestergaard P, Schwartz K, Pinholt EM, et al. Use of bisphosphonates and raloxifene and risk of deep venous thromboembolism and pulmonary embolism. *Osteoporos Int.* 2009.

91. Wysowski DK. Reports of esophageal cancer with oral bisphosphonate use. *N Engl J Med.* 2009;360:89–90.

92. Siris ES, Oster MW, Bilezikian JP. More on reports of esophageal cancer with oral bisphosphonate use. *N Engl J Med.* 2009;360:1791; author reply 1791–1792.

93. Hofbauer LC, Miehlke S. More on reports of esophageal cancer with oral bisphosphonate use. *N Engl J Med.* 2009;360:1790; author reply 1791–1792.

94. Shaheen NJ. More on reports of esophageal cancer with oral bisphosphonate use. *N Engl J Med.* 2009;360:1790–1791; author reply 1791–1792.

95. Robins HI, Holen KD. More on reports of esophageal cancer with oral bisphosphonate use. *N Engl J Med.* 2009;360:1790; author reply 1791–1792.

96. Solomon DH, Patrick A, Brookhart MA. More on reports of esophageal cancer with oral bisphosphonate use. *N Engl J Med.* 2009;360:1789–1790; author reply 1791–1782.

97. Abrahamsen B, Eiken P, Eastell R. More on reports of esophageal cancer with oral bisphosphonate use. *N Engl J Med.* 2009;360:1789; author reply 1791–1782.

98. Carmack SW, Vemulapalli R, Spechler SJ, et al. Esophagitis dissecans superficialis ("sloughing esophagitis"): a clinicopathologic study of 12 cases. *Am J Surg Pathol.* 2009;33:1789–1794.

99. Bayer O. A case of esophagitis dissecans. *Fortschr Geb Rontgenstr Nuklearmed.* 1955;82:551–552.

100. Beck RN. Oesophagitis dissecans superficialis. *Br Med J.* 1954;1:501–502.

101. Morgenstern M. Tube-like expulsion of esophageal mucosa (esophagitis exfoliativasive dissecans superficialis). *Zentralbl Allg Pathol.* 1952;89:17–22.

102. Ponsot P, Molas G, Scoazec JY, et al. Chronic esophagitis dissecans: an unrecognized clinicopathologic entity? *Gastrointest Endosc.* 1997;45:38–45.

103. Csikos M, Horvath O, Petri A, et al. Late malignant transformation of chronic corrosive oesophageal strictures. *Langenbecks Arch Chir.* 1985;365:231–238.

104. Shekitka KM, Helwig EB. Deceptive bizarre stromal cells in polyps and ulcers of the gastrointestinal tract. *Cancer.* 1991;67:2111–2117.

105. Jessurun J, Paplanus SH, Nagle RB, et al. Pseudosarcomatous changes in inflammatory pseudopolyps of the colon. *Arch Pathol Lab Med.* 1986;110:833–836.

106. Singh SP, Odze RD. Multinucleated epithelial giant cell changes in esophagitis: a clinicopathologic study of 14 cases. *Am J Surg Pathol.* 1998;22:93–99.

107. McDonald GB, Sullivan KM, Schuffler MD, et al. Esophageal abnormalities in chronic graft-versus-host disease in humans. *Gastroenterology.* 1981;80:914–921.

108. McDonald GB, Sullivan KM, Plumley TF. Radiographic features of esophageal involvement in chronic graft-vs.-host disease. *AJR Am J Roentgenol.* 1984;142:501–506.

109. Filipovich AH. Diagnosis and manifestations of chronic graft-versus-host disease. *Best Pract Res Clin Haematol.* 2008;21:251–257.

110. Abraham SC, Ravich WJ, Anhalt GJ, et al. Esophageal lichen planus: case report and review of the literature. *Am J Surg Pathol.* 2000;24:1678–1682.

111. Dickens CM, Heseltine D, Walton S, et al. The oesophagus in lichen planus: an endoscopic study. *BMJ.* 1990;300:84.

112. Quispel R, van Boxel OS, Schipper ME, et al. High prevalence of esophageal involvement in lichen planus: a study using magnification chromoendoscopy. *Endoscopy*. 2009;41:187–193.

113. Chryssostalis A, Gaudric M, Terris B, et al. Esophageal lichen planus: a series of eight cases including a patient with esophageal verrucous carcinoma. A case series. *Endoscopy*. 2008;40:764–768.

114. Calabrese C, Fabbri A, Benni M, et al. Squamous cell carcinoma arising in esophageal lichen planus. *Gastrointest Endosc*. 2003;57:596–599.

115. Schwartz MP, Sigurdsson V, Vreuls W, et al. Two siblings with lichen planus and squamous cell carcinoma of the oesophagus. *Eur J Gastroenterol Hepatol*. 2006;18:1111–1115.

116. Keate RF, Williams JW, Connolly SM. Lichen planus esophagitis: report of three patients treated with oral tacrolimus or intraesophageal corticosteroid injections or both. *Dis Esophagus*. 2003;16:47–53.

117. Reissmann A, Hahn EG, Faller G, et al. Sole treatment of lichen planus-associated esophageal stenosis with injection of corticosteroids. *Gastrointest Endosc*. 2006;63:168–169.

118. Gomi H, Akiyama M, Yakabi K, et al. Oesophageal involvement in pemphigus vulgaris. *Lancet*. 1999;354:1794.

119. Mignogna MD, Lo Muzio L, Galloro G, et al. Oral pemphigus: clinical significance of esophageal involvement: report of eight cases. *Oral Surg Oral Med Oral Pathol Oral Radiol Endod*. 1997;84:179–184.

120. Faias S, Lage P, Sachse F, et al. Pemphigus vulgaris with exclusive involvement of the esophagus: case report and review. *Gastrointest Endosc*. 2004;60:312–315.

121. Coelho LK, Troncon LE, Roselino AM, et al. Esophageal Nikolsky's sign in pemphigus vulgaris. *Endoscopy*. 1997;29:S35.

122. Isolauri J, Airo I. Benign mucous membrane pemphigoid involving the esophagus: a report of two cases treated with dilation. *Gastrointest Endosc*. 1989;35:569–571.

123. Monkemuller K, Neumann H, Fry LC. Esophageal blebs and blisters. *Gastroenterology*. 2010;138:e3–4.

124. Popovici Z, Deac M, Rotaru M, et al. Stenosis of the esophagus in cicatricial pemphigoid resolved by colon interposition: report of a case. *Surg Today*. 1997;27:234–237.

125. Fine JD, Eady RA, Bauer EA, et al. Revised classification system for inherited epidermolysis bullosa: Report of the Second International Consensus Meeting on diagnosis and classification of epidermolysis bullosa. *J Am Acad Dermatol*. 2000;42:1051–1066.

126. Ergun GA, Lin AN, Dannenberg AJ, et al. Gastrointestinal manifestations of epidermolysis bullosa. A study of 101 patients. *Medicine (Baltimore)*. 1992;71:121–127.

127. Tishler JM, Han SY, Helman CA. Esophageal involvement in epidermolysis bullosa dystrophica. *AJR Am J Roentgenol*. 1983;141:1283–1286.

128. Fine JD, Johnson LB, Weiner M, et al. Gastrointestinal complications of inherited epidermolysis bullosa: cumulative experience of the National Epidermolysis Bullosa Registry. *J Pediatr Gastroenterol Nutr*. 2008;46:147–158.

129. Ray A, Bhattacharya S, Kumar A, et al. Rare occurrence of carcinoma esophagus in a case of epidermolysis bullosa. *Indian J Cancer*. 2009;46:72–73.

130. Greenson JK, Beschorner WE, Boitnott JK, et al. Prominent mononuclear cell infiltrate is characteristic of herpes esophagitis. *Hum Pathol*. 1991;22:541–549.

131. Greenson JK. Macrophage aggregates in cytomegalovirus esophagitis. *Hum Pathol*.1997;28:375–378.

132. Walsh TJ, Belitsos NJ, Hamilton SR. Bacterial esophagitis in immunocompromised patients. *Arch Intern Med*. 1986;146:1345–1348.

133. Ezzell JH Jr., Bremer J, Adamec TA. Bacterial esophagitis: an often forgotten cause of odynophagia. *Am J Gastroenterol*. 1990;85:296–298.

134. Penfield JD, Lang DM, Goldblum JR, et al. The role of allergy evaluation in adults with eosinophilic esophagitis. *J Clin Gastroenterol*. 2010;44:22–27.

135. Almansa C, Krishna M, Buchner AM, et al. Seasonal distribution in newly diagnosed cases of eosinophilic esophagitis in adults. *Am J Gastroenterol.* 2009;104:828–833.

136. Moawad FJ, Veerappan GR, Lake JM, et al. Correlation between eosinophilic oesophagitis and aeroallergens. *Aliment Pharmacol Ther.* 2010;31:509–515.

137. Wang FY, Gupta SK, Fitzgerald JF. Is there a seasonal variation in the incidence or intensity of allergic eosinophilic esophagitis in newly diagnosed children? *J Clin Gastroenterol.* 2007;41:451–453.

138. Veerappan GR, Perry JL, Duncan TJ, et al. Prevalence of eosinophilic esophagitis in an adult population undergoing upper endoscopy: a prospective study. *Clin Gastroenterol Hepatol.* 2009;7:420–426, e421–422.

139. Franciosi JP, Tam V, Liacouras CA, et al. A case-control study of sociodemographic and geographic characteristics of 335 children with eosinophilic esophagitis. *Clin Gastroenterol Hepatol.* 2009;7:415–419.

140. Steiner SJ, Kernek KM, Fitzgerald JF. Severity of basal cell hyperplasia differs in reflux versus eosinophilic esophagitis. *J Pediatr Gastroenterol Nutr.* 2006;42:506–509.

141. Cohen MS, Kaufman AB, Palazzo JP, et al. An audit of endoscopic complications in adult eosinophilic esophagitis. *Clin Gastroenterol Hepatol.* 2007;5:1149–1153.

142. Dellon ES, Gibbs WB, Rubinas TC, et al. Esophageal dilation in eosinophilic esophagitis: safety and predictors of clinical response and complications. *Gastrointest Endosc.* 2010;71:706–712.

143. Nantes O, Jimenez FJ, Zozaya JM, et al. Increased risk of esophageal perforation in eosinophilic esophagitis. *Endoscopy.* 2009;41(Suppl 2):E177–178.

144. Shim LS, Grehan M. Education and Imaging. Gastrointestinal: oesophageal perforation during endoscopy for food impaction in eosinophilic oesophagitis. *J Gastroenterol Hepatol.* 2010;25:428.

145. Gomez Senent S, Adan Merino L, Froilan Torres C, et al. Spontaneous esophageal rupture as onset of eosinophilic esophagitis. *Gastroenterol Hepatol.* 2008;31:50–51.

146. Robles-Medranda C, Villard F, Bouvier R, et al. Spontaneous esophageal perforation in eosinophilic esophagitis in children. *Endoscopy.* 2008;40(Suppl 2):E171.

147. Furuta GT, Liacouras CA, Collins MH, et al. Eosinophilic esophagitis in children and adults: a systematic review and consensus recommendations for diagnosis and treatment. *Gastroenterology.* 2007;133:1342–1363.

148. Dellon ES, Aderoju A, Woosley JT, et al. Variability in diagnostic criteria for eosinophilic esophagitis: a systematic review. *Am J Gastroenterol.* 2007;102:2300–2313.

149. Rodrigo S, Abboud G, Oh D, et al. High intraepithelial eosinophil counts in esophageal squamous epithelium are not specific for eosinophilic esophagitis in adults. *Am J Gastroenterol.* 2008;103:435–442.

150. Kephart GM, Alexander JA, Arora AS, et al. Marked deposition of eosinophil-derived neurotoxin in adult patients with eosinophilic esophagitis. *Am J Gastroenterol.* 2010;105:298–307.

151. Decker GA, Loftus EV Jr, Pasha TM, et al. Crohn's disease of the esophagus: clinical features and outcomes. *Inflamm Bowel Dis.* 2001;7:113–119.

152. D'Haens G, Rutgeerts P, Geboes K, et al. The natural history of esophageal Crohn's disease: three patterns of evolution. *Gastrointest Endosc.* 1994;40:296–300.

153. Alcantara M, Rodriguez R, Potenciano JL, et al. Endoscopic and bioptic findings in the upper gastrointestinal tract in patients with Crohn's disease. *Endoscopy.* 1993;25:282–286.

154. Ruuska T, Vaajalahti P, Arajarvi P, et al. Prospective evaluation of upper gastrointestinal mucosal lesions in children with ulcerative colitis and Crohn's disease. *J Pediatr Gastroenterol Nutr.* 1994;19:181–186.

155. Ramaswamy K, Jacobson K, Jevon G, et al. Esophageal Crohn disease in children: a clinical spectrum. *J Pediatr Gastroenterol Nutr.* 2003;36:454–458.

156. Lenaerts C, Roy CC, Vaillancourt M, et al. High incidence of upper gastrointestinal tract involvement in children with Crohn disease. *Pediatrics*. 1989;83:777–781.

157. Rudolph I, Goldstein F, DiMarino AJ Jr. Crohn's disease of the esophagus: Three cases and a literature review. *Can J Gastroenterol*. 2001;15:117–122.

158. Tobin JM, Sinha B, Ramani P, et al. Upper gastrointestinal mucosal disease in pediatric Crohn disease and ulcerative colitis: a blinded, controlled study. *J Pediatr Gastroenterol Nutr*. 2001;32:443–448.

159. Rubio CA, Sjodahl K, Lagergren J. Lymphocytic esophagitis: a histologic subset of chronic esophagitis. *Am J Clin Pathol*. 2006;125:432–437.

160. Purdy JK, Appelman HD, Golembeski CP, et al. Lymphocytic esophagitis: a chronic or recurring pattern of esophagitis resembling allergic contact dermatitis. *Am J Clin Pathol*. 2008;130:508–513.

161. Primary immunodeficiency diseases. Report of a WHO Scientific Group. *Clin Exp Immunol*. 1995;99(Suppl 1):1–24.

162. Cunningham-Rundles C, Bodian C. Common variable immunodeficiency: clinical and immunological features of 248 patients. *Clin Immunol*. 1999;92:34–48.

163. Daniels JA, Lederman HM, Maitra A, et al. Gastrointestinal tract pathology in patients with common variable immunodeficiency (CVID): a clinicopathologic study and review. *Am J Surg Pathol*. 2007;31:1800–1812.

164. Hermans PE, Diaz-Buxo JA, Stobo JD. Idiopathic late-onset immunoglobulin deficiency. Clinical observations in 50 patients. *Am J Med*. 1976;61:221–237.

165. Washington K, Stenzel TT, Buckley RH, et al. Gastrointestinal pathology in patients with common variable immunodeficiency and X-linked agammaglobulinemia. *Am J Surg Pathol*. 1996;20:1240–1252.

166. Estrada CA, Lewandowski C, Schubert TT, et al. Esophageal involvement in secondary amyloidosis mimicking achalasia. *J Clin Gastroenterol*. 1990;12:447–450.

167. Lazaraki G, Nakos A, Katodritou E, et al. A rare case of multiple myeloma initially presenting with pseudoachalasia. *Dis Esophagus*. 2009;22:E21–E24.

168. Lopez-Cepero Andrada JM, Jimenez Arjona J, Amaya Vidal A, et al. Pseudoachalasia and secondary amyloidosis in a patient with rheumatoid arthritis. *Gastroenterol Hepatol*. 2002;25:398–400.

169. Rekhtman N, Hash KS, Moresi JM. Mucocutaneous bullous amyloidosis with an unusual mixed protein composition of amyloid deposits. *Br J Dermatol*. 2006;154:751–754.

170. Rubinow A, Burakoff R, Cohen AS, et al. Esophageal manometry in systemic amyloidosis. A study of 30 patients. *Am J Med*. 1983;75:951–956.

171. Bhavani RS, Lakhtakia S, Sekaran A, et al. Amyloidosis presenting as postcricoid esophageal stricture. *Gastrointest Endosc*. 2010;71:180–181; discussion 181.

172. Tada S, Iida M, Iwashita A, et al. Endoscopic and biopsy findings of the upper digestive tract in patients with amyloidosis. *Gastrointest Endosc*. 1990;36:10–14.

2

STOMACH

The stomach has four main zones with divergent types of mucosae. The cardia and antrum are similar histologically and are at the proximal and distal ends, respectively. In the middle are the fundus and body, which share the same histology. The fundus is the part above the gastroesophageal (GE) junction and the body lies below it.

A simple way to think about the lining of the different parts of the stomach is that the ends (cardia and antrum) have the function of protecting the esophagus and duodenum from acid and enzymes, whereas the middle of the stomach produces the acid and enzymes.

The empty stomach is thrown into rugae (folds). Tiny surface invaginations are termed gastric pits and are the conduits of secretions. The gastric glands, regardless of site, have an isthmus, neck, and base. These glands are not straight structures, but complex and convoluted in three dimensions. Thus, on a two-dimensional slide, there are not clear demarcations of the three regions. Histologically, the entire stomach has a surface of foveolar cells that secrete neutral mucin, which appears from magenta to pink on the periodic acid-Schiff (PAS) stain. In the isthmus region of the body and fundus, parietal cells (oxyntic cells) dominate, but mucous neck cells are also present. Mucous neck cells are seen in the neck, whereas chief cells dominate in the base. Endocrine cells are in the deep isthmus toward the base. In the cardia and antrum, things are simpler because all the layers predominantly produce mucin, although the antrum has G cells that produce gastrin whereas the cardia does not. Gastrin is secreted by the antrum, but not the body, fundus, or cardia. This finding can be exploited occasionally when assessing atrophic gastritis, a case in which marked atrophy results in an "antralized" appearance in the fundus or body. The lamina propria of the stomach should contain only a small population of lymphocytes, plasma cells, mast cells, and eosinophils. In the intestines, however, these constituents are more abundant. Bacteria are usually not seen in the normal gastric mucus, whereas they are normally present in the colon (Fig. 2.1, e-Figs. 2.1–2.4).

When assessing biopsies from the stomach, features that help in diagnosis often involve correlation with clinical information. Here are a few general points:

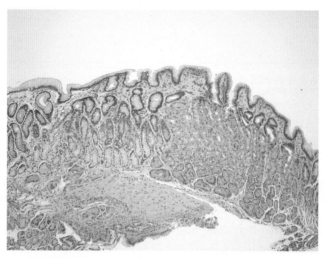

FIGURE 2.1 **Normal gastric mucosa.** This particular example is from the transitional antral/oxyntic mucosa. Note antral-type mucosa to the left and oxyntic mucosa to the right.

a. Noting the age and gender of the subject can be of value. For example, autoimmune metaplastic atrophic gastritis (AMAG) tends to affect patients predominantly in their 6th decade of life and is twice as common in females as in males (55).

b. In a busy gastrointestinal (GI) biopsy service, there are frequently many biopsies to review, and time efficiency is critical. So, it is critical to know which biopsies require the greatest attention. In gastric biopsies, the "snake in the grass" is always signet-ring cell carcinoma, which is often focal and subtle in mucosal biopsies. Any clinical concern (such as a stomach that distends poorly on insufflation) by the endoscopist merits a careful review of all biopsy fragments from gastric biopsies. Because gastric hyperplastic polyps occasionally harbor cancers, these should all be reviewed carefully (1). Most do not house a cancer, but all should be assessed for this possibility. In contrast, fundic gland polyps are not "red flag" lesions. All cases showing ulcers also should be studied carefully. Areas appearing fibrotic at scanning magnification are always reviewed at higher magnification. At our institution, all upper tract biopsies are stained with periodic acid-Schiff/Alcian blue (PAS/AB), and we find this stain helpful when evaluating any atypical cells in the lamina propria.

c. There are also sources of concern for carcinoma that are not neoplastic. In occasional cases, crushed oxyntic glands, in which mucous neck cells predominate, can resemble signet-ring cell carcinoma (Figs. 2.2, 2.3, e-Figs. 2.5–2.11). The epithelial changes in acute hemorrhagic gastritis and in iron pill gastritis can raise the possibility of carcinoma or dysplasia (2) (Figs. 2.4, 2.5). Lastly, gastric xanthoma can also be a source of concern and is further discussed in Volume 2 (e-Figs. 2.12, 2.13).

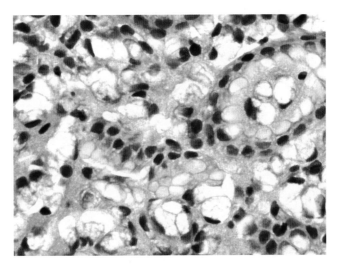

FIGURE 2.2 **Distorted mucous neck cells**. These may be mimickers of signet-ring cell carcinoma. In this case, note that the cells of concern are located within the lumina of the glands. Compare with Figure 2.3, a case of signet-ring cell carcinoma.

ACUTE HEMORRHAGIC GASTRITIS

Acute hemorrhagic gastritis is prototypically associated with alcohol abuse (3,4), but other agents that are injurious to the gastric mucosa can also be responsible (5–7) and infectious agents can result in this pattern of injury. Occasionally, a hemorrhagic gastropathy is encountered in association with phosphasoda bowel preparations for colonoscopy (8). Typically such lesions

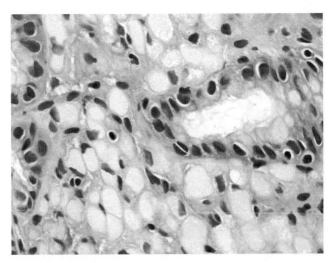

FIGURE 2.3 **A case of signet-ring cell carcinoma**. Note that the signet-ring cells are located within the lamina propria.

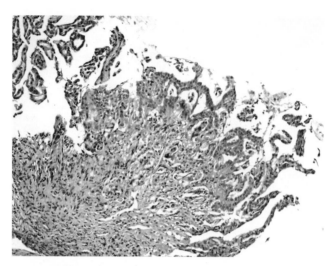

FIGURE 2.4 **Iron pill gastritis, hematoxylin and eosin (H&E) stain.** While there are nuclear alterations and marked reactive changes, the overall architecture is intact. Iron pigment also is apparent in this field.

are not biopsied in order to avoid further exacerbation of the mucosal injury. In early literature, it was difficult to separate the effects of *Helicobacter* gastritis from pure alcohol injury, but we currently believe that the acute injury from alcohol is similar to a corrosive one with little inflammation, but with abundant edema, hemorrhage, and reactive epithelial changes (Fig. 2.6, e-Fig. 2.14).

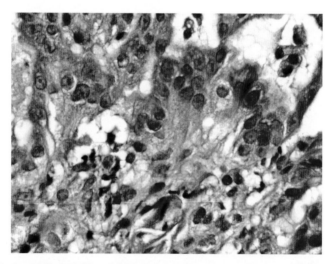

FIGURE 2.5 **Iron pill gastritis.** This higher magnification of Figure 2.4 shows iron deposition within the lamina propria in the left part of the field. The epithelial cell nuclei are small and regular with prominent nucleoli, a reactive change.

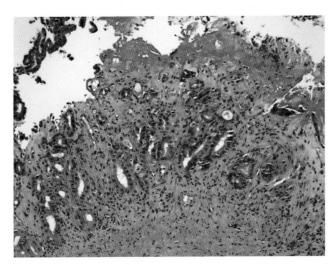

FIGURE 2.6 **Acute hemorrhagic gastritis.** There is little inflammation, but with abundant hemorrhage and reactive epithelial changes.

CHEMICAL GASTRITIS/REACTIVE GASTROPATHY

Chemical gastritis, also referred to as reactive gastropathy or previously as reflux gastritis, is seen mostly in the antrum and is common in our material. It is usually attributed to bile reflux and, thus, is usually seen in patients being evaluated for GE reflux disease (which, in reality, is duodenogastroesophageal reflux disease) (9). Bile reflux is injurious to the gastric antrum, as well as to the esophagus. In patients in whom the antrum has been removed, bile reflux injures the gastric body and is probably responsible for the so-called stump cancers found in the postantrectomy setting. In the intact stomach, this type of injury is largely associated with the use of nonsteroidal anti-inflammatory drugs (NSAIDs) (10,11). In a study by Sobala et al. (10), an association with heavy alcohol consumption was observed; however, this did not reach statistical significance. Other implicated medications, particularly in the pediatric setting, include anticonvulsants, psychiatric, and chemotherapeutic drugs (12). The general features of reactive gastropathy are foveolar hyperplasia, lamina propria edema, muscular stranding, and vascular ectasia (Fig. 2.7, e-Figs. 2.15–2.18). Active and chronic inflammation is minimal, which is why some prefer the term "reactive gastropathy" instead of "chemical gastritis." We use the latter term simply as a matter of institutional habit (i.e., it is understood by our clinicians) and with a comment that likely associations are both NSAIDs and bile reflux. In daily practice, it is known that neutrophils can be a component of acute chemical injury. Similarly, acute inflammatory cells can be seen if biopsies are taken in the vicinity of an NSAID-associated ulcer. They can be considered part of this condition when present in the absence of a lamina propria expanded with lymphoplasmacytic cells (infected by *Helicobacter*

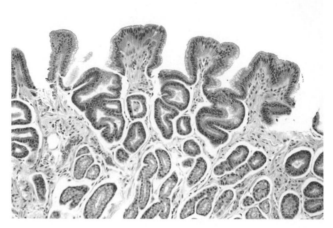

FIGURE 2.7 **Chemical gastritis/reactive gastropathy.** This particular example shows some surface mucin loss, corkscrewing of the gastric pits, and reactive epithelial changes. There is minimal lamina propria inflammation.

pylori [*H. pylori*]). A minimal lymphoplasmacytic component can similarly be dismissed. Of course, some patients who take NSAIDs have treated *H. pylori* and may manifest features of both conditions. Identical changes can be seen in patients with gastric antral vascular ectasia (GAVE; "watermelon stomach"). In the setting of GAVE, the endoscopist may offer a history of iron deficiency anemia and provide information regarding the endoscopic appearance (antral linear erythema or "watermelon stomach"). A search for fibrin thrombi may prove fruitful in this instance. GAVE is further discussed on page 88.

MUCOSAL CALCINOSIS

Mucosal calcinosis is seen in some renal failure patients (Fig. 2.8, 2.9, e-Figs. 2.19–2.22) and has been attributed to antacid use in these patients (13), but probably mostly reflects disorders of calcium metabolism and the "metastatic" calcium deposits that are typical in such patients (14). In addition to the wide variety of hypercalcemia- and/or hyperphosphatemia-causing clinical conditions, gastric mucosal calcinosis has also been associated with atrophic gastritis, hypervitaminosis A, organ transplantation, gastric neoplasia, uremia with eucalcemia/euphosphatemia, the use of citrate-containing blood products, isotretinoin, and sucralfate (15). Typically, the deposits of calcium are "metastatic" calcification.

Regardless, mucosal calcinosis itself seems to be of no immediate clinical significance except as an incidental finding in patients with renal failure. However, its presence in gastric biopsies should be reported, as it may serve as an indicator for generalized "metastatic" calcification, especially

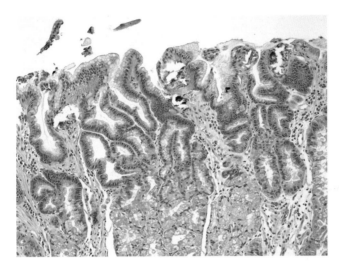

FIGURE 2.8 Mucosal calcinosis. This is essentially an incidental finding, usually noted in renal failure patients.

in organs where it may be fatal, such as the heart. Furthermore, some examples of systemic calcification are reversible with normalization of biochemical parameters. On biopsies, the deposits are tinctorially similar to cytomegalovirus (CMV) inclusions, a bluish purple color, ranging from 40 to 250 μm in diameter, and are present just beneath the surface epithelium at the tips of the foveolae. An x-ray microanalysis showed that these mucosal deposits contained such elements as aluminum, phosphorus, calcium, and chlorine (13).

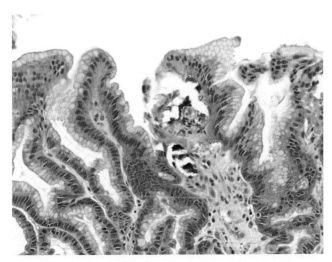

FIGURE 2.9 Mucosal calcinosis. A higher magnification of Figure 2.8.

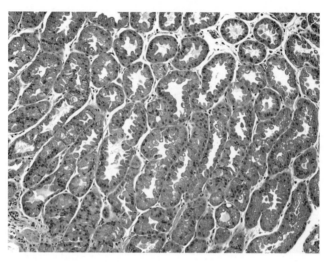

FIGURE 2.10 **Proton pump inhibitor effect.** The parietal cells appear hyperplastic with granular cytoplasm and apical snouts.

PROTON PUMP INHIBITOR EFFECTS

Proton pump inhibitors (PPI) are commonly taken by patients having gastric biopsies. Examples of these medications are omeprazole (Prilosec), lansoprazole (Prevacid), and esomeprazole (Nexium). These medications reduce acid secretion by gastric parietal cells and have a morphologic correlate of an appearance of apocrine-like cytoplasmic swelling and/or vacuolation of parietal cells (Figs. 2.10, 2.11, e-Figs. 2.23, 2.24). These findings

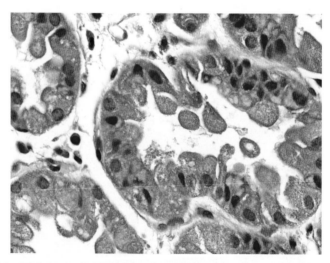

FIGURE 2.11 **Proton pump inhibitor effect on oxyntic mucosa.** Note the parietal cells with protrusions reminiscent of those in apocrine cells.

may be reported, or their absence noted, if there is a clinical concern about medication compliance. However, occasionally, patients not receiving these medications display such changes, so we report them as "changes of the type seen in patients taking proton pump inhibitors."

INJURY DUE TO CHEMICAL AGENTS AND IATROGENIC INJURY

Iron

In our material, iron-related mucosal injury is found in about 1% of biopsies from upper endoscopic examination (2); thus, it is not uncommon. It is more commonly encountered in the stomach than in the esophagus. Approximately half of the patients have underlying infectious, mechanical, toxic, or systemic medical conditions that could have initiated or exacerbated tissue injury.

Biopsies demonstrate crystalline iron deposition in the lamina propria, either covered by an intact epithelium, subjacent to small superficial erosions, or admixed with granulation tissue. Occasionally, iron-containing thrombi are seen in mucosal blood vessels. Erosive or ulcerative mucosal injury is seen in most cases. Iron pill gastritis appears similar to iron pill esophagitis (2), as discussed in Chapter 1, but it is of particular note since striking epithelial changes in the setting of iron pill gastritis sometimes mimic gastric carcinoma or dysplasia (Figs. 2.12, 2.13, e-Figs. 2.25–2.28). The epithelial changes found in "iron pill ulcers" lack the architectural changes of gastric cancer, but can be severe. The key is noting the yellow-brown hue at scanning magnification, which assumes a blue-black

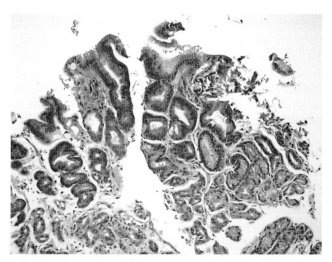

FIGURE 2.12 Iron pill gastritis. This H&E stain shows golden-brown iron deposits within the lamina propria and the surface epithelium.

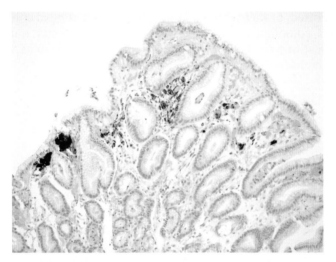

FIGURE 2.13 **Iron pill gastritis.** This iron stain highlights iron deposits within both the epithelium and lamina propria.

appearance in areas where the iron residue is thick. Of course, there is no reason why iron could not lodge in an ulcerated carcinoma, but the scenario of iron in a nonneoplastic ulcer is more commonly encountered.

Gastric Siderosis

In patients with hemochromatosis or other causes of iron overload (such as multiple transfusions), it is typically the reticuloendothelial system rather than the mucosa that houses the excess iron, so the pattern of epithelial (and even endothelial) iron deposition is more likely attributable to an exogenous source. However, occasionally a gastric siderosis pattern can be encountered in which the deep gastric glands (rather than the surface epithelium) appear brownish on H&E; the finding can be extremely subtle. This pattern of iron deposition in antral and fundic glands is rare, encountered in about 0.5% of gastric biopsies (16). When identified, it suggests the possibility of hemochromatosis (or iron overload due to other causes such as multiple transfusions).

Kayexalate

Kayexalate can be found associated with gastric mucosa and gastric erosions/ulcerations, just as in the case of the esophagus (see Chapter 1). As noted in Chapter 1, kayexalate is a cation-exchange resin. When administered orally or by nasogastric tube, sodium cations are released from the resin and exchanged for hydrogen ions. As the resin then passes through the intestines, hydrogen is exchanged for potassium, which is then eliminated in the feces along with the remainder of the altered resin, thereby lowering the serum potassium concentration.

In the early use of kayexalate, the resin was suspended in water and then administered. Although it was generally well tolerated, some patients were reported to develop gastric and bowel opacifications as a result of concretions of crystalline resin. Therefore, it became increasingly popular to administer kayexalate in a suspension with hypertonic sorbitol. This solution reduces both the frequency of kayexalate bezoar formation and colonic impaction by promoting an osmotic diarrhea. However, this hyperosmotic effect results in mucosal injury in a subset of patients, as discussed in Chapter 1.

Kayexalate also can be associated with severe mucosal injury in the upper GI tract, and a series of such cases has been reported by Abraham et al. (17). In most instances, kayexalate is easy to recognize in endoscopic biopsies and the clinician can be alerted if there is associated ischemic GI tract disease or erosive lesions.

As in other sites, kayexalate crystals found in the stomach are lightly basophilic on hematoxylin and eosin stain, red on PAS/AB and acid-fast stains, and blue on Diff-Quik staining. The crystals, usually found in an ulcer bed, display a characteristic mosaic pattern that resembles fish scales. The pattern is faintly present in many cases on routine hematoxylin and eosin stain but is better demonstrated on acid-fast, PAS/AB, and Diff-Quik stains. It is this mosaic pattern that distinguishes kayexalate crystals from histologically similar cholestyramine crystals. Kayexalate crystals are refractile but not polarizable. In the stomach, kayexalate bezoars may form (17) (Figs. 2.14, 2.15, e-Figs. 2.29, 2.30).

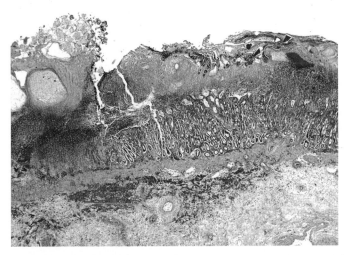

FIGURE 2.14 Ischemic gastritis with kayexalate bezoar formation. Refractile pill material is seen in the upper left, whereas the kayexalate crystals appear on the upper right.

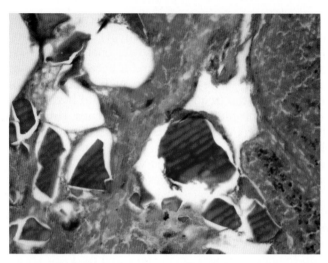

FIGURE 2.15 **Kayexalate crystals.** This high magnification image shows crystals embedded in necroinflammatory debris.

Colchicine and Taxol-Associated Changes

Colchicine is an alkaloid with antimitotic ability used to treat a variety of medical conditions, especially gout. Colchicine toxicity can result in multiorgan failure and death. If patients are taking colchicine in therapeutic doses, there are no abnormal biopsies. However, in patients who are colchicine-toxic (which typically occurs in the setting of renal insufficiency), one observes the following features in biopsy material: metaphase mitoses, epithelial pseudostratification, loss of nuclear polarity, and abundant crypt apoptotic bodies (18). These morphologic features are best seen in the biopsies from the duodenum and gastric antrum (Figs. 2.16, 2.17, e-Figs. 2.31–2.36), with relative sparing of the gastric body in the upper GI tract. Ki67 staining demonstrates an expansion of the proliferating region. Recognition of these features is important because colchicine toxicity can be fatal if undiagnosed clinically. The findings can occasionally be subtle with overlapping features with reactive gastropathy (e-Figs. 2.31–2.36).

Very similar findings can be encountered in patients who are taking paclitaxel (Taxol). Taxol chemotherapy has been associated with dramatic GI mucosal changes, accompanied by an increase in apoptosis (19) and has been discussed in more detail in Chapter 1.

Patients taking Taxol show changes in their gastric mucosa that are similar to those from colchicine toxicity. However, whereas colchicine changes are best seen in the antrum, Taxol-associated changes can be encountered anywhere in the stomach. The histologic hallmarks are arrested mitoses with ring forms. The ring mitoses are accompanied by prominent apoptosis in all GI tract sites and, regardless of the site, the

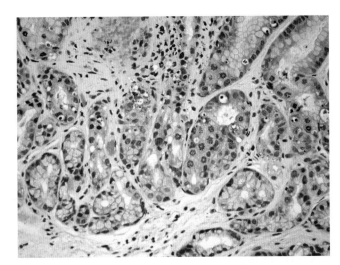

FIGURE 2.16 **Colchicine toxicity.** Epithelial apoptosis and ring mitoses are seen within the proliferative compartment. Awareness of the epithelial changes associated with this process (loss of polarity, mucin loss) avoids a diagnosis of dysplasia.

alterations are found in the proliferative compartment; thus, they are found in the gastric pits rather than the deeper glands. It was initially believed that finding this pattern of injury in a patient taking Taxol indicated clinical toxicity. However, if the patient happens to have a GI tract biopsy or resection within 4 days of the administration of the medication, the histologic changes are encountered even in asymptomatic patients (20). Thus, the histologic changes are an *effect* and correlation must be made with

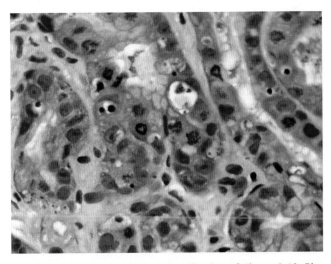

FIGURE 2.17 **Colchicine toxicity.** Higher magnification of Figure 2.16. Ring mitoses are seen in the center of the field.

clinical parameters to learn whether the patient has toxicity. Since biopsies are sometimes taken from the gastric cardia in patients with a history of esophageal cancer, the changes can at times be mistaken for columnar epithelial dysplasia (20). A clue in separating Taxol effect from dysplasia (besides the prominent ring mitoses found in patients taking Taxol) is that most [but not all (21)] examples of columnar epithelial dysplasia show epithelial changes on the surface, whereas Taxol-associated changes do not extend to the surface (20).

Mycophenolate

Mycophenolic acid (MPA) has been discussed in Chapter 1. It is an immunosuppressive drug used mainly in patients with solid organ transplants (kidney, liver, heart, lung) to maintain their grafts, but this medication is also administered to patients with a wide range of other conditions. In the United States, there are two available preparations for this compound: mycophenolate mofetil (MMF; Cellcept, Roche Pharmaceuticals) and mycophenolate sodium (Myfortic, Novartis Inc.). The principal difference between the two preparations is that Myfortic is an enteric-coated drug while MMF is not. Myfortic is therefore absorbed in the intestine while MMF is absorbed in the stomach. Their efficacy and toxicity profiles are similar.

MPA functions by inhibiting the *de novo* pathway of purine synthesis. In general, almost 100% of B and T lymphocytes depend on the *de novo* pathway for purine synthesis, while this dependency is lower for enterocytes (about 50%). Therefore, by inhibiting guanosine synthesis in lymphocytes, cytotoxic T lymphocytes responsible for cellular rejection and antibody production by B lymphocytes are suppressed in transplanted patients. Although the dependency of enterocytes on the *de novo* pathway for purine genesis is lower than that of lymphocytes, MPA can inhibit the proliferation of enterocytes, leading to epithelial injury.

The side effects of MPA predominantly involve the GI tract and hematopoiesis and include diarrhea, nausea, vomiting, gastritis, ulcers, opportunistic infections, and anemia. Changes in the lower GI tract were initially studied, consisting of graft versus host disease (GVHD)-like findings. Parfitt et al. (22) described upper GI tract injury caused by MPA and noted the following features: active esophagitis with ulceration or erosion, chemical gastropathy and Crohn-like features in the stomach, and GVHD-like changes and Crohn-like features in the duodenum. We have further studied the pathologic features of the upper GI tract in patients taking MPA and noted that clinical symptoms tended to correlate with apoptotic counts (23). In the stomach, there are normally very few apoptotic bodies, so finding >3 apoptotic bodies per 100 glands is in keeping with mycophenolate injury and can be diagnosed as such (23) in the correct clinical setting (Figs. 2.18, 2.19, e-Figs. 2.37, 2.38). Finding apoptosis is not specific for mycophenolate-associated injury. The findings are essentially identical to those of GVHD such that clinical correlation is always required–if the patient has had a bone marrow rather than solid organ transplant, then

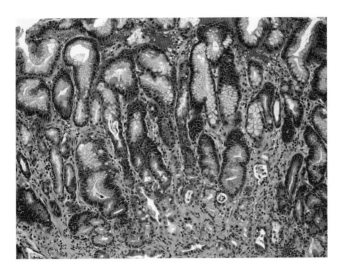

FIGURE 2.18 **Mycophenolate-associated gastric injury.** There is prominent apoptosis in deep glands.

prominent apoptosis is generally a reflection of GVHD. CMV infection (and other viral infections) are also associated with apoptosis. If a patient taking mycophenolate has CMV gastritis as well, there is no way to determine the cause of any apoptotic bodies that may be encountered.

Corrosive Injury

Injury from corrosive ingestion is more of an issue in the developing world than in wealthier countries, especially in children, who accidentally ingest

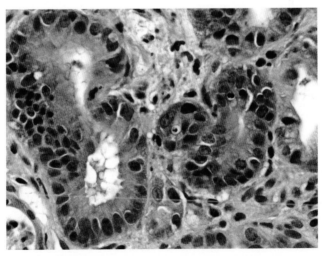

FIGURE 2.19 **Mycophenolate-associated gastric injury.** Apoptotic bodies are easy to find in this high-power field.

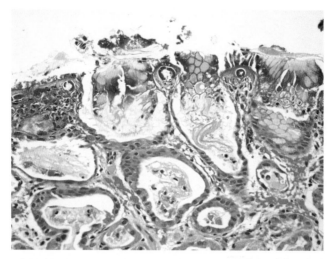

FIGURE 2.20 **Gastric injury associated with calcium pill fragments.** Pill fragments are seen embedded here in the superficial epithelium and lamina propria and associated with reactive epithelial changes.

caustic substances (lye, household bleach, acids, alkaline liquids from chafing dishes, etc.) (24–28). In adults, such ingestions are typically related to suicide attempts (29). Patients are usually not biopsied at the time of initial intervention but are instead given supportive care. If there are biopsies, these are likely to show a hemorrhagic gastritis pattern.

Other Forms of Injury

As in the esophagus, pills can embed themselves in the gastric mucosa and result in mucosal damage (Fig. 2.20, e-Fig. 2.39). Radiation damage will be discussed in more detail in the small and large intestine (Chapters 3 and 4), but radiation injury in the gastric mucosa displays the same features as such damage elsewhere. Lamina propria vessels are thickened and oriented parallel to the surface and the lamina propria becomes hyalinized. Occasionally, gastric radiation injury can be attributable to selective internal radiation with yttrium microspheres (30). In such cases, black, spherical foreign material can be seen on biopsies in damaged mucosa.

HELICOBACTER GASTRITIS

Helicobacter gastritis (Figs. 2.21, 2.22, e-Figs. 2.40–2.45) has, of course, been a source of gastritis for years, but was not recognized until Barry Marshall called attention to it (31) and ultimately fulfilled Koch postulates by swallowing a pure culture of the organism and acquiring gastritis (32). Based on a computer search, there have been over 28,000 publications devoted to this organism in the ensuing 25 years. *H. pylori* is now recognized as a curved, flagellated, gram-negative rod that has variant forms

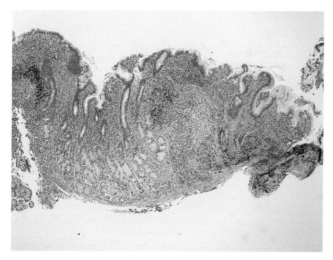

FIGURE 2.21 *Helicobacter pylori* gastritis. This classic, low-magnification view displays a lymphoid follicle and lamina propria lymphoplasmacytosis in a diffuse distribution (in contrast to the patchy inflammation of autoimmune gastritis or Crohn gastritis). There are many neutrophils in the epithelium.

(especially a coccoid form seen in treated patients) and that is now known to be associated with both gastric carcinoma and mucosa-associated lymphoid tissue (MALT) lymphoma. Another variant, called *H. heilmannii* (Figs. 2.23, 2.24, e-Figs. 2.45–2.52), is more tightly coiled and rare (<1% of *Helicobacter* isolates). But, *H. heilmannii* cross-reacts with the immunohistochemical stain for *H. pylori* and is fully capable of producing gastritis

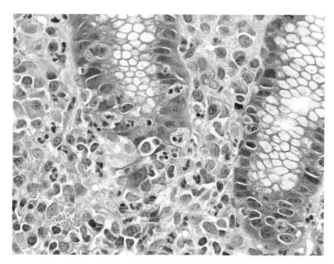

FIGURE 2.22 **Helicobacter gastritis.** Note Lamina propria and intraepithelial neutrophils.

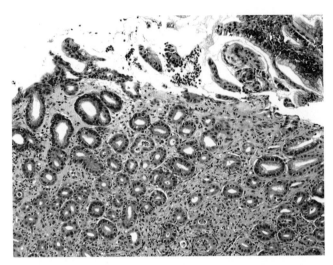

FIGURE 2.23 *Helicobacter heilmannii* **gastritis.** This organism also produces active, chronic gastritis with all its complications, although many observers note a less severe pattern. If immunohistochemistry is performed, this organism stains with preparations designed for *H. pylori*.

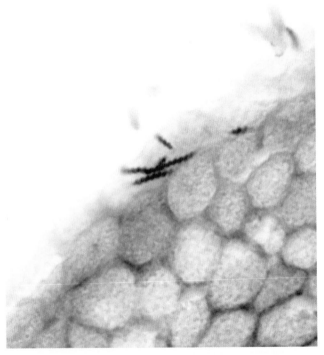

FIGURE 2.24 *Helicobacter heilmannii* organisms are seen here in a Diff Quik stain. Compared to *Helicobacter pylori*, they are longer and tightly coiled.

and associating with MALT lymphoma and gastric adenocarcinoma. Like *H. pylori*, it produces antral-predominant gastritis, but this gastritis is less severe than *H. pylori* gastritis (33). *Helicobacter* gastritis was formerly known as "diffuse antral gastritis," type B gastritis (whereas autoimmune gastritis was type A), and "superficial gastritis." In modern practice of pathology, of course, all gastric biopsy reports should include a statement on *Helicobacter* status. At our hospital, all gastric biopsies are stained with Diff-Quik for this, but any such stain is appropriate. H&E staining alone is not regarded as sufficient, although *Helicobacter* organisms can certainly be recognized on routine H&E stains (34). We seldom use immunohistochemistry, as it is not cost-effective in our practice (serology is less expensive), but some observers perform immunohistochemistry in every case. One situation in which it is extremely helpful to do so is when considering gastric Crohn disease. It is reassuring to have a negative immunohistochemical test for *H. pylori* prior to suggesting a diagnosis of Crohn disease on an upper tract biopsy that displays patchy, active gastritis but lacks granulomas, particularly in children. Another scenario where immunohistochemistry might prove useful is when biopsies from the gastric mucosa show a pattern of inflammation that is classic for *Helicobacter* gastritis but the organisms are not readily identified by H&E or special stains. This can occur as a result of prior antibiotic therapy or use of PPIs (35). Immunohistochemistry highlights organisms embedded in tissue (e-Figs. 2.43, 2.44, 2.49–2.52), specifically in parietal cells and is valuable in identifying small coccoid forms present in partially treated patients. Alternatively, a comment suggesting correlation with other, noninvasive methods (serology, stool antigen test, urease test) may be prudent.

In the United States, there are no screening guidelines for identifying patients with *H. pylori*. This is in contrast to countries with populations at high risk such as Japan, where both the high prevalence of *H. pylori* infection and incidence of gastric cancer call for such programs. For example, in 2008 the Asian-Pacific Gastric Cancer Consensus Conference recommended serology screening in high-risk countries starting 10 to 20 years before the incidence of gastric cancer begins to increase in a given population (36). Another screening method used in high-risk areas is measurement of serum pepsinogen levels, which have been shown to be a marker for *H. pylori* infection. Increased levels of pepsinogen II correlate well with infection and histologic gastritis, while decreased levels of pepsinogen I are associated with significant atrophy (37–39).

In contrast to biopsies in the esophagus, in which the endoscopist usually recognizes the pathologic process grossly, the endoscopic findings in *H. pylori* gastritis are usually not useful and correlate poorly with pathologic findings. However, Yan et al. report that mucosal mosaic appearance with or without areas of hyperemia identifies *Helicobacter* gastritis with a sensitivity, specificity, positive, and negative predictive values of 100%, 86%, 94%, and 100%, respectively (40), and some observers are able to detect organisms endoscopically using confocal laser endomicroscopy (41). Histologically, *H. pylori* organisms are seen in gastric mucus and overlying surface and foveolar epithelium. There is typically abundant, lymphoplasmacytic, chronic inflammation of the lamina propria. The presence of lymphoid follicles (MALT) is almost always indicative of infection. There is often abundant, active inflammation (neutrophils) concentrated in the upper mucosa, hence the old term "superficial gastritis." Granulomas can be seen on occasion. Following successful treatment, the neutrophilic constituent resolves, but the chronic, inflammatory component may persist from months to more than 5 years in approximately 20% of the patients and serology may remain positive in approximately 33% (42). The organisms do not colonize non-surface or foci of intestinal metaplasia and the latter could be a source of histologic false negatives.

Helicobacter sp. may have a particular predilection to damage D cells in the antrum, which secrete somatostatin. Since somatostatin usually keeps gastrin secretion in check, loss of these D cells causes excess gastrin, which stimulates excess acid secretion in infected patients. This, in turn, may be responsible for the duodenal ulcers that often accompany *Helicobacter* gastritis (43).

INACTIVE CHRONIC GASTRITIS

There is extensive literature on grading chronic gastritis, complete with published pictograms akin to the Gleason diagram in prostatic cancer (44). However, in contrast to the Gleason diagram, the pictograms for chronic gastritis are seldom valued in daily practice. However, they are a useful construct for considering chronic gastritis and allow standardization in research studies. Chronic gastritis is generally attributable to prior *Helicobacter* infection, based on serologic studies, and is a common finding in biopsy material. However, the threshold for diagnosing it is not entirely clear and is a subjective matter. Some observers provide a diagnosis of inactive chronic gastritis when as few as one or two plasma cells are encountered on high-power examination. In an approach more practical than evidence based, we diagnose inactive chronic gastritis at 4× and confirm at higher magnification. At low magnification, the lamina propria of the stomach should have only a few inflammatory cells, which appear as small dots. We essentially use a slight prominence in "dot density" as the criterion for a low-magnification diagnosis of inactive chronic gastritis (Figs. 2.25, 2.26, e-Figs 2.53–2.56). If there is no increased "dot density" on low power exam but there are a few scattered plasma cells on close inspection, some observers diagnose "mild chronic inflammation." However, this finding is of no clinical significance and the same biopsies may be called "normal" by others. As a rule of thumb, the normal number of lamina propria plasma cells is up to 5 per high-power field or two or three plasma cells between foveolae (the area in which chronic inflammatory cells are most often found).

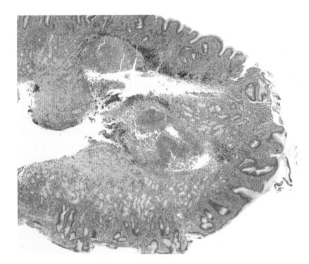

FIGURE 2.25 Inactive chronic gastritis. Increased "dot density" (lymphocytes and plasma cells) in the lamina propria is evident at scanning magnification. When germinal centers are identified, a search for Helicobacter organisms should be performed because they are almost invariably present.

PHLEGMONOUS GASTRITIS

Phlegmonous gastritis (e-Figs. 2.57–2.62), a rare suppurative inflammation of the gastric wall analogous to necrotizing fasciitis of the soft tissues, is caused by a myriad of microorganisms including *Streptococcus*, *Staphylococcus*, *Enterococcus*, and *E. coli*, among others. Patients are usually debilitated with conditions such as human immunodeficiency virus (HIV) infection, lymphoma, myeloid sarcoma, diabetes, rheumatoid

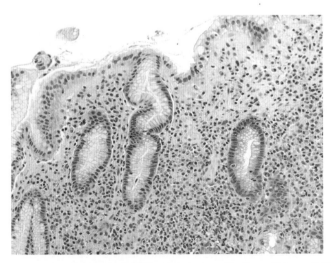

FIGURE 2.26 Inactive chronic gastritis. Higher magnification of Figure 2.25.

arthritis, and Kaposi sarcoma (45–48). It has been reported following endoscopic mucosal resection, possibly as a result of a contaminated endoscope (49) and following ingestion of large quantities of alcohol (50). Presenting symptoms include epigastric/abdominal pain, nausea, anorexia, hiccups, foul-smelling vomit, and hematemesis (45,46,51). CT scan may show a thick gastric wall with hypodense areas with or without peripheral rim enhancement, which indicates an intramural abscess (52,53). Endoscopic evaluation may reveal thickened folds, mass effect, ulcerations, and surface necrotic material. Involvement of the esophageal wall is possible (52,54). Biopsies show an acutely inflamed, necrotic mucosa and submucosa. A Gram stain may disclose the presence of bacteria within the tissue. Awareness of the clinical and radiologic scenarios is helpful when examining these specimens. Early diagnosis is key as the overall mortality rate is high, reported at 67% in a review of 23 cases (50). Treatment consists of antibiotic therapy or gastrectomy.

Emphysematous gastritis is a form of phlegmonous gastritis characterized by gastric pneumatosis, caused by gas-forming bacteria such as *Proteus* or *Clostridium*. One interesting organism associated with emphysematous gastritis is *Sarcina ventriculi* (56). A gram-positive, anaerobic, sugar-fermenting bacterium, *S. ventriculi* was first observed in the human stomach in 1842 by Goodsir (57). The microorganism is readily found in soil and is known to cause a similar type of gastric injury in animals (58). It thrives in acidic environments and ferments carbohydrates with production of ethyl alcohol and CO_2 (59). The pathogenetic mechanism is uncertain but delayed gastric emptying and carbohydrate stasis in association with acidic gastric juices may provide an ideal culture medium for the organism (59). Lam-Himlin et al. have further studied gastric lesions in which *Sarcina ventriculi* was detected. The studied patients all had underlying delayed gastric emptying (one had a bezoar) from diabetic neuropathy, narcotic use, and pyloric stenosis secondary to malignancy (60). The organism may simply colonize preexisting lesions, but there are too few cases to draw firm conclusions as to whether the organism is truly a pathogen.

Microscopically, the organism is seen in packets of 4, 8, or more cells with characteristic flattening or molding in areas of contact with one another with or without associated giant cells (Figs. 2.27, 2.28, e-Figs. 2.63–2.65). The differential diagnosis is with *Micrococcus* (e-Fig. 2.66, 2.67).

METAPLASTIC ATROPHIC GASTRITIS

Metaplastic atrophic gastritis occurs in two distinct types and, because of this, it is best if the pathologist reviews biopsies from both the gastric antrum and the body. These two types are termed "autoimmune" and "environmental." Some authors have published studies with cartoons as templates for grading the degree of inflammation and atrophy in gastritis, but these are of little value in daily practice (61).

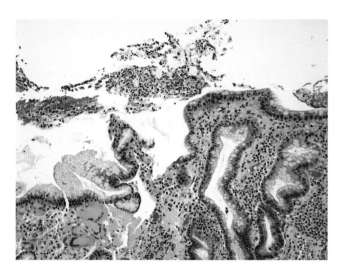

FIGURE 2.27 *Sarcina ventriculi* **gastritis.** At low magnification, one sees suppurative inflammation and lamina propria giant cells.

Autoimmune Metaplastic Atrophic Gastritis

AMAG (Figs. 2.29–2.35, e-Figs. 2.68–2.73) was called "type A" gastritis in the past (before the role of *Helicobacter* was elucidated). A frequently underrecognized entity, AMAG is a disease in which antibodies attack parietal cells and is typically seen in biopsies from older female patients. Autoimmune gastritis is the precursor and etiologic cause of the majority of

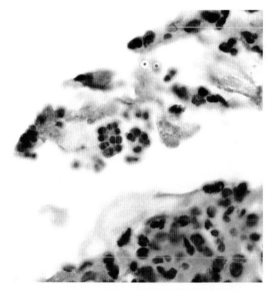

FIGURE 2.28 *Sarcina ventriculi* **gastritis.** This higher magnification image of Figure 2.27 shows *Sarcina ventriculi* arranged in cell packets with characteristic flattening or molding in areas of contact with one another.

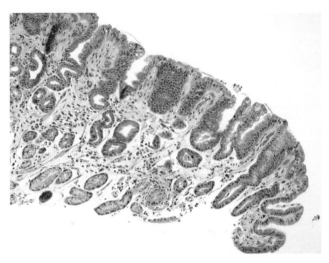

FIGURE 2.29 **Gastric antrum biopsy from a patient with autoimmune metaplastic atrophic gastritis.** This biopsy has little inflammation and essentially displays the features of chemical gastritis, presumably from bile reflux.

cases of pernicious anemia and may precede pernicious anemia by years to decades (62). In the past, the condition was believed to preferentially affect Northern Europeans and their ancestors (63), but this has been shown to be untrue and, in fact, all races are affected (64). Little is known regarding disease etiology. In an interesting report by Hershko et al., the authors studied 160 patients with autoimmune gastritis identified by hypergastrinemia and the presence of antiparietal antibodies. Eighty-three, forty-eight,

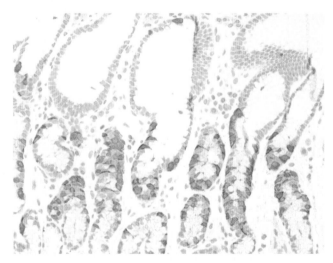

FIGURE 2.30 **Gastric antrum biopsy in a patient with autoimmune metaplastic atrophic gastritis,** same case as Figure 2.29. G cells are immunoreactive with a gastrin stain, confirming the biopsy is indeed from the antrum.

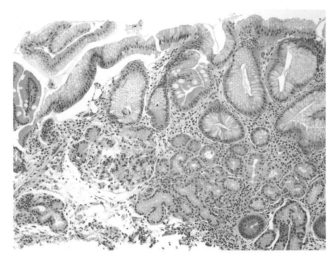

FIGURE 2.31 **Gastric body biopsy from a patient with autoimmune metaplastic atrophic gastritis.** There is loss of oxyntic cells, and the presence of deep glands, which resemble those found in the antrum ("antralized" mucosa). In the middle portion, there is a focus of intestinal metaplasia of the complete type. There is a nodule composed of small, round cells in the lower left portion, which is probably an endocrine cell nest, although it is best to confirm this finding with immunohistochemical stains.

and twenty-nine patients presented with iron deficiency anemia, normal indices, and macrocytic anemia, respectively. Patients with iron deficiency anemia were 21 years younger (and mostly females) than patients with macrocytic anemia. Additionally, stratification by age from those younger

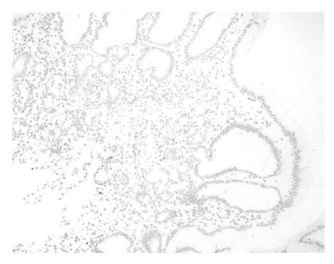

FIGURE 2.32 **Gastric body biopsy in a patient with autoimmune metaplastic atrophic gastritis, same case shown in Figure 2.31.** A gastrin stain shows absence of G cells, confirming this biopsy is indeed from the gastric body.

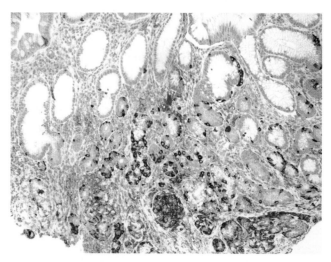

FIGURE 2.33 **Autoimmune metaplastic atrophic gastritis.** A chromogranin stain in the gastric body shows nodular and linear hyperplasia of endocrine cells. "Linear" hyperplasia implies that there are five to six immunoreactive cells in a row in a gastric gland.

than 20 to those older than 60 showed an increasing trend in mean corpuscular volume and a decrease in vitamin B12 levels. Finally, the prevalence of *H. pylori* infection decreased from 87.5% at age younger than 20 to 12.4% at age older than 60. Thus, the authors challenged the notion that AMAG is a disease of the elderly (although it may present in the elderly), suggesting that vitamin B12 deficiency may be the end result of a long-standing process triggered initially by *H. pylori* and that may present in

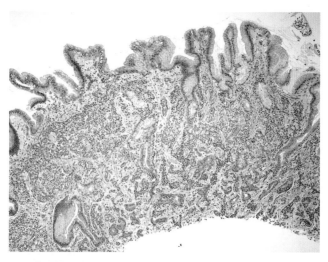

FIGURE 2.34 **Well differentiated neuroendocrine tumor (carcinoid tumor).** These tumors can arise in patients with autoimmune metaplastic atrophic gastritis as a result of constant ECL cell stimulation by gastrin.

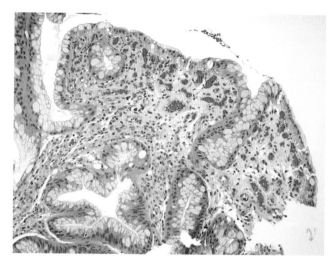

FIGURE 2.35 **Hyperplastic gastric polyp.** These hyperplastic polyps are often a consequence of atrophic gastritis.

its initial stages in younger patients (particularly females) with microcytic iron deficiency anemia and in its later stages in older patients with macrocytic pernicious anemia (65). It is possible that, via molecular mimicry, *H. pylori* may be able to induce production of antiparietal/anti-intrinsic factor antibodies in susceptible individuals (66).

Patients with AMAG are at threefold risk of developing gastric cancer. But they are not at risk for ulcers because their parietal cells are reduced in number to absent, thus producing little-to-no acid. Since parietal cells are the type affected, the changes occur only in zones where parietal cells are found. Thus, there is metaplasia and atrophy only in the body and fundus. An affected patient with biopsies from the antrum and the fundus will show no significant inflammatory disease in the antrum (hence the importance of taking biopsies from both sites [Fig 2.29–2.32, e-Fig. 2.68–2.72]). Fundus biopsies show extensive loss of parietal cells and metaplasia (Fig 2.31, e-Fig. 2.70). In some cases, there are residual nests of parietal cells with chronic inflammatory cells (T cells) in the process of destroying them. In fact, the residual, more normal mucosa sometimes appears polypoid to the endoscopist when seen in a sea of severe atrophy (67,68). Alternatively, the endoscopist may see a flat, thin mucosa, devoid of rugae. Metaplasia is usually of the intestinal type or the "pseudopyloric" type. Pancreatic acinar cell metaplasia is not uncommon (Fig. 2.36, e-Fig. 2.74). In fact, this type of metaplasia in a biopsy of the oxyntic mucosa should prompt the pathologist to consider the possibility of autoimmune gastritis as it has been observed in 50% of patients with AMAG and is rare in other

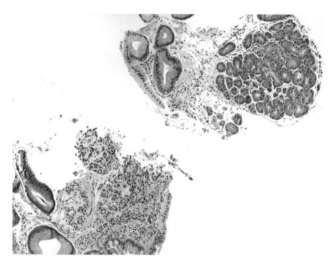

FIGURE 2.36 Pancreatic acinar cell metaplasia associated with autoimmune meta-plastic atrophic gastritis. ECL cell hyperplasia is evident on the lower left hand side.

gastritides (69). In "pseudopyloric metaplasia," the oxyntic mucosa resembles antral mucosa, in that it lacks parietal and chief cells (oxyntic glands), but differs from it by not secreting gastrin. Only the real antrum secretes gastrin (Fig. 2.30, e-Fig. 2.69). Thus, immunohistochemistry for gastrin in biopsies from the body lacks reactive cells (Fig. 2.32, e-Fig. 2.71), a finding that can be exploited both to establish a diagnosis and to exclude inaccurate sampling (i.e., the endoscopist has biopsied the antrum and labeled it as "body"). In AMAG, there is typically no metaplasia in the antrum, which often shows reactive features that are possibly secondary to bile reflux. Because the patients are hypoacidic due to loss of parietal cell mass, a feedback loop causes the antral G cells to produce abundant gastrin to stimulate acid secretion. As there are few-to-no parietal cells, gastrin levels become progressively elevated in these patients, and this gastrin stimulates proliferation of endocrine cells in the gastric body as a side effect. Thus, chromogranin stains show linear and nodular endocrine cell hyperplasia in the body, neither of which is attributable to G cells (Fig. 2.33, e-Fig. 2.72). If this condition persists, small indolent carcinoid tumors can result (Fig. 2.34, e-Fig. 2.73, discussed further in Volume 2, Chapter 2).

To summarize, one can determine the presence of AMAG in a biopsy by looking for the following features in the gastric body and then noting that the patient's antrum is unaffected:

Body and Fundus in Autoimmune Gastritis
Loss of parietal cells
Intestinal metaplasia
"Pseudopyloric metaplasia"
Pancreatic acinar cell metaplasia

Negative gastrin stain (or scattered cells especially if the sample is from transition zone between antrum and body)

Nodular and linear enterochromaffin cell-like (ECL) cell hyperplasia on chromogranin stain

Antrum in Autoimmune Gastritis

Essentially normal biopsy

No intestinal metaplasia

G cells present on gastrin stain

Normal number of cells on chromogranin stain

"EARLY" AMAG. Autoimmune gastritis can be easily recognized when the histologic features are fully developed, but recognizing it before the complete loss of the oxyntic mucosa is more challenging. One feature of fully developed, autoimmune gastritis is ECL cell hyperplasia. Torbenson et al. studied biopsy specimens from 40 patients diagnosed with possible autoimmune gastritis, based on the presence of lymphocytic infiltration and damage to oxyntic glands and/or the presence of metaplastic epithelium that disproportionately involved the body mucosa (70). Nineteen cases had follow-up serologic studies for antiparietal cells and/or anti-intrinsic factor antibodies: 13 were positive and 6 were negative. The remaining 21 cases were indeterminate because of incomplete testing. The histologic findings were similar in the patients who were serologically positive and those who were indeterminate. In all of these cases, the oxyntic mucosa showed lymphoplasmacytic infiltrates within the lamina propria, with focal gland infiltration and damage. Sixty-five percent (22 of 34) of the cases showed intestinal and/or pyloric metaplasia, and 85% (29 of 34) showed parietal cell pseudohypertrophy. Chromogranin stains were performed in 11 of 13 cases with positive serologic markers for autoimmune gastritis, and all showed at least linear ECL cell hyperplasia. In contrast, none of the 6 cases with negative serologic studies had linear ECL cell hyperplasia ($p < 0.001$). The authors concluded that (a) the combination of deep or diffuse lymphoplasmacytic infiltrates within the lamina propria with foci of gland infiltration and damage, (b) epithelial metaplasia, (c) parietal cell pseudohypertrophy, and (d) ECL cell hyperplasia at the linear or greater level all support a diagnosis of autoimmune gastritis before the complete loss of oxyntic mucosa.

Environmental Metaplastic Atrophic Gastritis

Helicobacter gastritis is probably the most important cause of environmental gastritis that we know, but it is probably not the cause of all cases. Other associations include various dietary factors such as excessive salt, smoked foods, nitrites, paucity of green vegetables and fruits (lack of vitamins C, E, β-carotene, selenium), and nitrosamines. Nitrosamines can be produced from nitrites, in the setting of colonization by anaerobic bacteria in a hypoacidic stomach. This type of gastritis has been called "type B gastritis" and "multifocal atrophic gastritis."

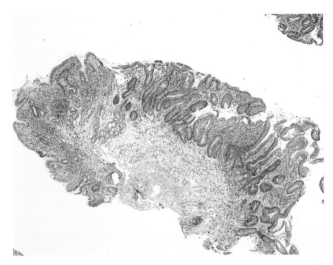

FIGURE 2.37 Environmental atrophic gastritis. This low power magnification shows increased "dot density" of the lamina propria and some loss of glands. Even at scanning magnification, intestinal metaplasia is visible.

The key feature is that environmental atrophic gastritis is most marked in the antrum (Fig. 2.37, 2.38, e-Figs. 2.75, 2.76). Multiple foci first appear in the transition zone between antrum and body (incisura angularis) at the area of the lesser curvature. Over time, the entire antrum is affected, but the body is relatively spared. While there is less disease in the body, it first appears in the distal body and affects more of the body over many years. The body can display pseudopyloric and intestinal metaplasia, just

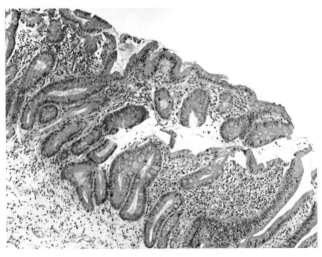

FIGURE 2.38 Environmental atrophic gastritis. Higher magnification of Figure 2.37 highlighting intestinal metaplasia.

as in autoimmune gastritis, but, of course, the antrum is affected as well. These patients retain enough parietal cell mass that they do not develop pernicious anemia. They can become hypochlorhydric, but achlorhydria is rare. Their serum gastrin is usually normal and they can have both ulcers and develop cancers. In the United States, environmental atrophic gastritis is usually seen in patients older than 50 years, but in certain parts of the world, atrophy appears in patients in their 3rd or 4th decades (e.g., Japan, Andean South America).

Gastric Changes in Autoimmune enteropathy/Immune dysfunction, Polyendocrinopathy, Enteropathy, and X-Linked Inheritance and Related Conditions

Autoimmune enteropathy (AIE), further discussed in Chapter 3, is a rare cause of intractable diarrhea associated with circulating gut autoantibodies and a predisposition to autoimmunity. The diagnostic criteria for AIE include (a) severe villous atrophy not responding to any dietary restriction, (b) circulating gut autoantibodies and/or associated autoimmune conditions, and (c) lack of severe immunodeficiency (71). Although it is primarily considered to be a disease of children, adult-onset AIE is known (72–75). AIE must be distinguished from refractory sprue, which is a form of celiac disease (CD) no longer responsive to a gluten-free diet. The term AIE was classically applied to a form of "intractable diarrhea" with serum gut autoantibodies, characterized by male predominance, early onset, poor response to parenteral nutrition and association with type 1 diabetes. In recent years, AIE has become better defined as the molecular underpinnings have been elucidated (76,77). The FOXP3 molecule governs generation and maturation of regulatory T cells (Treg) expressing CD4+ and CD25+ molecules. Mutations of the FOXP3 gene, located in X chromosome, produce a syndrome with Immune dysfunction, Polyendocrinopathy, Enteropathy, and X-linked inheritance (IPEX). The majority of the AIE cases probably correspond to the newly delineated IPEX syndrome, even in female patients who presumably have some autosomal genetic variants. Besides FOXP3, other molecules are likely to be involved in the generation and function of regulatory T cells and their deficiency may also enhance autoimmune disease and IPEX-like syndromes. Not surprisingly, such patients can display changes throughout the GI tract (78).

Gastric biopsies from these patients may present findings similar to those in AMAG, namely, glandular atrophy accompanied by a dense lymphoplasmacytic infiltrate with or without intestinal metaplasia (Figs. 2.39, 2.40, e-Figs. 2.77, 2.78) (72–74,78). Increased intraepithelial lymphocytes may be present. Patients may have a multitude of additional circulating autoantibodies, among them, antiparietal cell and anti-intrinsic factor antibodies (72,74). Unlike in AMAG, the antrum is equally affected and ECL cell hyperplasia is often absent (78).

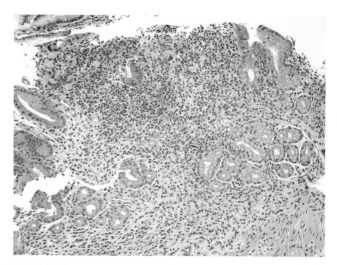

FIGURE 2.39 **Gastric biopsy in a patient with a autoimmune enteropathy.** This image shows destruction of oxyntic mucosa of the gastric body in a patient with IPEX.

Atrophic Autoimmune Pangastritis

In 2006, Jevremovic et al. (79) described eight patients with a unique form of atrophic pangastritis. Characteristic features included (a) moderate-to-marked, "bottom heavy" lymphoplasmacytic and neutrophilic lamina propria infiltrates persisting into the phase of glandular atrophy, (b) involvement of both antrum and body, (c) lack of ECL cell hyperplasia, (d) lack of *H. pylori* infection, and (e) an autoimmune basis as evidenced by

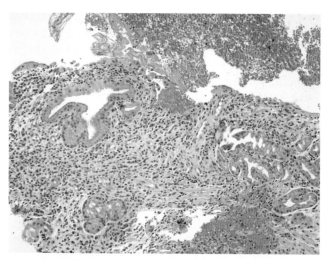

FIGURE 2.40 **Gastric biopsy in a patient with autoimmune enteropathy.** Higher magnification of Figure 2.39. Note the pyloric metaplasia.

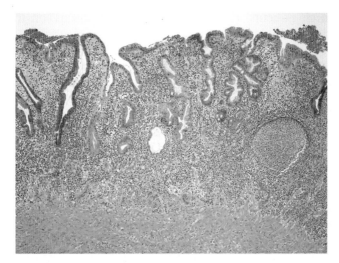

FIGURE 2.41 **Atrophic autoimmune pangastritis.** This image is from the gastric body but lacks oxyntic glands. Note the striking expansion of the lamina propria with inflammatory cells.

associated systemic autoimmune diseases in seven of the studied patients (Figs. 2.41, 2.42, e-Figs. 2.79–2.82). The histologic picture is therefore more similar to gastric biopsies from patients with AIE than to those with AMAG. Indeed, four of the eight studied patients had a diagnosis of autoimmune enterocolitis, two of whom also had documented antigoblet cell and antienterocyte antibodies. This process may pose a risk for neoplastic transformation as evidenced by development of persistent low-grade dysplasia

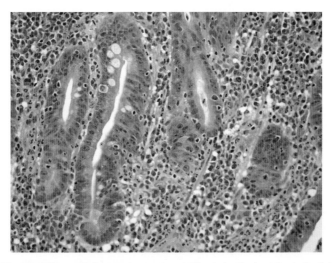

FIGURE 2.42 **Atrophic autoimmune pangastritis.** Intestinal metaplasia, intraepithelial neutrophils and lymphocytes, and lamina propria inflammation are seen here.

in one of their patients. It seems clear from this discussion that definite histologic diagnosis of autoimmune pangastritis is difficult if not impossible in the absence of clinical information. Awareness of this entity and its associations allows proposal as a diagnostic possibility to a puzzled clinician. Patients may improve after treatment with immunosuppressive therapy.

GASTRIC ANTRAL VASCULAR ECTASIA

GAVE, also known as "watermelon stomach," was first described by Jabbari et al. in 1984 (80) and refers to an endoscopic appearance. In this condition, longitudinal antral folds have visible, reddened vessels radiating from the pylorus in a distribution resembling a watermelon rind. Patients present with iron deficiency, secondary to chronic gastric bleeding. The typical patient is an elderly woman with hypochlorhydria; chronic liver disease; calcinosis, Raynaud phenomenon, esophageal motility disorders, sclerodactyly, and telangiectasia (CREST) syndrome; or lymphoma. Some cases are associated with scleroderma (81). In some cases, the endoscopic appearance is not prototypic but instead consists of diffuse gastric erythema. The etiology is not well understood, but it is probably an acquired lesion. Some patients have antral prolapse (80).

Histologic examination discloses features that reflect a mucosal prolapse component: there is foveolar hyperplasia, dilated mucosal capillaries, focal fibrin thrombi, and fibromuscular hypertrophy (82) (Fig. 2.43, e-Figs. 2.83, 2.84). Similar features may be seen in patients who have portal hypertension, but the dilated capillaries in portal hypertension lack fibrin thrombi (e-Fig. 2.85). Some observers have used CD61 immunolabeling (CD61 recognizes platelet glycoprotein IIIa) to highlight the thrombi in GAVE.

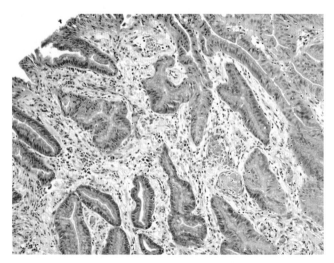

FIGURE 2.43 **A case of gastric antral vascular ectasia (GAVE).** This particular case shows marked reactive epithelial changes with mucin loss and fibrin thrombi.

Unfortunately, patients with "watermelon stomach" may also have portal hypertension (83). Treatment of "watermelon stomach" often entails mucosal ablation, since the patients have uncontrolled blood loss. Endoscopic therapy, including contact and noncontact thermal ablations of the ectatic vascular lesions, is the mainstay of conservative therapy. However, many patients fail endoscopic therapy and develop recurrent, acute, and chronic GI bleeding episodes. Surgical resection may be the only reliable method for achieving a cure and eliminating transfusion dependency. Traditionally, surgery was used only as a last resort after patients failed prolonged medical and/or endoscopic therapy. However, based on experience garnered from the literature, some authors have recommended a more aggressive surgical approach in patients who fail a short trial of endoluminal therapy (84).

PORTAL GASTROPATHY

Portal hypertensive gastropathy is the main differential diagnostic consideration with "watermelon stomach". Like GAVE, portal hypertensive gastropathy can be a cause of GI bleeding. In contrast to GAVE, it is not treated by endoscopic ablation but, rather, by measures to reduce the portal hypertension. Endoscopically, whereas GAVE is notable for a striped endoscopic appearance, the appearance of portal gastropathy has been described as a mosaic or "snakeskin" appearance (85). Unfortunately, some patients display nonspecific endoscopic appearances.

GAVE is associated with connective tissue disorders, and portal hypertensive gastropathy is associated with portal hypertension from cirrhosis associated with a host of liver diseases. Unfortunately, the two conditions can overlap. Patients with portal hypertensive gastropathy have increased numbers of lamina propria vessels and their vessels are of larger caliber than normal antral lamina propria vessels (e-Fig. 2.85). Interestingly, if microvessel density is measured by immunolabeling for CD31 in GAVE versus portal hypertensive gastropathy, both have similarly increased lamina propria microvessel density compared to normals (86). The vessels in portal hypertensive gastropathy lack fibrin thrombi, as noted above. Thrombi can be difficult to see on H&E stains, but if CD61 staining is used to assess for subtle thrombi (as above, CD61 recognizes platelet glycoprotein IIIa), staining seems to correlate with patients with clinical GAVE rather than portal hypertension (86).

DIEULAFOY LESION

Another source of gastric bleeding is Dieulafoy lesion (also known as exulceratio simplex, caliber-persistent artery, and gastric atherosclerotic aneurysm), an uncommon cause of recurrent, often massive, and potentially life threatening GI hemorrhage. The lesion accounts for approximately 2% of cases of acute GI hemorrhage (87) and was described initially in a small series by the French surgeon Georges Dieulafoy (1839–1911). He termed the lesion exulceratio simplex (literally meaning "simple aggravation"), as he thought it was the initial stage of a gastric ulcer.

The lesion typically presents as recurrent, often massive GI hemorrhage without preceding GI symptoms. It occurs in older adults (median age, 54 years) and is more common in men (male-to-female ratio is 2:1). Patients often have associated comorbid conditions such as hypertension and ischemic heart disease (87,88). The GI bleeding presentation is typically both hematemesis and melena, but, in a minority of cases, the patient may present solely with one or the other. The patients typically have no other contributing GI pathology and usually no significant use of alcohol or NSAIDs. The resulting anemia is typically severe, requiring red cell transfusions.

Dieulafoy lesion is a rare cause of upper GI bleeding. However, it should be seriously considered in the differential diagnosis when one has a patient with a massive GI hemorrhage without an endoscopically identifiable source. This lesion can be difficult to recognize on endoscopy, due to its typical proximal fundic location along the lesser curvature.

The majority (~80%) of these lesions can be identified by endoscopy. While most are recognized on initial exam, frequently, multiple endoscopies are needed to identify them due to associated excessive blood. Angiography may also be useful to identify those not recognized endoscopically. Dieulafoy lesions in the colon have not been as amenable to endoscopic diagnosis.

The endoscopic appearance is that of a 2- to 5-mm mucosal defect, and the protruding vessel may be visible. They are typically located within 6 cm of the GE junction on the lesser curvature. They can be easily missed due to this proximal gastric location, so endoscopic ultrasound may be useful in confirming the diagnosis.

The pathogenesis is believed to be the abnormal presence of large caliber arteries in the submucosa (Fig. 2.44, e-Figs. 2.86, 2.87) that subsequently cause thinning of the overlying mucosa, which then leads to erosion and exposure of the vessel wall to the lumen and eventual intraluminal hemorrhage. One third are extragastric (87), and lesions have been described in the small intestine, colon, and rectum.

Histologic examination is typically limited to resection and autopsy specimens, as endoscopic biopsy is typically not done. But when it is, the biopsy only reveals mucosal fibrin. The histology is that of an essentially normal artery, lacking atherosclerotic or aneurysmal dilatations, which is primarily located in the superficial submucosa and focally extends into and through the mucosa. The luminally exposed aspect of the vessel shows focal disruption of the wall covered by fibrin clot. The mucosa immediately adjacent to the imposing vessel is obliterated by fibrin. The mucosa farther from the vessel may show some chronic inflammation, but is generally unremarkable, typically without pathology.

Endoscopic therapeutic modalities are now used successfully and have significantly reduced the mortality of this lesion, but their long-term

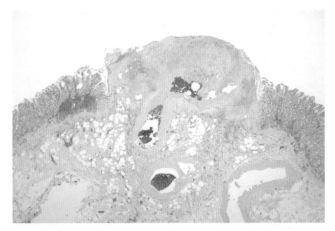

FIGURE 2.44 **Dieulafoy lesion.** Low magnification of a large, ectatic gastric vessel that produced profound gastric hemorrhage.

effectiveness in controlling recurrent bleeding is in some doubt, and surgical therapy may be required to ensure long-term bleeding control. Endoscopic therapies include electrocoagulation, injection sclerotherapy, heater probe, laser photocoagulation, epinephrine, hemoclipping, ethanol injection, and banding. Surgical therapies include gastrotomy (to identify the lesion, followed by ligation of the responsible vessel), proximal gastric resection, and large-wedge resection. Determining the precise location of the lesion, and thus allowing for a more limited gastric resection, might be enhanced by tattooing the lesion on initial endoscopy.

GASTRITIS CYSTICA POLYPOSA/PROFUNDA

This uncommon process typically occurs at gastroenterostomy stomas (89) and is essentially another mucosal prolapse condition. In gastritis cystica polyposa, 1- to 3-cm polyps form a circular ring, or simply a fullness, around the stoma. There is a grossly thickened mucosal layer, and numerous submucosal microcysts. Microscopically, there are elongated pits with serration, hyperplasia, cystic dilation of pyloric glands, which have herniated into submucosa, regenerative surface epithelial changes, and loss of fundic glands. Disorganized strands of muscularis mucosae are seen in irregular bundles (Fig. 2.45, e-Fig. 2.88).

LYMPHOCYTIC GASTRITIS

The term "lymphocytic gastritis" applies to a pattern of inflammation, rather than a specific etiology. This is yet another example of the limited repertoire of responses that the GI tract can mount to a host of different types of injury. Lymphocytic gastritis is an uncommon chronic gastritis, characterized by lymphocytosis of foveolar and surface epithelium

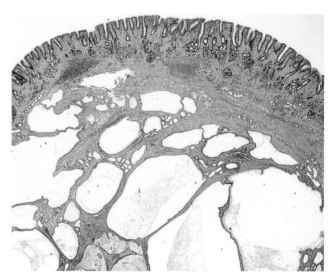

FIGURE 2.45 **Gastritis cystic polyposa profunda.** This lesion presented as a polyp in an anastomotic site. The glands in the submucosa are bland-appearing.

(Figs. 2.46, 2.47, e-Figs. 2.89–2.98). Lymphocytic gastritis is associated with celiac disease, *H. pylori* gastritis, and varioliform gastritis (an endoscopic form of gastropathy comprised of enlarged folds, nodules, and erosions). Wu et al. (90) studied 103 patients with lymphocytic gastritis classified according to the associated entities, including the distribution and severity of the

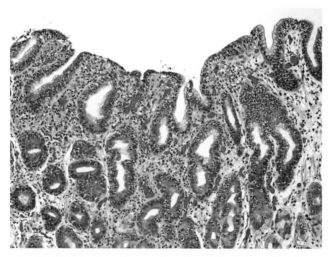

FIGURE 2.46 **Lymphocytic gastritis.** Striking intraepithelial lymphocytosis is seen here. This term describes a pattern of inflammation, rather than assigning an etiology. The patient from whom this biopsy was obtained has celiac disease, which is often associated with a lymphocytic gastritis pattern.

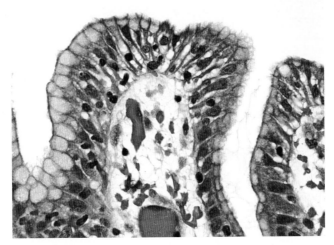

FIGURE 2.47 **Lymphocytic gastritis.** This is a high magnification image of the surface epithelium from the same patient depicted in Figure 2.46.

gastritis in the 70 patients from whom biopsy specimens of both antrum and body were available. In 84 patients (82%), a distinct associated entity was identified, including 39 with celiac disease, 30 with *H. pylori* infection, 4 with varioliform gastritis, 2 with inflammatory polyp, 2 with Crohn disease, 2 with HIV infection, 2 with lymphoma, 2 with esophageal carcinoma, and 1 with lymphocytic gastroenterocolitis. Lymphocytic gastritis was found in 33% of patients with celiac disease and 4.1% of those with histopathologically defined *H. pylori* gastritis. The severity of intraepithelial lymphocytosis was greater in antrum than in body in 83% (20 of 24) of lymphocytic gastritis associated with celiac disease, but in only 19% (4 of 21) of cases associated with *H. pylori* infection ($p < 0.00002$). All four patients with varioliform gastritis had more severe involvement of body. Lymphocytic colitis was common (38%, 5 of 13) in celiac disease with lymphocytic gastritis. The authors concluded that lymphocytic gastritis most commonly occurs in celiac disease and *H. pylori* infection, but rarely with other entities. Patients with antrum-predominant intraepithelial lymphocytosis may benefit from duodenal biopsies and/or serology for celiac disease. Similarly, antibiotic therapy for *H. pylori* may be beneficial irrespective of the microscopic identification of the organism as bacterial burden in these patients is often minimal or localized. Studies have shown that treatment leads to healing of the lymphocytic gastritis in a significant number of patients, irrespective of the histologic *H. pylori* status (91,92). There is no need to count lymphocytes to arrive at a diagnosis of lymphocytic gastritis; they should simply be "prominent." Remember that "lymphocytic gastritis" describes a pattern of injury rather than a diagnosis and the pathologist must consider the associated underlying type of damage (Table 2.1). For example, patients with common variable immunodeficiency

TABLE 2.1   Differential Diagnosis of Prominent Gastric Intraepithelial Lymphocytosis
Conditions Associated with a Lymphocytic Gastritis Pattern
Celiac disease
H. pylori gastritis
Common variable immunodeficiency
Autoimmune enteropathy (autoimmune gastroenteropathy)
Autoimmune pangastritis
Others

(CVID) or AIE can also have a lymphocytic gastritis pattern and we are aware of patients with a severe "lymphocytic gastroenterocolitis" who responded to antitumor necrosis factor treatment (93).

COLLAGENOUS GASTRITIS

This term describes a rare, poorly understood pattern of gastric injury in which prominent subepithelial collagen, intraepithelial lymphocytosis, and surface epithelial damage with flattening and detachment is present (Figs. 2.48, 2.49, e-Figs. 2.99–2.103). It has been associated with celiac and collagenous sprue, lymphocytic and collagenous colitis, lymphocytic gastritis, and other autoimmune diseases in adults. Extragastric manifestations,

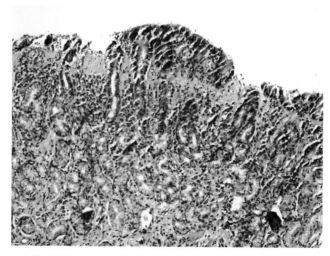

FIGURE 2.48 **Collagenous gastritis.** A thick and irregular collagen table with entrapped capillaries is seen here. Note detachment of the surface epithelium.

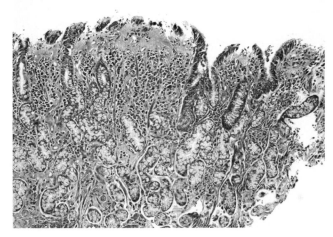

FIGURE 2.49 **Collagenous gastritis.** A trichrome stain highlights the thick and irregular collagen table.

while reported, are less common in pediatric patients (94–96). Adults usually present with nausea, vomiting, diarrhea, abdominal pain, or weight loss, while anemia is a common presenting symptom in pediatric patients (95,97,98). Endoscopic examination may disclose an atrophic or nodular mucosa (94,96,97,99). There is a female predominance and the changes may be found throughout the stomach. Management is difficult with only some patients achieving symptomatic relief after treatment with a gluten-free diet, budesonide, carafate, or steroids. There is no clear association with *H. pylori* infection.

GASTRIC CROHN DISEASE

In the absence of granulomas, it is difficult to know in gastric biopsies whether inflammatory changes reflect unspecified gastritis or are a manifestation of the patient's systemic disease (Fig. 2.50, e-Fig. 2.103). However, some observers have used the term "focally enhanced gastritis" (100) to refer to a pattern of gastritis seen in association with Crohn disease. In other words, small foci are inflamed (instead of a uniform distribution of inflammation) with a characteristic complement of inflammatory constituents and these foci are separated by more normal mucosa. In a prospective study, biopsy specimens from the antrum and body from 75 patients with established Crohn disease of the large and/or small bowel, and 200 Crohn disease-free controls were evaluated by histology and immunohistochemistry. *H. pylori*–associated gastritis was found in 25 patients with Crohn disease (33.3%) and 78 controls (39%). In *H. pylori*–negative patients with Crohn disease, a characteristic type of gastritis was found in antral biopsy specimens of 36 patients (48%) and in body biopsy specimens of 18 patients

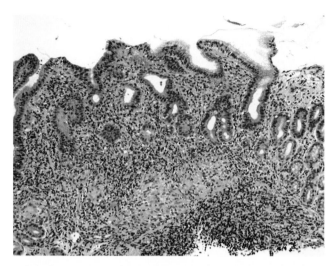

FIGURE 2.50 **Focally enhanced gastritis in a patient with Crohn disease.** There is active and chronic inflammation with an associated granuloma. Notice relative sparing of the mucosa to the right hand side of the field. Some observers refer to this pattern of gastritis associated with Crohn disease as "focally enhanced gastritis."

(24%). It was characterized by a focal infiltration of CD3+ lymphocytes, CD68R+ histiocytes, and, in 80% of cases, granulocytes. Granulomas were found in 11 patients. Overall, granulomas and/or focally enhanced gastritis were observed in 76% of *H. pylori*–negative patients with Crohn disease and in 0.8% of controls. There were no correlations between the occurrence of focally enhanced gastritis and clinical or laboratory findings. These authors concluded that focally enhanced gastritis is common in Crohn disease and that its recognition should guide the clinician to further investigate patients not yet known to have Crohn disease. We have also found that identifying this pattern of focally enhanced gastritis helps to distinguish upper tract Crohn disease. Unfortunately, however, such a pattern can also be seen in patients who do not have Crohn disease, so it is not specific (101).

GRANULOMATOUS GASTRITIS

"Granulomatous gastritis" is explained by Crohn disease in about half of cases seen in Western populations. It has been attributed to *Helicobacter* in populations with prevalent infection (102), but its etiology often remains unexplained and it seems to be of little clinical significance. In daily practice, when confronted with isolated granulomas in a gastric biopsy, we attempt to correlate with a history or Crohn disease or sarcoidosis, exclude infectious etiologies (including *Helicobacter* gastritis), and render a descriptive diagnosis. Rare cases of granulomatous gastritis have been associated with adenocarcinoma, so this is always sought (103). If a necrotizing appearance is present, rather than isolated small granulomas, vasculitis is considered. But, of course, we are reluctant to diagnose vasculitis definitively on any mucosal biopsy.

Sarcoidosis can manifest in the stomach just as it can elsewhere in the body and, like elsewhere, it is a diagnosis of exclusion. Generally, patients known to have sarcoidosis have small nonnecrotizing granulomas in their stomachs although, we are aware of a patient ultimately shown to have sarcoidosis who presented with necrotizing gastric granulomas (104).

OTHER INFLAMMATORY CONDITIONS

A discussion of every cause of gastric inflammation is beyond the scope of this text, but some of these conditions merit brief mention. Like the esophagus, the stomach can also be the epicenter of GI tract allergic disease (eosinophilic gastritis), and prominent eosinophilia involving epithelium and muscularis is sought (since scattered eosinophils are a normal lamina propria constituent). We do not count eosinophils in the stomach since there are no established counting methods but it is easy to assess whether they are where they do not belong, or to simply note that they are prominent in the lamina propria (Fig. 2.51, e-Fig. 2.104–2.107) and suggest correlation with other stigmata of allergic disease.

Syphilis Gastritis

Unfortunately syphilis-associated gastritis has a variety of appearances but should be considered in patients with striking gastritis with mixed inflammation and damage to gastric glands. In our limited experience, there is overwhelming inflammation reminiscent of the pattern seen in autoimmune pangastritis, with a mixed inflammatory pattern but the diagnosis

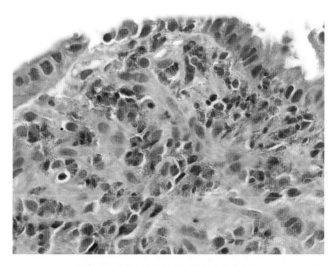

FIGURE 2.51 Eosinophilic gastritis.

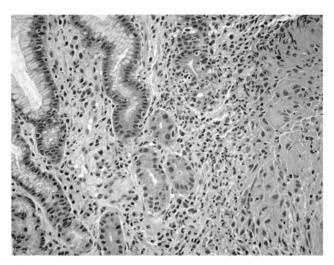

FIGURE 2.52 **Syphilitic gastritis.** Syphilis may manifest a variety of appearances. In this patient, granulomatous inflammation, mixed lamina propria and intra-epithelial inflammation, and prominent pit apoptosis are all present.

must be established on direct immunofluorescence (105) or, more recently, immunolabeling (106) (Fig. 2.52, e-Fig 2.108).

Cytomegalovirus Gastritis and Epstein-Barr–Associated Gastritis

CMV gastritis is not uncommon in inpatient material, where it can be found in both epithelial and endothelial cells (Figs. 2.53, 2.54, e-Figs. 2.109–2.114). A pitfall in diagnosis can be the monocytic reaction it can

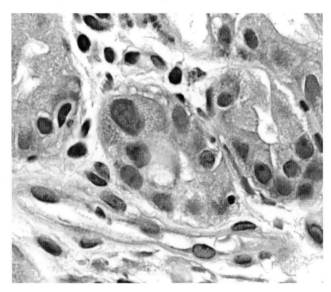

FIGURE 2.53 **Cytomegalovirus (CMV) gastritis.** A viral inclusion is seen here within an epithelial cell.

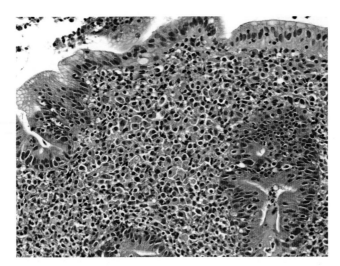

FIGURE 2.54 Cytomegalovirus (CMV) gastritis. Infection with CMV can invoke a striking monocytic reaction, provoking concern for a gastric lymphoma, a pitfall in diagnosis.

invoke, which can be mistaken for lymphoma (Fig. 2.54, e-Figs. 2.109, 2.110). This is also a potential pitfall with rare examples of Epstein-Barr virus (EBV) gastritis, which appears similar to large cell lymphoma in the manner that infectious mononucleosis simulates leukemia. When considering a diagnosis of large cell lymphoma in the setting of an active inflammatory backdrop, it is worthwhile to add EBV assessment to the workup panel.

Russell Body Gastritis

First described in 1998 by Tazawa and Tsutsumi (107), Russell body gastritis is a rare, inflammatory, poorly understood condition characterized by dense, mucosal accumulation of plasma cells containing intracytoplasmic, eosinophilic globules composed of immunoglobulins (Russell bodies) that push the nucleus aside, accompanied by a chronic inflammatory infiltrate (Figs. 2.55, 2.56, e-Figs. 2.115–2.120). It is generally best regarded as a benign incidental finding. The principal association is with *H. pylori* infection (107–109) although monoclonal gammopathy of uncertain significance and EBV-related gastric carcinoma have been reported in association with Russell body gastritis (110,111). Russell body gastritis is mostly important because the plasma cells can be mistaken for signet-ring carcinoma cells. Lack of nuclear atypia, along with mucin stain and/or immunohistochemical tests for cytokeratins and plasma cell markers (CD138, CD79a, κ and λ light chains) are helpful in this respect. Patients are usually treated with *H. pylori* eradication therapy.

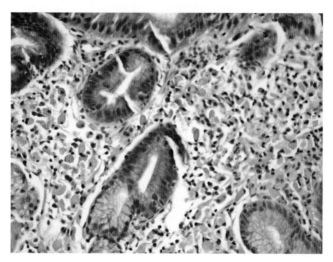

FIGURE 2.55 **Russell body gastritis.** Note the lamina propria plasma cells with prominent Russell bodies.

Gastric Findings in Common Variable Immunodeficiency

Like those in the esophagus, the gastric histologic findings in patients with this disease are nonspecific. Daniels et al. observed a lack of lamina propria plasma cells and the presence of lymphoid aggregates in approximately two thirds of these patients. Increased number of apoptotic bodies, granulomata, and a lymphocytic gastritis pattern may also be seen (112). When intraepithelial neutrophils are present, it is often in association with infections like CMV, *H. pylori*, or Cryptosporidium (112) (Figs. 2.57, 2.58,

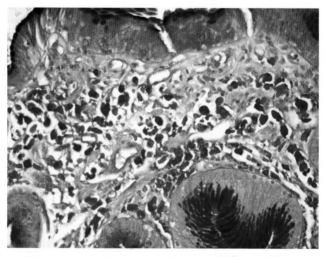

FIGURE 2.56 **Russell body gastritis.** Prominent PAS staining of Russell bodies can raise concern for signet ring cell carcinoma.

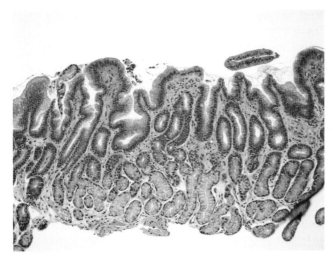

FIGURE 2.57 **Common variable immunodeficiency.** This sample appears unremarkable at scanning magnification.

e-Figs. 2.121, 2.122). The pathologist may suggest the possibility of CVID in a patient whose biopsy displays one or more of these features, provided a suitable clinical scenario.

Gastric Graft Versus Host Disease

Gastric graft versus host disease shows the same features as GVHD elsewhere in the GI tract, with epithelial apoptosis and ulcers/erosions to a varying degree. We make an attempt to grade these changes as mild,

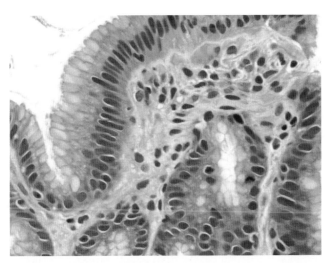

FIGURE 2.58 **Common variable immunodeficiency.** On higher magnification of the area in Figure 2.57, plasma cells are wholly absent.

moderate, and severe, in which severe changes include ulcers/erosions (e-Figs. 2.123–2.125). We try to compare current biopsies with prior ones and, when possible, to assess improvements (or lack thereof). Such biopsies are carefully studied for CMV inclusions as well.

HYPERPLASTIC/HYPERTROPHIC GASTRITIS

A simplistic approach to hyperplastic gastritis, or "giant folds" (Fig. 2.59, e-Figs. 2.126–2.129), is to consider whether the thickened folds (seen as "hypertrophic gastritis" by the endoscopist) are imparted by foveolar hyperplasia or hyperplasia of oxyntic glands.

Foveolar Hyperplasia

The syndrome of hypertrophic gastric folds, oxyntic gland loss (and thus achlorhydria), and protein loss is also termed "Ménétrier disease" (113–129). However, this term often describes a phenotype, rather than an etiology, when used to encompass the host of lesions that can display hyperplastic mucosa. When used this way, it is another example of the limited repertoire of mucosal response to a variety of insults and, in fact, probably the original cases reported by Ménétrier were not a single entity. However, some observers suggest isolating those cases that display massive diffuse foveolar hyperplasia in the absence of inflammation as the "true" disease (massive foveolar hyperplasia) (121). The mucin in this condition has a profile that differs from the mucin extracted from normal stomachs, but this pattern does not explain the etiology (124).

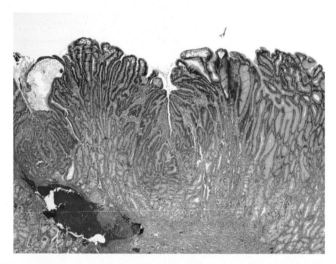

FIGURE 2.59 Hyperplastic gastropathy. Note diffuse hyperplasia of foveolar epithelium. This focus in isolation is indistinguishable from a gastric hyperplastic polyp, so diagnosis requires endoscopic correlation. This condition typically affects the gastric body. Note the loss of oxyntic glands.

Ménétrier disease is a rare disorder that has been described in adults, as well as children, on average in their 4th and 6th decades. It is three times more common in men than women. The disease course is usually chronic, with an unfavorable prognosis. Patients present with hypoproteinemia, due to nonselective protein loss across the gastric mucosal barrier and peripheral edema. Studies have shown loss of immunoglobulins, albumin, and transferrin. Other causes of protein loss, due to renal and liver disorders, need to be excluded. Patients may present with low or normal acid output. Symptoms appear insidiously and become progressive, consisting of epigastric pain, dyspepsia, anorexia, peripheral edema, hematemesis, and vomiting. The risk of developing carcinoma with Ménétrier disease is subject to debate. Approximately 15% of Ménétrier disease cases in the literature have been associated with carcinoma. In contrast to adults, children have a self-limited course for hyperplastic gastropathy, and CMV infection has been frequently implicated. Overexpression of transforming growth factor-α (TNF-α), one of various ligands that bind to the epidermal growth factor receptor (EGFR), has a possible role in the pathogenesis of Ménétrier disease. Transgenic mice that overproduce TNF-α in the stomach have many features of Ménétrier disease, such as foveolar hyperplasia, increased mucin content, decreased parietal cell mass, and reduced acid production. Erbitux, a monoclonal antibody that blocks EGFR, has been used with some success (128). Gastrectomy may be necessary in some cases.

On a mucosal biopsy, this condition appears no different from a gastric hyperplastic polyp or a polyp of the type seen in Cronkhite-Canada syndrome (see Volume 2, Chapter 2). Its features consist of hyperplastic foveolar epithelium, arranged in a disorderly fashion, with loss of oxyntic mucosa in biopsies from the body or fundus (Fig. 2.59, e-Fig. 2.127). It is impossible to diagnose this sort of hyperplastic gastropathy on mucosal biopsies without proper correlation with endoscopic and imaging findings.

Hyperplasia of Oxyntic Glands

Giant folds may be imparted by marked hyperplasia of the oxyntic component of the mucosa (Figs. 2.60, 2.61, e-Figs. 2.130–2.134). This happens as a result of hypergastrinemia in patients with normal parietal cells. As above, hypergastrinemia can occur in the setting of an interrupted feedback loop when there is loss of oxyntic mucosa in autoimmune gastritis. Of course, there cannot be hyperplasia of oxyntic mucosa if it has been destroyed by an autoimmune process. However, if there is intact gastric mucosa, hypergastrinemia can result from a gastrin-producing neoplasm (a "gastrinoma"). The resultant hypertrophic gastropathy is referred to as a component of Zollinger-Ellison syndrome. Since the gastrin in Zollinger-Ellison syndrome also stimulates endocrine cells, endocrine cell hyperplasia is also a component of this condition. On a mucosal biopsy, the oxyntic component is markedly expanded and thick. But, the key feature is that

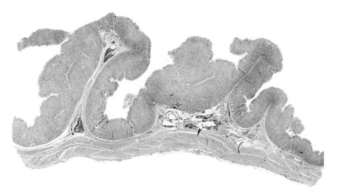

FIGURE 2.60 **Hyperplastic gastropathy in Zollinger-Ellison syndrome.** The patient had a gastrin-secreting tumor in the pancreas, and the oxyntic epithelium is the component that is hyperplastic.

parietal cells are seen insinuated in the epithelium nearly at, or just at, the surface between residual foveolar cells (rather than nested down deeper in the mucosa).

FINDINGS IN SYSTEMIC DISEASES

Major systemic diseases tend to affect the function of the stomach, rather than the morphology of gastric mucosa. Patients with scleroderma may have mural fibrosis that leads to pseudo-obstructive lesions, but these only affect the mucosa in terms of stasis changes and bacterial overgrowth. The same can be said for "diabetic gastropathy," which does not affect the mucosa *per se*, but leads to delayed gastric emptying. Vasculitis may lead to ischemic effects, but is difficult to diagnose confidently on mucosal

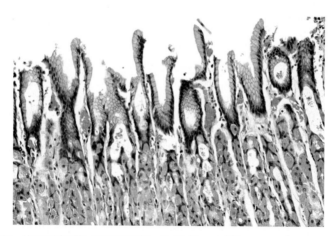

FIGURE 2.61 **Hyperplastic gastropathy in Zollinger-Ellison syndrome.** Parietal cells are seen almost up to the surface.

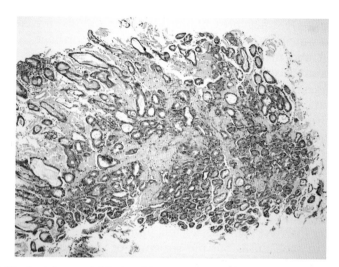

FIGURE 2.62 **Gastric amyloidosis.** This striking example shows acellular eosinophilic material surrounding many glands.

biopsies. Amyloidosis, however, can be recognized on mucosal biopsies and we have even seen a case associated with a hypertrophic gross appearance similar to other hypertrophic gastropathies. The endoscopic appearance from this case is seen in e-Figs. 2.135–2.137. Amyloidosis often results in friable mucosa and is thus associated with GI hemorrhage. The histologic features of gastric amyloidosis are like those anywhere in the body, with waxy material thickening vessel walls and basement membranes, which can be stained with Congo red (Figs. 2.62, 2.63, e-Figs. 2.137–2.140).

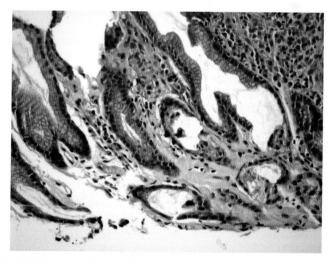

FIGURE 2.63 **Gastric amyloidosis.** Higher magnification showing more subtle deposition around gastric glands.

Overall, GI tract presentations of amyloidosis are nonspecific. Features can include macroglossia, dyspepsia, hemorrhage, a change in bowel habit and malabsorption. Endoscopic and radiologic features of amyloidosis are also nonspecific. The small intestine is most commonly affected. Since there are no specific treatments for GI amyloidosis, therapy is directed at eliminating the source of abnormal protein. Supportive measures (nutritional support and antidiarrheal agents) are the mainstay of care. Surgery is usually reserved for when the benefits clearly outweigh the risks, as there is a risk of decompensation of organs affected by systemic disease (130). For a comprehensive discussion, GI amyloidosis has been reviewed by Sattianayagam et al. (130–132).

Essentially, amyloidosis describes a disorder characterized by abnormal protein folding that results in deposition of insoluble fibrils in tissues. These fibrils interfere with tissue function. A large number of proteins may result in such fibrils but the structure of the fibrils is similar. They are embedded in nonfibrillary proteins consisting of glycosaminoglycans, proteoglycans, and serum amyloid P protein (a normal serum protein). Amyloidosis can be acquired or hereditary. Deposition of proteins can be either localized or systemic. Amyloidosis is classified on the basis of the type of proteins forming the deposits:

- Fibrils can form when there are persistently elevated levels of normal proteins (such as serum amyloid A in prolonged inflammatory states or β_2 microglobulin in persons undergoing long-term dialysis).
- Fibrils can form as a result of production of an abnormal protein that tends to form amyloid (immunoglobulins from plasma cell disorders).
- Fibrils can form from accumulation of normal transthyretin in elderly patients ("senile amyloidosis"), particularly in the heart, but such fibrils can be found in the GI tract.

The types of amyloid and their associated clinical manifestations are shown in Table 2.2.

In diagnosing gastric amyloidosis, or amyloidosis anywhere else in the body for that matter, ideally it is worthwhile to consider the type of amyloid and make an attempt to classify the amyloid, particularly if the patient has features of systemic disease. This can be a cumbersome process and it is sometimes most efficient to forward samples to a laboratory specializing in this endeavor but a panel of immunolabeling using antibodies against serum amyloid protein, serum amyloid A, albumin, transthyretin, κ light chain, and λ light chain can be effective. For the pathologist in a small center, some commercial laboratories and other centers offer such panels. For example, Mayo Medical Laboratories is able to perform amyloid testing (using mass spectrometry on receipt of a paraffin block). Information on centers with expertise in amyloidosis is available through the Amyloidosis Foundation at http://www.amyloidosis.org/faqs.asp.

TABLE 2.2 Amyloidosis Classification, Common Types		
Amyloidosis Type	**Protein Type**	**Key Clinical Features**
AA	Amyloid A protein (serum)	Reactive; associated with chronic inflammatory conditions
AL	Immunoglobulin light chains	Systemic disease associated with plasma cell disorders
$A\beta_2M$	β_2-microglobulin	Usually associated with long-term dialysis
ATTR	Plasma transthyretin (normal)	"Senile amyloidosis"; often systemic, cardiac disease common
ATTR	Genetically altered transthyretin	Autosomal dominant systemic amyloidosis and familial amyloid polyneuropathy

REFERENCES

1. Abraham SC, Singh VK, Yardley JH, et al. Hyperplastic polyps of the stomach: associations with histologic patterns of gastritis and gastric atrophy. *Am J Surg Pathol.* 2001;25:500–507.

2. Abraham SC, Yardley JH, Wu TT. Erosive injury to the upper gastrointestinal tract in patients receiving iron medication: an underrecognized entity. *Am J Surg Pathol.* 1999;23:1241–1247.

3. Laine L, Marin-Sorensen M, Weinstein WM. Campylobacter pylori in alcoholic hemorrhagic "gastritis". *Dig Dis Sci.* 1989;34:677–680.

4. Laine L, Weinstein WM. Histology of alcoholic hemorrhagic "gastritis": a prospective evaluation. *Gastroenterology.* 1988;94:1254–1262.

5. Dyer S, Mycyk MB, Ahrens WR, et al. Hemorrhagic gastritis from topical isopropanol exposure. *Ann Pharmacother.* 2002;36:1733–1735.

6. Takeda K, Nakamoto M, Yasunaga C, et al. Acute hemorrhagic gastritis associated with acetazolamide intoxication in a patient with chronic renal failure. *Clin Nephrol.* 1997;48:266–268.

7. Yabuki K, Maekawa T, Satoh K, et al. Extensive hemorrhagic erosive gastritis associated with acute pancreatitis successfully treated with a somatostatin analog. *J Gastroenterol.* 2002;37:737–741.

8. Nam SY, Choi IJ, Park KW, et al. Risk of hemorrhagic gastropathy associated with colonoscopy bowel preparation using oral sodium phosphate solution. *Endoscopy.* 2010;42:109–113.

9. Haber MM, Lopez I. Reflux gastritis in gastroesophageal reflux disease: a histopathological study. *Ann Diagn Pathol.* 1999;3:281–286.

10. Sobala GM, King RF, Axon AT, et al. Reflux gastritis in the intact stomach. *J Clin Pathol.* 1990;43:303–306.

11. Haber MM, Lopez I. Gastric histologic findings in patients with nonsteroidal anti-inflammatory drug-associated gastric ulcer. *Mod Pathol.* 1999;12:592–598.

12. Pashankar DS, Bishop WP, Mitros FA. Chemical gastropathy: a distinct histopathologic entity in children. *J Pediatr Gastroenterol Nutr.* 2002;35:653–657.

13. Greenson JK, Trinidad SB, Pfeil SA, et al. Gastric mucosal calcinosis. Calcified aluminum phosphate deposits secondary to aluminum-containing antacids or sucralfate therapy in organ transplant patients. *Am J Surg Pathol.* 1993;17:45–50.

14. Stroehlein KB, Stroehlein JR, Kahan BD, et al. Gastric mucosal calcinosis in renal transplant patients. *Transplant Proc.* 1999;31:2124–2126.

15. Gorospe M, Fadare O. Gastric mucosal calcinosis: clinicopathologic considerations. Adv Anat Pathol 2007;14:224–228.

16. Marginean EC, Bennick M, Cyczk J et al. Gastric siderosis: patterns and significance. *Am J Surg Pathol.* 2006;30:514–520.

17. Abraham SC, Bhagavan BS, Lee LA, et al. Upper gastrointestinal tract injury in patients receiving kayexalate (sodium polystyrene sulfonate) in sorbitol: clinical, endoscopic, and histopathologic findings. *Am J Surg Pathol.* 2001;25:637–644.

18. Iacobuzio-Donahue CA, Lee EL, Abraham SC, et al. Colchicine toxicity: distinct morphologic findings in gastrointestinal biopsies. *Am J Surg Pathol.* 2001;25:1067–1073.

19. Hruban RH, Yardley JH, Donehower RC, et al. Taxol toxicity. Epithelial necrosis in the gastrointestinal tract associated with polymerized microtubule accumulation and mitotic arrest. *Cancer.* 1989;63:1944–1950.

20. Daniels JA, Gibson MK, Xu L, et al. Gastrointestinal tract epithelial changes associated with taxanes: marker of drug toxicity versus effect. *Am J Surg Pathol.* 2008;32:473–477.

21. Lomo LC, Blount PL, Sanchez CA, et al. Crypt dysplasia with surface maturation: a clinical, pathologic, and molecular study of a Barrett's esophagus cohort. *Am J Surg Pathol.* 2006;30:423–435.

22. Parfitt JR, Jayakumar S, Driman DK. Mycophenolate mofetil-related gastrointestinal mucosal injury: variable injury patterns, including graft-versus-host disease-like changes. *Am J Surg Pathol.* 2008;32:1367–1372.

23. Nguyen T, Park JY, Scudiere JR, et al. Mycophenolic acid (CellCept and Myofortic) induced injury of the upper GI tract. *Am J Surg Pathol.* 2009;33:1355–1363.

24. Ozokutan BH, Ceylan H, Ertaskin I, et al. Pediatric gastric outlet obstruction following corrosive ingestion. *Pediatr Surg Int.* 2010;26:615–618.

25. Al-Binali AM, Al-Shehri MA, Abdelmoneim I, et al. Pattern of corrosive ingestion in southwestern Saudi Arabia. Saudi J Gastroenterol. 2009;15:15–17.

26. Kar H, Batuk G, Cekin N, et al. Deaths due to corrosive ingestion: a 10-year retrospective study. *Toxicol Mech Methods.* 2006;16:405–409.

27. Havanond C. Clinical features of corrosive ingestion. *J Med Assoc Thai.* 2003;86:918–924.

28. Fyfe AH, Auldist AW. Corrosive ingestion in children. *Z Kinderchir* 1984;39:229–233.

29. Ramasamy K, Gumaste VV. Corrosive ingestion in adults. *J Clin Gastroenterol.* 2003;37:119–124.

30. Ulenaers M, Dedeurwaerdere F, Christiaens P. Gastric ulceration complicating selective internal radiation therapy of liver metastases. *Clin Gastroenterol Hepatol.* 2010;8:A18.

31. Marshall BJ, Warren JR. Unidentified curved bacilli in the stomach of patients with gastritis and peptic ulceration. *Lancet.* 1984;1:1311–1315.

32. Marshall BJ, Armstrong JA, McGechie DB, et al. Attempt to fulfil Koch's postulates for pyloric Campylobacter. *Med J Aust.* 1985;142:436–439.

33. Jhala D, Jhala N, Lechago J, et al. Helicobacter heilmannii gastritis: association with acid peptic diseases and comparison with Helicobacter pylori gastritis. *Mod Pathol.* 1999;12:534–538.

34. Montgomery EA, Martin DF, Peura DA. Rapid diagnosis of Campylobacter pylori by Gram's stain. *Am J Clin Pathol.* 1988;90:606–609.

35. Dickey W, Kenny BD, McConnell JB. Effect of proton pump inhibitors on the detection of Helicobacter pylori in gastric biopsies. *Aliment Pharmacol Ther.* 1996;10:289–293.

36. Talley NJ, Fock KM, Moayyedi P. Gastric Cancer Consensus conference recommends Helicobacter pylori screening and treatment in asymptomatic persons from high-risk populations to prevent gastric cancer. *Am J Gastroenterol.* 2008;103:510–514.

37. Di Mario F, Cavallaro LG, Moussa AM, et al. Usefulness of serum pepsinogens in Helicobacter pylori chronic gastritis: relationship with inflammation, activity, and density of the bacterium. *Dig Dis Sci.* 2006;51:1791–1795.

38. Di Mario F, Moussa AM, Cavallaro LG, et al. Clinical usefulness of serum pepsinogen II in the management of Helicobacter pylori infection. *Digestion.* 2004;70;167–172.

39. Kiyohira K, Yoshihara M, Ito M, et al. Serum pepsinogen concentration as a marker of Helicobacter pyloriinfection and the histologic grade of gastritis; evaluation of gastric mucosa by serum pepsinogen levels. *J Gastroenterol.* 2003;38:332–338.

40. Yan SL, Wu ST, Chen CH, et al. Mucosal patterns of Helicobacter pylori-related gastritis without atrophy in the gastric corpus using standard endoscopy. *World J Gastroenterol.* 2010;16:496–500.

41. Kiesslich R, Goetz M, Burg J, et al. Diagnosing Helicobacter pylori in vivo by confocal laser endoscopy. *Gastroenterology.* 2005;128:2119–2123.

42. Veijola L, Oksanen A, Linnala A et al. Persisting chronic gastritis and elevated Helicobacter pylori antibodies after successful eradication therapy. *Helicobacter.* 2007;12:605–608.

43. Moss SF, Legon S, Bishop AE, et al. Effect of Helicobacter pylori on gastric somatostatin in duodenal ulcer disease. *Lancet.* 1992;340:930–932.

44. Dixon MF, Genta RM, Yardley JH, et al. Histological classification of gastritis and Helicobacter pylori infection: an agreement at last? The International Workshop on the Histopathology of Gastritis. Helicobacter. 1997;2 (Suppl 1):S17–24.

45. Guo J, Young SK, Lorenzo CR, et al. Phlegmonous gastritis in a patient with myeloid sarcoma: a case report. *Appl Immunohistochem Mol Morphol.* 2009;17:458–462.

46. Harikumar R, Pramod K, Pushpa M, et al. Gastric lymphoma presenting as phlegmonous gastritis. *J Gastrointest Cancer.* 2007;38:24–27.

47. Kavalar R, Skok P, Kramberger KG. Phlegmonous gastritis in a patient with rheumatoid arthritis. *Wien Klin Wochenschr.* 2005;117:364–368.

48. Yu QQ, Tariq A, Unger SW, et al. Phlegmonous gastritis associated with Kaposi sarcoma: a case report and review of the literature. *Arch Pathol Lab Med.* 2004;128:801–803.

49. Lee BS, Kim SM, Seong JK, et al. Phlegmonous gastritis after endoscopic mucosal resection. *Endoscopy.* 2005;37:490–493.

50. Miller AI, Smith B, Rogers AI. Phlegmonous gastritis. *Gastroenterology.* 1975;68:231–238.

51. Munroe CA, Chen A. Suppurative (phlegmonous) gastritis presenting as a gastric mass. *Dig Dis Sci.* 2010;55:11–13.

52. Jung C, Choi YW, Jeon SC, et al. Acute diffuse phlegmonous esophagogastritis: radiologic diagnosis. *AJR Am J Roentgenol.* 2003;180:862–863.

53. Sood BP, Kalra N, Suri S. CT features of acute phlegmonous gastritis. *Clin Imaging.* 2000;24:287–288.

54. Wakayama T, Watanabe H, Ishizaki Y, et al. A case of phlegmonous esophagitis associated with diffuse phlegmonous gastritis. *Am J Gastroenterol.* 1994;89:804–806.

55. Park JY, Cornish TC, Lam-Himlin D, et al. Gastric lesions in patients with autoimmune metaplastic atrophic gastritis (AMAG) in a tertiary care setting. *Am J Surg Pathol.* 2010;34(11):1591-1598.

56. Laass MW, Pargac N, Fischer R, et al. Emphysematous gastritis caused by Sarcina ventriculi. *Gastrointest Endosc* 2010;72:1101-1103.

57. Crowther JS. Sarcina ventriculi in human faeces. *J Med Microbiol.* 1971;4:343–350.

58. DeBey BM, Blanchard PC, Durfee PT. Abomasal bloat associated with Sarcina-like bacteria in goat kids. *J Am Vet Med Assoc.* 1996;209:1468–1469.

59. Canale-Parola E. Biology of the sugar-fermenting Sarcinae. *Bacteriol Rev.* 1970;34:82–97.

60. Lam-Himlin D, Anders R. Sarcina ventriculi. 2010 (in press at the time of this writing in The American Journal of Surgical Pathology).

61. Dixon MF, Genta RM, Yardley JH, et al. Classification and grading of gastritis. The updated Sydney System. International Workshop on the Histopathology of Gastritis, Houston 1994. *Am J Surg Pathol.* 1996;20:1161–1181.

62. Hurst A. Addison's (pernicious) anemia and subacute combined degeneration of the spinal cord. *BMJ.* 1924;1:93–100.

63. Chanarin I. Historical review: a history of pernicious anaemia. *Br J Haematol.* 2000; 111:407–415.

64. Park J, Cornish T, Lam-Himlin D, et al. Gastric lesions in patients with autoimmune metaplastic atrophic gastritis (AMAG) in a tertiary care setting. *Am J Surg Pathol.* 2010;34(11):1591–1598.

65. Hershko C, Ronson A, Souroujon M, et al. Variable hematologic presentation of autoimmune gastritis: age-related progression from iron deficiency to cobalamin depletion. *Blood* 2006;107:1673–1679.

66. D'Elios MM, Bergman MP, Amedei, A et al. Helicobacter pylori and gastric autoimmunity. *Microbes Infect.* 2004;6:1395–1401.

67. Krasinskas AM, Abraham SC, Metz DC, et al. Oxyntic mucosa pseudopolyps: a presentation of atrophic autoimmune gastritis. *Am J Surg Pathol.* 2003;27:236–241.

68. Okano A, Takakuwa H, Matsubayashi Y. Parietal-cell hyperplasia mimicking sporadic fundic gland polyps in the atrophic mucosa of autoimmune gastritis. *Gastrointest Endosc* 2007;66:394–395; discussion 395.

69. Jhala NC, Montemor M, Jhala D, et al. Pancreatic acinar cell metaplasia in autoimmune gastritis. *Arch Pathol Lab Med.* 2003;127:854–857.

70. Torbenson M, Abraham SC, Boitnott J, et al. Autoimmune gastritis: distinct histological and immunohistochemical findings before complete loss of oxyntic glands. *Mod Pathol.* 2002;15:102–109.

71. Unsworth DJ, Walker-Smith JA. Autoimmunity in diarrhoeal disease. *J Pediatr Gastroenterol Nutr.* 1985;4:375–380.

72. Casis B, Fernandez-Vazquez I, Barnardos E, et al. Autoimmune enteropathy in an adult with autoimmune multisystemic involvement. *Scand J Gastroenterol.* 2002;37: 1012–1016.

73. Leon F, Olivencia P, Rodriguez-Pena R, et al. Clinical and immunological features of adult-onset generalized autoimmune gut disorder. *Am J Gastroenterol.* 2004;99:1563–1571.

74. Mitomi H, Tanabe S, Igarashi M, et al. Autoimmune enteropathy with severe atrophic gastritis and colitis in an adult: proposal of a generalized autoimmune disorder of the alimentary tract. *Scand J Gastroenterol.* 1998;33:716–720.

75. Akram S, Murray JA, Pardi DS, et al. Adult autoimmune enteropathy: Mayo Clinic Rochester experience. Clin Gastroenterol Hepatol 2007;**5**;1282–1290; quiz 1245.

76. Blanco Quiros A, Arranz Sanz E, Bernardo Ordiz D et al. From autoimmune enteropathy to the IPEX (immune dysfunction, polyendocrinopathy, enteropathy, X-linked) syndrome. Allergol Immunopathol (Madr) 2009;**37**;208–215.

77. d'Hennezel E, Ben-Shoshan M, Ochs HD et al. FOXP3 forkhead domain mutation and regulatory T cells in the IPEX syndrome. N Engl J Med 2009;**361**;1710–1713.

78. Oliva-Hemker M, Berkenblit GV, Anhalt GJ, et al. Pernicious anemia and widespread absence of gastrointestinal endocrine cells in a patient with autoimmune polyglandular syndrome type I and malabsorption. *J Clin Endocrinol Metab.* 2006;91: 2833–2838.

79. Jevremovic D, Torbenson M, Murray JA, et al. Atrophic autoimmune pangastritis: A distinctive form of antral and fundic gastritis associated with systemic autoimmune disease. *Am J Surg Pathol.* 2006;30:1412–1419.

80. Jabbari M, Cherry R, Lough JO, et al. Gastric antral vascular ectasia: the watermelon stomach. *Gastroenterology.* 1984;87:1165–1170.

81. Manolios N, Eliades C, Duncombe V, et al. Scleroderma and watermelon stomach. J Rheumatol 1996;23:776–778.

82. Gilliam JH, 3rd, Geisinger KR, Wu WC, et al. Endoscopic biopsy is diagnostic in gastric antral vascular ectasia. The ""watermelon stomach"". *Dig Dis Sci.* 1989;34:885–888.

83. Dulai GS, Jensen DM, Kovacs TO, et al. Endoscopic treatment outcomes in watermelon stomach patients with and without portal hypertension. *Endoscopy.* 2004;36:68–72.

84. Novitsky YW, Kercher KW, Czerniach DR, et al. Watermelon stomach: pathophysiology, diagnosis, and management. *J Gastrointest Surg.* 2003;7:652–661.

85. Thuluvath PJ, Yoo HY. Portal Hypertensive gastropathy. *Am J Gastroenterol.* 2002;97:2973–2978.

86. Westerhoff M, Tretiakova M, Hovan L, et al. CD61, CD31, and CD34 improve diagnostic accuracy in gastric antral vascular ectasia and portal hypertensive gastropathy: an immunohistochemical and digital morphometric study. *Am J Surg Pathol.* 2010;34:494–501.

87. Norton ID, Petersen BT, Sorbi D, et al. Management and long-term prognosis of Dieulafoy lesion. *Gastrointest Endosc.* 1999;50:762–767.

88. Sone Y, Kumada T, Toyoda H, et al. Endoscopic management and follow up of Dieulafoy lesion in the upper gastrointestinal tract. *Endoscopy.* 2005;37:449–453.

89. Littler ER, Gleibermann E. Gastritis cystica polyposa. (Gastric mucosal prolapse at gastroenterostomy site, with cystic and infiltrative epithelial hyperplasia). *Cancer.* 1972;29:205–209.

90. Wu TT, Hamilton SR. Lymphocytic gastritis: association with etiology and topology. *Am J Surg Pathol.* 1999;23:153–158.

91. Madisch A, Miehlke S, Neuber F, et al. Healing of lymphocytic gastritis after Helicobacter pylori eradication therapy–a randomized, double-blind, placebo-controlled multicentre trial. *Aliment Pharmacol Ther.* 2006;23:473–479.

92. Muller H, Volkholz H, Stolte M. Healing of lymphocytic gastritis by eradication of Helicobacter pylori. *Digestion.* 2001;63:14–19.

93. Aram G, Bayless TM, Chen ZM, et al. Refractory lymphocytic enterocolitis and tumor necrosis factor antagonist therapy. *Clin Gastroenterol Hepatol.* 2010;8:391–394.

94. Billiemaz K, Robles-Medranda C, Le Gall C, et al. A first report of collagenous gastritis, sprue, and colitis in a 9-month-old infant: 14 years of clinical, endoscopic, and histologic follow-up. *Endoscopy.* 2009;41(Suppl 2):E233–E234.

95. Leung ST, Chandan VS, Murray JA, et al. Collagenous gastritis: histopathologic features and association with other gastrointestinal diseases. *Am J Surg Pathol.* 2009;33:788–798.

96. Wilson C, Thompson K, Hunter C. Nodular collagenous gastritis. *J Pediatr Gastroenterol Nutr.* 2009;49:157.

97. Dray X, Reignier S, Vahedi K, et al. Collagenous gastritis. *Endoscopy.* 2007;39 (Suppl 1):E292–293.

98. Kori M, Cohen S, Levine A, et al. Collagenous gastritis: a rare cause of abdominal pain and iron-deficiency anemia. *J Pediatr Gastroenterol Nutr.* 2007;45:603–606.

99. Kamimura K, Kobayashi M, Narisawa R, et al. Collagenous gastritis: endoscopic and pathologic evaluation of the nodularity of gastric mucosa. *Dig Dis Sci.* 2007;52: 995–1000.

100. Oberhuber G, Puspok A, Oesterreicher C, et al. Focally enhanced gastritis: a frequent type of gastritis in patients with Crohn's disease. *Gastroenterology.* 1997;112:698–706.

101. Xin W, Greenson JK. The clinical significance of focally enhanced gastritis. *Am J Surg Pathol.* 2004;28:1347–1351.

102. Maeng L, Lee A, Choi K, et al. Granulomatous gastritis: a clinicopathologic analysis of 18 biopsy cases. *Am J Surg Pathol.* 2004;28:941–945.

103. Rashid AM, Williams RM. A new differential diagnosis in granulomatous gastritis. *Histopathology* 1992;20:280–281.

104. Liang DB, Price JC, Ahmed H, et al. Gastric sarcoidosis: case report and literature review. *J Natl Med Assoc.* 2010;102:348–351.

105. Chen CY, Chi KH, George RW, et al. Diagnosis of gastric syphilis by direct immunofluorescence staining and real-time PCR testing. *J Clin Microbiol.* 2006;44:3452–3456.

106. Buffet M, Grange PA, Gerhardt P, et al. Diagnosing Treponema pallidum in secondary syphilis by PCR and immunohistochemistry. *J Invest Dermatol.* 2007;127:2345–2350.

107. Tazawa K, Tsutsumi Y. Localized accumulation of Russell body-containing plasma cells in gastric mucosa with Helicobacter pylori infection: 'Russell body gastritis'. *Pathol Int.* 1998;48:242–244.

108. Ensari A, Savas B, Okcu Heper A, et al. An unusual presentation of Helicobacter pylori infection: so-called "Russell body gastritis". *Virchows Arch.* 2005;446:463–466.

109. Licci S, Sette P, Del Nonno F, et al. Russell body gastritis associated with Helicobacter pylori infection in an HIV-positive patient: case report and review of the literature. *Z Gastroenterol.* 2009;47:357–360.

110. Shinozaki A, Ushiku T, Fukayama M. Prominent Mott cell proliferation in Epstein-Barr virus-associated gastric carcinoma. *Hum Pathol.* 2010;41:134–138.

111. Wolkersdorfer GW, Haase M, Morgner A, et al. Monoclonal gammopathy of undetermined significance and Russell body formation in Helicobacter pylori gastritis. *Helicobacter.* 2006;11:506–510.

112. Daniels JA, Lederman HM, Maitra A, et al. Gastrointestinal tract pathology in patients with common variable immunodeficiency (CVID): a clinicopathologic study and review. *Am J Surg Pathol.* 2007;31:1800–1812.

113. Balfour DC Jr., Hightower NC Jr., Gambill EE, et al. Giant hypertrophy of the gastric rugae (Menetrier's disease) associated with severe hypoproteinemia relieved only by total gastrectomy; report of case. *Gastroenterology.* 1950;16:773–781.

114. Burns B, Gay BB, Jr. Menetrier's disease of the stomach in children. *Am J Roentgenol Radium Ther Nucl Med.* 1968;103:300–306.

115. Chang KW, Lin SJ, Hsueh C, et al. Menetrier's disease associated with cytomegalovirus infection in a child. *Acta Paediatr Taiwan.* 2000;41:339–340.

116. Cieslak TJ, Mullett CT, Puntel RA, et al. Menetrier's disease associated with cytomegalovirus infection in children: report of two cases and review of the literature. *Pediatr Infect Dis J.* 1993;12:340–343.

117. Di Vita G, Patti R, Aragona F, et al. Resolution of Menetrier's disease after Helicobacter pylori eradicating therapy. *Dig Dis Sci.* 2001;19:179–183.

118. Eisenstat DD, Griffiths AM, Cutz E, et al. Acute cytomegalovirus infection in a child with Menetrier's disease. *Gastroenterology.* 1995;109:592–595.

119. Fishbein M, Kirschner BS, Gonzales-Vallina R, et al. Menetrier's disease associated with formula protein allergy and small intestinal injury in an infant. *Gastroenterology.* 1992;103:1664–1668.

120. Hamlin M, Shepherd K, Kennedy M. Resolution of Menetrier's disease after Helicobacter pylori eradication therapy. *N Z Med J.* 2001;114:382–383.

121. Hendrix TR, Yardley JH. Menetrier's disease. *Gut.* 1995;36:945–946.

122. Hoffer V, Finkelstein Y, Balter J, et al. Ganciclovir treatment in Menetrier's disease. *Acta Paediatr.* 2003;92:983–985.

123. Ibarrola C, Rodriguez-Pinilla M, Valino C, et al. An unusual expression of hyperplastic gastropathy (Menetrier type) in twins. *Eur J Gastroenterol Hepatol.* 2003;15:441–445.

124. Mall AS, Dent DM, McLeod H, et al. Extraction, isolation, and SDS-PAGE analysis of purified gastric mucin in a patient with Menetrier's disease. *Am J Gastroenterol.* 2002;97:752–755.

125. Mitchell RE Jr. Giant hypertrophy of the gastric mucosa (Menetrier's disease). *Va Med Mon (1918).* 1965;92:99–100.

126. Reese DF, Hodgson JR, Dockerty MB. Giant hypertrophy of the gastric mucosa (Menetrier's disease): a correlation of the roentgenographic, pathologic, and clinical findings. *Am J Roentgenol Radium Ther Nucl Med.* 1962;88:619–626.

127. Sandberg DH. Hypertrophic gastropathy (Menetrier's disease) in childhood. *J Pediatr.* 1971;78:866–868.

128. Settle SH, Washington K, Lind C, et al. Chronic treatment of Menetrier's disease with Erbitux: clinical efficacy and insight into pathophysiology. *Clin Gastroenterol Hepatol.* 2005;3:654–659.

129. Sharma RN. Giant hypertrophic gastritis (Menetrier's disease). *J Indian Med Assoc.* 1967;49:77–78.

130. Sattianayagam P, Hawkins P, Gillmore J. Amyloid and the GI tract. *Expert Rev Gastroenterol Hepatol.* 2009;3:615–630.

131. Sattianayagam P, Gibbs S, Hawkins P, et al. Systemic AL (light-chain) amyloidosis and the gastrointestinal tract. *Scand J Gastroenterol.* 2009;44:1384–1385.

132. Sattianayagam PT, Hawkins PN, Gillmore JD. Systemic amyloidosis and the gastrointestinal tract. *Nat Rev Gastroenterol Hepatol.* 2009;6:608–617.

3

SMALL INTESTINE

The small intestine, like the rest of the gastrointestinal (GI) tract, reacts to injury with a limited number of responses. Consequently, diagnosis of nonneoplastic, small intestinal diseases requires correlation with clinical parameters. When reviewing small bowel biopsies, it is important to examine each compartment in a systematic fashion, especially in children. This theme of systematic examination continues in evaluating nonneoplastic colon, particularly in the immunosuppressed patient. The fragments of debris on the slide are scanned for organisms (*Giardia*, in particular) and the appearance of mucus noted; it may appear thick and inspissated in children with cystic fibrosis (Fig. 3.1, e-Fig. 3.1). The epithelium should be assessed for the presence of the brush border and intraepithelial inflammatory cells (Figs. 3.2 and 3.3). It is normal to have scattered intraepithelial lymphocytes (IELs) (T cells), but they should not be a prominent feature. The lamina propria should be scanned for abnormal inflammatory constituents and dilated lymphatic spaces. In adults, tumors may metastasize to the small bowel and the malignant cells may be seen exclusively and focally within lamina propria lymphatics (Fig. 3.4, e-Fig. 3.2). In other cases, lymphatic dilation due to extrinsic compression from an impinging neoplasm is the primary issue. In children, the issue is congenital lymphangiectasia (1,2), a potentially lethal condition with subtle biopsy findings. Plasma cells, lymphocytes, and a few eosinophils are normal, but neutrophils and numerous histiocytes/macrophages are not. The lamina propria may house too many histiocytes (consider *Mycobacterium avium* complex [MAI], Whipple disease [WD]), too many mast cells (consider mastocytosis) (Figs. 3.5 and 3.6, e-Figs. 3.3 and 3.4), or lack plasma cells (consider common variable immunodeficiency [CVID]). Unlike the colon, the lamina propria of the small bowel has sufficient lymphatic access to sustain metastases like that of the esophagus and stomach. Tumors that invade the lamina propria are staged as T1.

In assessing the surface epithelium, sometimes the cytoplasm of the enterocytes appears bubbly and lipid-laden (Figs. 3.7 and 3.8), as noted by the lack of cytoplasmic staining on the periodic acid-Schiff/Alcian blue (PAS/AB) staining preparation (Fig. 3.8). The differential diagnosis is between ingestion of lipids (such as coffee with cream/milk) just prior to the procedure versus abetalipoproteinemia (which is associated with acanthocytes

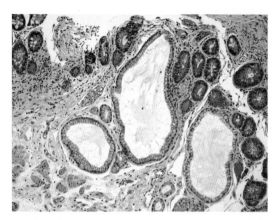

FIGURE 3.1 **Cystic fibrosis.** There is prominent inspissated mucus in Brunner glands in this duodenal biopsy.

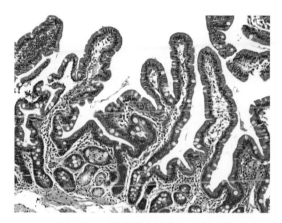

FIGURE 3.2 **Normal intestinal mucosa.** Note the scattered intra-epithelial lymphocytes.

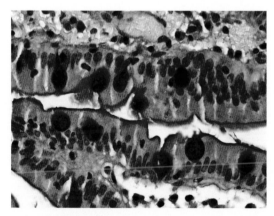

FIGURE 3.3 **Normal intestinal mucosa, PAS/AB stain.** PAS/AB stain highlights goblet cells in purple and the brush border is accentuated in pink.

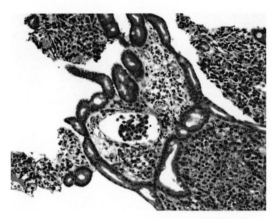

FIGURE 3.4 Metastatic melanoma, small intestine. This patient's biopsy shows metastatic melanoma both within the lamina propria and the lamina propria lymphatics.

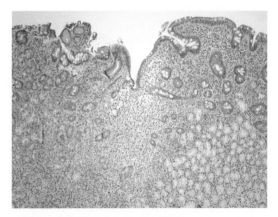

FIGURE 3.5 Systemic mastocytosis, small intestine. Lamina propria expansion is striking in this case of systemic mastocytosis.

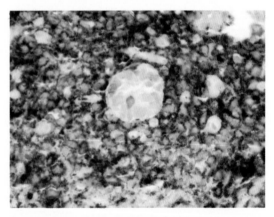

FIGURE 3.6 Systemic mastocytosis, CD117 immunostain. Notice how the neoplastic mast cells aggregate within the lamina propria and around glands.

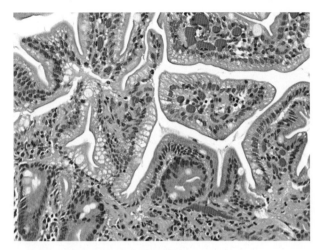

FIGURE 3.7 **Intracytoplasmic lipids in absorptive enterocytes.** It is more likely that the patient "cheated" by ingesting lipids during the preprocedural fasting period than that a fat absorption disorder is involved.

on the peripheral smear). Ingestion of lipids is, of course, the more common scenario and we see this fairly frequently on our biopsy material. However, we comment on cytoplasmic lipids in our report if there is a history of malabsorption.

"ARTIFACT" MISTAKEN FOR OTHER LESIONS

Crushed Brunner glands are easily mistaken for pathologic conditions. We have seen them mistaken for myxoid nerve sheath tumors (Figs. 3.9 and 3.10, e-Figs. 3.5 and 3.6). In our material, this is obviated by noting the strongly

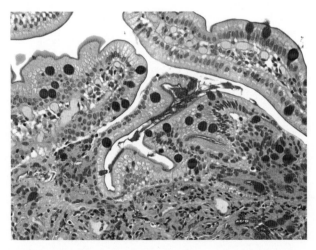

FIGURE 3.8 **Intracytoplasmic lipid in enterocytes.** Absorptive enterocytes with intracellular lipid lack cytoplasmic staining on the PAS/AB staining preparation.

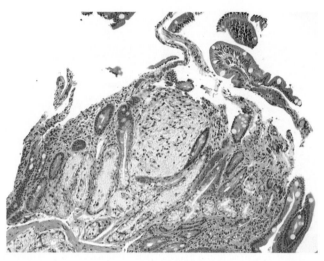

FIGURE 3.9 **Duodenum, crushed Brunner glands.** These are sometimes mistaken for nerve sheath tumors.

reactive PAS stain (Fig. 3.10, e-Fig. 3.6). On the other hand, crushed Brunner glands may occasionally raise the possibility of WD owing to their strong PAS reactivity (e-Figs. 3.5 and 3.6). Any doubt can be resolved by immunohistochemistry (3), but it is most easily resolved by comparing to adjacent intact and partially crushed Brunner glands. Another peculiar incidental finding in mucosal biopsies is the presence of tiny black flecks of titanium (from toothpaste and some foodstuffs [e-Fig. 3.7]), which may be found in lymphoid aggregates in both the small intestine and the colon (e-Fig. 3.8) (4).

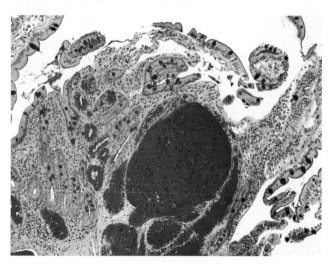

FIGURE 3.10 **Duodenum, crushed Brunner glands.** Submucosal brunner glands are strongly reactive with a PAS stain.

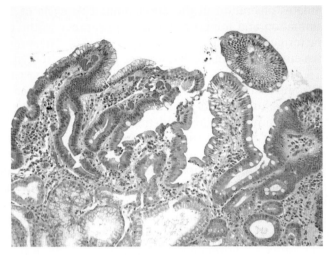

FIGURE 3.11 **Peptic duodenitis.** The lesion displays gastric mucin cell metaplasia.

REACTIVE LESIONS

When the esophagus and stomach are injured, metaplasia ensues, and often it is intestinal-type metaplasia. When the duodenum is injured, it also can undergo metaplasia, transforming to gastric-type mucosa. Originally, *Helicobacter* gastritis was strongly associated with duodenal ulceration (5,6), since *Helicobacter pylori* infection may upregulate gastric acid secretion by damaging D cells that secrete somatostatin (which normally reduces gastric secretion). It is predominantly the bulb (the area just beyond the pyloric sphincter) that is damaged. Gastric mucin cell metaplasia supervenes with Brunner gland hyperplasia and displacement into the mucosa (Figs. 3.11 and 3.12, e-Figs. 3.9–3.17). In addition, the area of metaplastic duodenum is then able to support *H. pylori* (e-Figs. 3.14 and 3.15), which

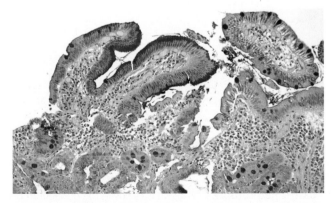

FIGURE 3.12 **Peptic duodenitis.** Gastric mucin cell metaplasia is usually apparent on H&E stains but it is highlighted by the PAS/AB stain.

further stimulates ulceration in the duodenum. This cycle of events may attract inflammation and impart a nodular appearance to the duodenum, which can be termed "nodular peptic duodenitis" (7,8). There may be striking reparative epithelial changes that are occasionally mistaken for adenomas (e-Figs. 3.11–3.13, 3.16, 3.17). If PAS staining is done, these foci usually have at least some gastric mucin cell metaplasia (e-Fig. 3.17) as a clue that the process is reparative, rather than neoplastic. Compare, e.g., e-Figures 18 and 19, which show a duodenal adenoma with e-Figures 3.16 and 3.17. When in doubt, repeat biopsy can be requested following treatment. The pathologist should not hesitate to ask for additional samples as the clinical consequences of such diagnoses can be profound. Peptic duodenitis appears similar to gastric heterotopia, which occurs as a nodule in an uninjured small bowel and often consists of oxyntic mucosa (Fig. 3.13, e-Figs. 3.20–3.24). It must be noted, though, that in many cases it is impossible to suggest whether the endoscopically noted nodule consists of a heterotopic or metaplastic process; fortunately, both are benign. The important point is that gastric-type tissue in the duodenal bulb is not a finding that should necessarily cause the pathologist to consider a diagnosis of Crohn disease. In contrast, pyloric metaplasia in the terminal ileum is commonly seen in the setting of Crohn disease. Of course, the atypical stromal cells that can be found in ulcer beds in any GI tract site are also found in the small bowel (9) (Fig. 3.14, e-Fig. 3.25).

Enteric mucosal calcinosis is a rare finding and, like its gastric counterpart, is seen in the setting of renal failure, usually in association with gastric mucosal calcinosis (Fig. 3.15, e-Figs. 3.26–3.29).

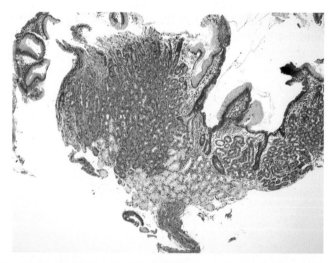

FIGURE 3.13 **Gastric heterotopia.** This lesion is clearly in the duodenum because of the presence of Brunner glands. Otherwise, it appears identical to gastric oxyntic mucosa. Note that this lesion produced a nodule.

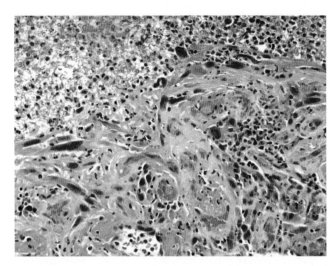

FIGURE 3.14 Atypical stromal cells. As in other parts of the GI tract, atypical stromal cells associated with ulcer beds are seen in the small bowel. Note striking nuclear atypia associated with a low nuclear-to-cytoplasmic ratio.

INFECTIOUS ENTERITIS

A host of etiologic agents may affect small bowel mucosa and they should be identified. It is impossible to be exhaustive, but some merit comment.

Mycobacterium avium Complex

In immunocompetent hosts, atypical mycobacteria show little virulence. However, MAI is a significant cause of opportunistic infection in

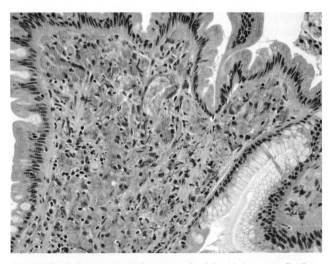

FIGURE 3.15 Mucosal calcinosis. Enteric mucosal calcinosis is a rare finding and, like its gastric counterpart, is seen in the setting of renal failure, usually in association with gastric mucosal calcinosis. Note the classic location underneath the surface epithelium.

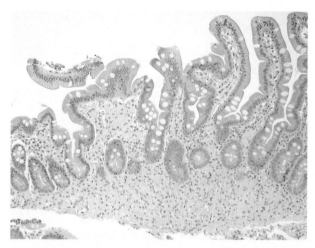

FIGURE 3.16 *Mycobacterium avium complex.* This image illustrates infiltration of small intestinal villi by histiocytes loaded with acid-fast bacilli. Note the absence of granulomas. This may impart a granular mucosal appearance on endoscopic exam.

immunocompromised patients, especially patients with acquired immuno-deficiency syndrome (AIDS). Patients with CD4 cell counts of <100 per μL are at risk for developing MAI. Symptoms include abdominal pain, fever, weight loss, chronic malabsorption, diarrhea, and so on. Disseminated GI tract infection with MAI is common in AIDS patients. Clarithromycin and azithromycin are the preferred agents for MAI prophylaxis.

MAI usually affects both the small and large bowels. Endoscopically, the small bowel mucosa either appears normal or shows a coarse granularity without significant exudate (implying an attenuated local immunologic response). The granular mucosa corresponds to massive infiltration of small intestinal villi by histiocytes loaded with acid-fast bacilli (Figs. 3.16 and 3.17, e-Figs. 3.30–3.35).

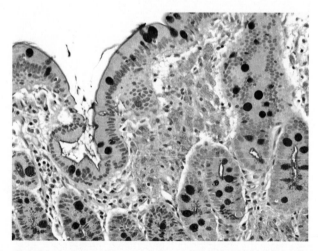

FIGURE 3.17 *Mycobacterium avium complex.* A PAS/AB stain highlights intracytoplasmic mycobacteria.

Unlike the response to *Mycobacterium tuberculosis*, well-defined granulomas are not usually elicited in MAI. Instead, loose clusters of foamy histiocytes appear with little other accompanying inflammation. Apart from the GI tract, MAI infection can affect a wide range of organs, including lungs, lymph nodes, spleen, liver, bone marrow, brain, etc.

Strongyloides Infection

Strongyloides stercoralis is a nematodal infection with a worldwide distribution affecting 30 to 100 million people. It is endemic to Africa, Southeast Asia, South America, and parts of the United States (e.g., Kentucky and Eastern Tennessee).

The life cycle of this worm is as follows: The female lays eggs without fertilization (parthenogenesis) in small intestinal crypts. The embryonated eggs hatch into rhabditiform larvae, which pass into the lumen and are expelled with feces. The rhabditiform larvae develop into filariform larvae (infective form), which penetrate human skin, then pass through blood vessels to the lungs and into the upper airways. When the patient coughs, the larvae are swallowed and ultimately reach the small intestine and mature into adult worms. The males are rapidly expelled after fertilizing the females. The female worms can remain in the intestine for decades— and are known in some cases to be present for up to 30 years. In immunosuppressed patients, autoinfection is a major threat as the rhabditiform larvae undergo a transformation, penetrate intestinal mucosa, and disseminate throughout the body. Autoinfection/hyperinfection carries a high mortality rate (up to 80%). Unlike hookworm, in which eggs are a means of identifying the parasite during stool exams, eggs are not present in the stool of those infected by *Strongyloides*. Diagnosis is based most frequently on identification of rhabditiform larvae in stool. Intestinal biopsies are used less often for diagnosis. Characteristic findings in the biopsy are the presence of all stages of the worm embedded in mucosal crypts (Figs. 3.18 and 3.19, e-Figs. 3.36–3.40). Thus, larvae, eggs, and, rarely, adult worms (recognized by one intestinal tract and a pair of reproductive tubes) can all be seen. Additional changes include villous flattening, crypt hyperplasia, and an inflammatory reaction consisting of lymphocytes, plasma cells, and eosinophils. Finding a prominent eosinophilic infiltrate and Charcot-Leyden crystals should prompt a search for a parasitic infestation. Treated worms invoke a brisk immunologic response (e-Fig. 3.40). The small intestine is the most commonly affected site, but in rare cases, the stomach and the colon can also be involved.

Patients can remain asymptomatic or present with nausea, vomiting, diarrhea, constipation, malabsorption, abdominal pain, and weight loss. Depending on worm burden and site of infestation, the presentations can be varied. Thiabendazole and ivermectin are used to treat strongyloidiasis.

We have also occasionally encountered *Trichuris trichuria* in the small bowel (e-Figs. 3.41–3.44).

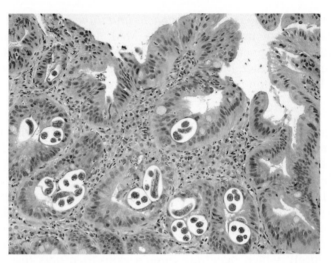

FIGURE 3.18 *Strongyloides stercoralis.* Organisms are seen here embedded in mucosal crypts.

Whipple Disease

WD is a rare systemic bacterial infection caused by *Tropheryma whippleii* (an actinomycete). There is a striking male predominance in the ratio of 8 to 10:1, with white males between the 4th and 5th decade to be most commonly affected. Patients present with diarrhea, low-grade fever, weight loss, malabsorption, abdominal pain, arthralgia, anemia, lymphadenopathy (50%), cardiac conditions, and central nervous system symptoms (10%). Most patients respond dramatically to antibiotics (trimethoprim and sulfamethoxazole). However, some patients can have a chronic relapsing

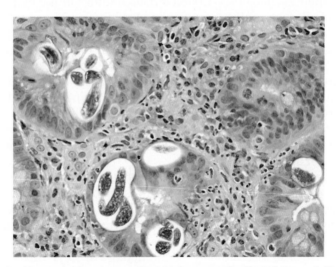

FIGURE 3.19 *Strongyloides stercoralis.* A higher magnification of Figure 3.18.

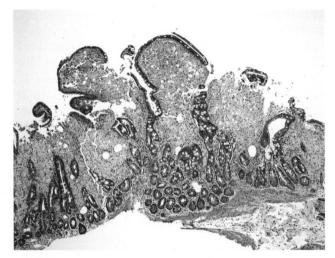

FIGURE 3.20 **Whipple disease.** Blunted and rounded villi are seen here in association with distention of lamina propria by foamy, pink macrophages. Lymphatic obstruction gives rise to dilated lacteals and lipid deposits, a helpful feature that suggests the diagnosis on H&E stain. This latter feature is seldom encountered in cases of *M. avium* complex.

course, with organisms persisting in affected tissues for a long time despite extended antibiotic treatment.

WD was first described by Dr. George Whipple at Johns Hopkins Hospital in 1907 as "intestinal lipodystrophy" due to the prominent accumulation of lipids in intestinal mucosa and lymph nodes (Figs. 3.20 and 3.21, e-Figs. 3.45–3.58). The bacterial etiology of this condition was confirmed by electron microscopy in 1961 (10) (e-Fig. 3.53).

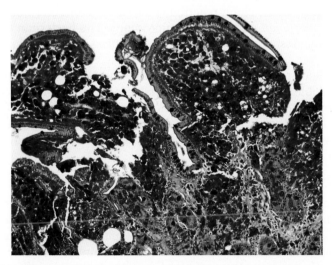

FIGURE 3.21 **Whipple disease.** Intensely PAS-positive foamy macrophages and dilated lacteals are seen here.

WD usually involves the postbulbar duodenum and jejunum. Thus, biopsies should be taken both from proximal and distal duodenum and also the jejunum. The characteristic appearance of a small intestinal biopsy consists of blunted and rounded villi, with distention of lamina propria by foamy, pink macrophages. The macrophages contain PAS-positive, diastase-resistant rod- or sickle-shaped bacterial inclusions. The bacterial inclusions can also be present in the extracellular space of lamina propria, as well as in epithelial cells, fibroblasts, endothelial cells, and smooth muscle. Lymphatic obstruction gives rise to dilated lacteals containing lipid deposits—a helpful feature that suggests the diagnosis of WD on hematoxylin and eosin (H&E) stain (Fig. 3.20, e-Figs. 3.45–3.48). Endoscopically, the lesions can present as yellowish-white plaques, as pale yellow shaggy mucosa, or have an erythematous friable appearance.

Characteristics of WD are the classic histologic features of intensely PAS-positive, foamy macrophages, and dilated lacteals with large lipid droplets (Fig. 3.21, e-Figs. 3.51 and 3.52).

Some diagnostic challenges to identifying WD include (a) the macrophages can be distributed in a patchy manner and may be present only in submucosa, which is usually minimally represented in biopsies; (b) partial treatment with antibiotics can cause a dramatic reduction in the number of macrophages (e-Figs. 3.59 and 3.60); and (c) the disease may only affect extraintestinal organs such as brain or heart, with no intestinal manifestation.

Apart from histology and special stains, the Whipple antigen can be detected by immunohistochemical analysis, using a polyclonal rabbit antibody produced against a cultured strain of *T. whippleii* (e-Figs. 3.49, 3.50, 3.56, 3.57) (3,11). The antigen is a component of the bacterial cell wall. This is both a sensitive and specific method of detecting WD. Other tests consist of polymerase chain reaction (PCR) assays for 16S ribosomal RNA genes of *T. whippleii* and electron microscopy. The bacterium of WD has also been successfully grown in human fibroblast cell line using shell-vial assays.

With electron microscopy, PAS stain, and Whipple immunostain, it is still possible to see retained bacterial products for months and even years after initiation of therapy, despite clinical improvement. Thus, PCR may be a better tool to monitor treatment response, as the bacterium has been shown to become undetectable shortly after initiation of antibiotic treatment.

Other Agents and Granulomatous Enteritis

Other infectious agents known to affect the small bowel are *Yersinia* sp., which produce necrotizing granulomas and adenovirus (e-Figs. 3.61 and 3.62), which results in marked lymphoid hyperplasia that can, in turn, lead to obstruction or intussusception (12). Yersiniosis is more likely to be detected on resection specimens than on biopsies because the necrotizing granulomas tend to be deep, whereas adenovirus is found affecting epithelial cells.

Various other unusual agents can be found in immunosuppressed individuals. An example of cryptococcal enteritis is depicted in e-Figures 3.63 and 3.64. Histoplasmosis is also rarely encountered (e-Figs. 3.65–3.67).

Histoplasmosis is the most prevalent endemic infection in the United States and a common opportunistic infection (13). Immunosuppressed individuals are at high risk for severe infection. Murine models have shown that cell-mediated immunity, including that mediated by tumor necrosis factor-α, is critical for host defense against *Histoplasma capsulatum* (14).

GI histoplasmosis is not exclusively a disease of the immunodeficient but can also mimic Crohn disease in immunocompetent individuals, a phenomenon to which Lamps et al. (15) called attention. They evaluated 56 specimens from 52 patients with H&E and silver stains. The presentation was with GI rather than pulmonary disease in 43% of their patients. Gross GI features included ulcers (49% of patients), nodules (21%), hemorrhage (13%), obstructive masses (6%), and normal mucosa (23%). Microscopic GI findings included diffuse lymphohistiocytic infiltration (83%), ulceration (45%), lymphohistiocytic nodules (25%), or minimal inflammatory reaction (15%) but only rare well-formed granulomas (8.5%). The most common hepatic finding was portal lymphohistiocytic inflammation; discrete hepatic granulomas were seen in <20% of involved livers. In their series, about half of patients were immunocompetent, underscoring the need to consider this possibility before making a new diagnosis of Crohn disease.

The differential diagnosis of granulomatous enterocolitis includes enterocolitis from the range of processes that result in granuloma formation elsewhere in the body, but some infections are relatively specific to the GI tract. These processes include primarily yersiniosis (either with *Yersinia enterocolitica* or *pseudotuberculosis*) and some examples of salmonellosis. The granulomatous process in yersiniosis is centered around Peyer patches and there may be histologic features of chronicity in specimens, although features of acute self-limiting enterocolitis may similarly accompany yersiniosis (16,17). *Yersinia* genetic material has been detected from specimens from patients with Crohn disease where it may better reflect an accomplice than a perpetrator (17). Of course, tuberculosis also sometimes affects the GI tract. Malakoplakia is also a possibility.

Several forms of immunodeficiency disease can also result in granulomatous enterocolitis. Chronic granulomatous disease, discussed further in Chapter 4, is an inherited disorder manifesting as immune deficiency caused by mutations in any of the genes, which encode the various subunits of the superoxide-generating phagocyte NADPH oxidase system responsible for the respiratory burst involved in organism killing. This disease affects around 1 in 250,000 children and is associated with significant morbidity and mortality, with the predicted life expectancy reduced to around 25 to 30 years of age, with recurrent severe bacterial and fungal infections with granuloma formation. Treatment usually involves the use of prophylactic and therapeutic antibiotics, and newer therapies have been developed such as interferon (IFN)-γ, bone marrow transplantation, and gene therapy. Chronic granulomatous disease can affect the GI tract in about a third of patients (18) and displays prominent macrophages and eosinophils. Granulomas, if present, are often poorly formed. Macrophages are often pigmented (19). Occasional cases of CVID also show granuloma formation, but of course, the hallmark is the absence of lamina propria plasma cells and apoptosis (20,21).

Once the remainder of other granulomatous lesions are considered and excluded, sarcoidosis can rarely be diagnosed in the lower GI tract (e-Figs. 3.68–3.70).

Cytomegalovirus (CMV) displays the same features in the small bowel as it does elsewhere in the body (e-Fig. 3.71).

Giardiasis is the most commonly encountered parasitic infection in the United States. Cysts of the organism are transmitted by the fecal-oral route either through person-to-person or animal to animal, or in contaminated food or water (sometimes animal to person) (22). Surface water becomes contaminated through the discharge of human sewage or drainage from animal feces. For example, large numbers of cattle and sheep excrete high loads of Giardia cysts, which can contaminate water sources. Such cysts can survive for months in surface water and soil. The organisms (cysts, especially) can be detected in stool by both ELISA and an immunofluorescence test. The flagellated protozoans can be detected in small bowel biopsies (Figs. 3.22 and 3.23, e-Figs. 3.72–3.77). However, biopsies from infected patients may lack organisms (e-Figs. 3.78–3.81) (presumably based on sampling error), whereas Giardia organisms as well as other types of organisms are plentiful in biopsies from immune deficient patients (e-Figs. 3.82–3.85) (21).

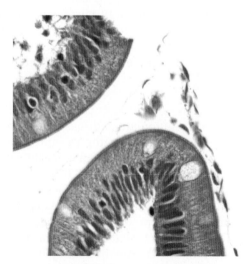

FIGURE 3.22 **Giardiasis, H&E stain.** Details of the organisms are apparent.

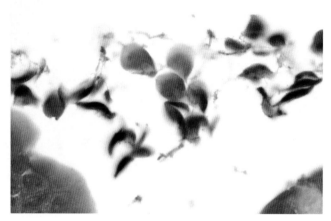

FIGURE 3.23   Giardiasis.

ISCHEMIC DISEASE

In contrast to ischemic colitis, ischemic enteritis usually results from mechanical alterations (leading to resections) rather than chronic vascular insufficiency. It is seldom seen on endoscopic biopsies. A possible scenario in which one might encounter an ischemic picture in the duodenum involves the utilization of selective internal radiation spheres (SIRSs). Used as a local ablative procedure in patients with inoperable primary or metastatic liver tumors, SIRSs consist of Yttrium-90–incorporated microspheres that are embolized into the arterial supply of the liver with the goal of selectively targeting tumors, which receive most of their blood supply from the hepatic artery. If there is a significant degree of shunting from the liver to the GI tract, the spheres may become lodged in the duodenal circulation resulting in ulceration and ischemic changes (Fig. 3.24, e-Figs. 3.86 and 3.87). The spheres appear as round, black structures found within submucosal vessels. Other adverse effects include radiation cholecystitis, pneumonitis, or hepatitis (23).

MEDICATION-ASSOCIATED INJURY AND OTHER IATROGENIC FORMS OF INJURY

Nonsteroidal Anti-inflammatory Drugs

Nonsteroidal anti-inflammatory drugs (NSAIDs) are well-known to be associated with mucosal damage in the small intestine. They may even lead to a peculiar form of strictures called "diaphragm disease," based on their macroscopic appearance (24–26). The typical injury consists of ulcers, which may lead to strictures (e-Fig. 3.88). Unfortunately, the histologic features of NSAID-associated ulcers are not specific, although they are usually not associated with abundant chronic inflammation.

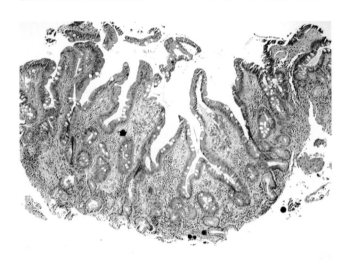

FIGURE 3.24 **Radiation enteritis associated with Yttrium-90 microspheres.** The microspheres are the black particles in the deeper portions of the biopsy. The damage in the tips of the villi is similar to the pattern seen in ischemic enteritis.

Graft Versus Host Disease

Patients with graft versus host disease (GVHD) present with secretory diarrhea, abdominal pain, and, at times, hemorrhage. There is also a syndrome of upper GI GVHD, presenting clinically as anorexia, dyspepsia, food intolerance, nausea, and vomiting. These syndromes were first recognized in the early 1990s (27–29), and endoscopic criteria for recognizing the lesions of GVHD are now available (30). Of course, patients who have had bone marrow transplants are prone to many infectious causes of enteritis, but many also have upper tract GVHD. The original grading criteria were published by Snover et al. (28) and are summarized as follows:

> Grade 1 = increased crypt apoptosis (Fig. 3.25)
> Grade 2 = apoptosis with crypt abscess (Fig. 3.26)
> Grade 3 = individual crypt necrosis (Fig. 3.27)
> Grade 4 = total denudation of areas of mucosa

These criteria are simple to apply and correlate well with clinical findings. Unfortunately, chronic GVHD results in nonspecific features of lamina propria fibrosis, mucosal atrophy, and crypt distortion without basal plasmacytosis. When confronted with such biopsies, we attempt to grade the active component and note the features of the chronic component. We also compare the biopsies to any prior ones.

Mycophenolate-associated Injury

Mycophenolic acid (MPA) and its mechanism of action have been discussed in some detail in Chapters 1 and 2, and the findings in the small intestine are akin to the findings in other sites. Papadimitriou et al. (31)

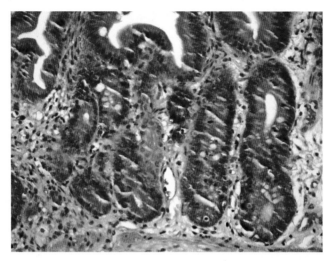

FIGURE 3.25 **Graft-versus-host-disease (GVHD), mild.** Apoptotic bodies are easily identified but the mucosa is essentially intact.

initially reported a GVHD-like response, namely striking apoptosis, to CellCept (mycophenolate mofetil) in colon biopsies and others have documented similar findings in the upper GI tract (including the duodenum) in patients taking the same medication (32,33). CellCept is widely used for maintenance immunosuppression in solid organ transplantation. GI toxicity, usually manifested as diarrhea, is its most common side effect. The key finding is crypt apoptosis, which it shares with GVHD. As a rule of thumb, it is abnormal to encounter more than 2 apoptotic bodies per 100 crypts, which roughly corresponds to one relatively generous mucosal

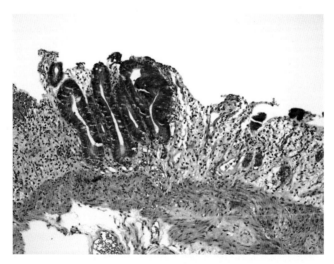

FIGURE 3.26 **Graft-versus-host-disease (GVHD).** Apoptosis is prominent and there is loss of glands. Note that the endocrine cells are more resilient to apoptotic injury.

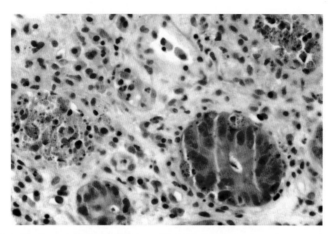

FIGURE 3.27 Graft-versus-host-disease (GVHD), severe. There is extensive apoptotic damage and crypt necrosis.

biopsy fragment. Put another way, if it is easy to find apoptotic bodies, there are too many. It is reasonable to count both "halo" cells (Fig. 3.28) and cells with popcorn-like nuclei (Fig. 3.29); there is no need to stain with cleaved caspase 3 immunostaining (which marks apoptotic bodies), but such immunolabeling correlates with a looser definition of apoptosis that includes "halo" cells (34).

If a patient is taking mycophenolate and has also had a bone marrow transplant, it is essentially impossible to sort out the cause of prominent apoptosis. Mycophenolate drug levels can be tested, but the correlation between blood levels and clinical toxicity is imperfect (32). Similarly, infections

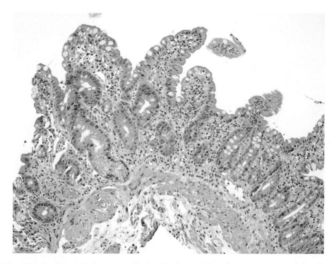

FIGURE 3.28 Mycophenolate-associated injury. The features are virtually identical to those of GVHD. Separating them required knowledge of the clinical history. In this biopsy, crypt apoptosis is the key feature.

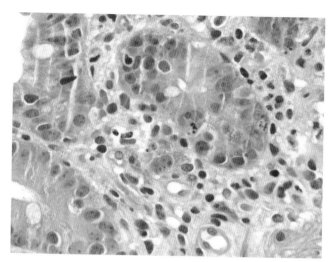

FIGURE 3.29 Mycophenolate-associated injury, high magnification. Crypt apoptosis is striking.

(especially with CMV) can result in prominent crypt apoptosis, so biopsies must be carefully assessed. At our institutions, we have a low threshold for ordering CMV immunostains in transplant patients whose biopsies display erosions/ulcerations as well as prominent apoptosis. A partial listing of conditions associated with prominent apoptosis appears in Table 3.1.

Ipilimumab-associated Injury

Monoclonal antibodies (mAbs) against the cytotoxic T lymphocyte antigen-4 (CTLA-4) molecule are used as an adjuvant to experimental tumor immunization protocols in the treatment of a growing number of malignant neoplasms (e.g., melanomas, ovarian carcinomas, and pancreatic carcinoma). Among adverse effects associated with these medications, severe gastroenteritis has been reported. Oble et al. (35) have reported their observations of five patients who developed severe GI toxicity affecting the gastric, small intestinal, and colonic mucosa. The endoscopic findings

TABLE 3.1 Small Intestinal Crypt Apoptosis
Conditions Associated with Prominent Small Intestinal Crypt Apoptosis
GVHD
Mycophenolate (CellCept, Myofortic)
CMV enteritis
Common variable immunodeficiency
Autoimmune enteropathy
Other viruses and medications

were variable, ranging from normal to diffusely erythematous and ulcerated mucosa. The constant histologic findings included a lymphoplasmacytic expansion of the lamina propria with increase in IELs and prominent apoptosis. Samples displayed cryptitis and glandular inflammation in the colon, ileum, and stomach, whereas villous blunting was present in the ileal and duodenal mucosa (e-Figs. 3.89 and 3.90). Immunohistochemical analysis revealed a marked increase of all T-cell subsets (CD3$^+$, CD4$^+$, and CD8$^+$) and of CD4$^+$CD25$^+$ regulatory T cells. The authors pointed out that the findings resembled those seen in autoimmune enteropathy (discussed below).

Colchicine Toxicity

Colchicine is an alkaloid with an antimitotic ability used to treat a variety of medical conditions. Colchicine toxicity can result in multiorgan failure and death, so it is worthwhile to learn to spot these changes in routine biopsies. Iacobuzio-Donahue et al. (36) reported findings in 21 GI mucosal biopsies from nine patients receiving oral colchicine therapy. All patients had a history of gout. Four patients with chronic renal failure also had clinical evidence of colchicine toxicity, and the other five patients did not. Distinct morphologic changes—seen as metaphase mitoses, epithelial pseudostratification, and loss of polarity—were seen in biopsy material from four of four (100%) patients with clinical colchicine toxicity (Figs. 3.30 and 3.31, e-Figs. 3.91–3.98). Three of these four cases (75%) also contained abundant crypt apoptotic bodies. These morphologic features were best seen in the biopsies from duodenum and gastric antrum, with relative sparing of the gastric body in the upper GI tract. Ki67 staining demonstrated an expansion of the proliferating region in three available cases with clinical colchicine toxicity (e-Fig. 3.93). Probably the most important finding in

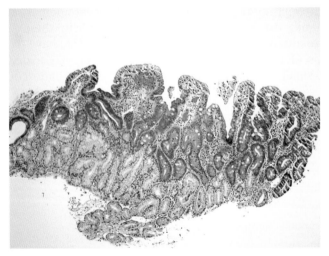

FIGURE 3.30 **Colchicine toxicity.** Note the expanded proliferative compartment. Mitotic arrest can be seen at this power.

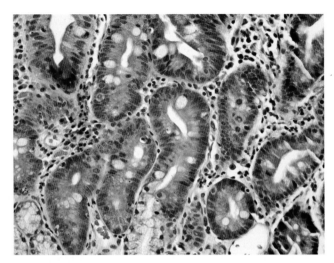

FIGURE 3.31 **Colchicine toxicity.** Ring mitoses are seen here within the proliferative compartment.

this study was that the distinctive morphologic features were absent in the five patients without clinical colchicine toxicity.

MALABSORPTION

Patients who do not properly absorb intestinal contents can have bloating, cramping, "gas", bulky stools, chronic diarrhea, steatorrhea, failure to thrive, muscle wasting, and weight loss. Treatment includes replacing nutrients and vitamins but should be directed at an underlying cause.

Other entities discussed in this chapter can present with malabsorption, but the classic considerations for patients with malabsorption include celiac disease, refractory and collagenous sprue/enteritis, tropical sprue, and small bowel bacterial overgrowth (SBBO). Patients with cystic fibrosis (Fig. 3.1, e-Fig. 3.1) have malabsorption as do patients with cholestasis and patients who have undergone bariatric surgery. Patients with lactose intolerance malabsorb but there are no findings on mucosal biopsies.

Celiac Disease

Celiac disease is a relatively common (far more common than previously realized) systemic autoimmune disorder induced by gluten proteins found in wheat, barley, and rye. Injury to the small intestine is the hallmark of disease, but manifestations are systemic. Sites of extraintestinal injury include, but are not limited to, the skin (classically with dermatitis herpetiformis), joints, and uterus, such that clinical presentations can be subtle and not GI-tract related. Certain human leukocyte antigens (HLAs) confer the highest risk, i.e., HLA-DQ2 and HLA-DQ8 (37), and certain subsets of patients similarly are at high risk, e.g., family members of those with celiac disease, type I diabetics, children with Down syndrome (38), and individuals with iron deficiency anemia. Prevalence of celiac disease has been reported as high as 1.5% in Finnish school children (39) and only slightly less in the general population of the United States (40), such that some observers suggest that there might be some utility in screening large numbers of individuals for this condition (41). The incidence of celiac disease appears nil to low in Southeast Asians, while there are endemic populations in the Sahara/Middle East with a high incidence of celiac disease (42,43). Undiagnosed celiac disease is responsible for growth retardation in some children (44) and has been associated with fetal wastage, infertility, and osteoporosis. A National Institutes of Health (NIH) conference was held on this topic and a statement is available at *http://consensus.nih.gov.*

When assessing biopsies, it is worthwhile to remember that antigliadin tests are no longer recommended because they produce too many false positives. For example, patients with Crohn disease may have both false-positive antigliadin tests and prominent IELs, a combination likely to result in misdiagnosis. Presently, antitissue transglutaminase and antiendomysial tests are recommended. These are IgA-based tests, in general, so they yield false-negative results in IgA-deficient patients. IgG-based tests exist for this situation.

Certain duodenal endoscopic findings may provide a clue to the diagnosis, namely scalloped folds with or without mosaic pattern mucosa, reduction in number of folds, or nodular mucosa (45). It is best to evaluate biopsies from beyond the bulb (first portion), since these are less prone to injury from gastric contents. Several biopsies should be obtained because characteristic features may be patchy (46,47). Review is easiest in well-oriented samples.

There is a range of appearances in biopsies obtained from patients with celiac disease. The constellation of findings has been classified by Marsh (48) and further modified by Rostami et al. (49); their grading schemes appear in Table 3.2. What is important about these classifications is that they provide a framework for recognizing celiac disease lesions that fall short of mucosal atrophy. In the past, these observers published their findings in the gastroenterology literature, rather than pathology literature, so many pathologists remained unaware of subtle findings that suggest celiac disease (50,51), although such findings are by no means specific (52,53). Essentially, subtle lesions display only intraepithelial lymphocytosis (Fig. 3.32, e-Fig. 3.99), either similar in density or more prominent in the tips of the villi than in the bases (where IELs are physiologic). In the normal small bowel biopsy, the number of IELs decreases in the tips of the villi when compared to the bases. The finding of prominent "tip heavy" intraepithelial lymphocytosis may be subtle and not wholly diagnostic, but its presence can prompt the pathologist to suggest celiac disease serology as patients with mild enteropathy and positive serology benefit from early dietary treatment (54). As a quick method to assess

TABLE 3.2 **Schemes for Assessment of Biopsies in Patients with Celiac Disease**

Lesion Type	Rostami Modification	Marsh Classification
Marsh 0	Same as original	Preinfiltrative: normal mucosal and villous architecture
Marsh I	Same as original	Infiltrative: normal mucosal and villous architecture Prominent intraepithelial lymphocytes
Marsh II	Same as original	Hyperplastic: same as "infiltrative" but also with enlarged crypts and increased crypt Mitoses
Marsh III	A. Partial villous atrophy B. Subtotal villous atrophy C. Total villous atrophy	Destructive lesion: flat mucosa–complete loss of villi lymphocyte infiltration Enlarged hyperplastic crypts
Marsh IV	Same as original	Hypoplastic: total villous atrophy normal intraepithelial lymphocyte count believed to reflect severe malnutrition and be nonspecific

From Rostami K, Kerckhaert JP, Tiemessen R, et al. The relationship between antiendomysium antibodies and villous atrophy in coeliac disease using both monkey and human substrate. *Eur J Gastroenterol Hepatol.* 1999;11(4):439–442; Marsh MN. Gluten, major histocompatibility complex, and the small intestine. A molecular and immunobiologic approach to the spectrum of gluten sensitivity ("celiac sprue"). *Gastroenterology.* 1992;102(1):330–354.

whether there are too many lymphocytes in the tips of the villi, count 20 enterocyte nuclei in the very tip of a villus (10 on one side to the tip and 10 on the other) and (on H&E) count the lymphocytes in this area. If there are six or more, this is too many. It is not necessary to immunolabel T cells to assess these biopsies, although some colleagues routinely order CD3 stains on small intestinal biopsies based on reports of their utility in patients with intraepithelial lymphocytosis (51). If this practice is introduced, remember that initially CD3 labeling will highlight more IELs than are typically apparent on H&E such that one might consider celiac disease in every case. In addition, most treated patients who are clinically improved still retain intraepithelial lymphocytosis, despite regrowth of damaged villi (which can take years following the implementation of a gluten-free diet) (55). As the injury of celiac disease progresses, the lamina propria becomes expanded with numerous lymphocytes and plasma cells, the villi become progressively attenuated with epithelial damage,

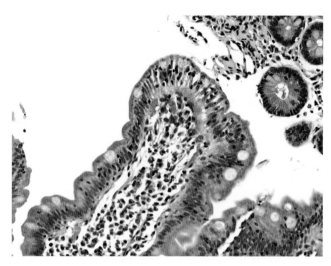

FIGURE 3.32 "Latent" celiac disease. Intraepithelial lymphocytes (IELs) are prominent in the tips of the villi. This finding is not specific but is worth noting in biopsy reports and suggesting correlation with pertinent serology.

and the crypts become hyperplastic (Fig. 3.33, e-Figs. 3.100–3.102). The cells accounting for the infiltrate are T cells (e-Fig. 3.102), and there is extensive literature devoted to the phenotype of these cells, most of which is valuable for research purposes only.

Of course, celiac disease is not unique in causing villous atrophy (Table 3.3). Diseases that may produce villous atrophy include dermatitis

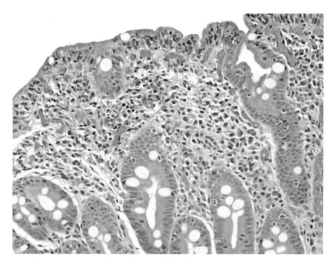

FIGURE 3.33 Celiac disease. This illustration shows a lamina propria expanded with numerous lymphocytes and plasma cells, attenuated villi, and increased IELs.

TABLE 3.3	Associations with Villous Atrophy

Celiac disease

Dermatitis herpetiformis

Refractory sprue

Collagenous sprue

Cow's milk intolerance

Giardiasis

"Peptic duodenitis"

Crohn disease

Small bowel bacterial overgrowth

Eosinophilic enteritis

Radiation enteropathy

Tropical sprue

Amyloidosis

Lymphoma

Graft versus host disease

Autoimmune enteropathy

Common variable immunodeficiency

Whipple disease

Abetalipoproteinemia

Malnutrition

Ischemia

herpetiformis, a condition related to and a variant of celiac disease; cow's milk protein intolerance (pediatric); giardiasis; peptic duodenitis; Crohn disease; SBBO (stasis and overgrowth, usually of anaerobes); eosinophilic gastroenteritis (Fig. 3.34, e-Fig. 3.103), radiation enteritis; tropical sprue; lymphoma; GVHD (Figs. 3.25–3.27); autoimmune enteropathy; hypogammaglobulinemia/CVID syndrome; and α chain disease. Villous atrophy, usually in association with a thin mucosa, can also be seen in the setting of severe malnutrition as a result of malignant or nonmalignant conditions (Figs. 3.35 and 3.36 e-Figs. 3.104–3.106). A rule of thumb in considering atrophic enteritis is that neutrophils and histiocytes are not a typical inflammatory constituent in celiac disease; their presence should prompt other considerations, particularly bacterial overgrowth (stasis changes), Crohn disease, and autoimmune enteropathy. In reality, there are biopsies for which it is difficult to offer a precise etiology and, in that situation, a descriptive report and dialogue with the endoscopist is indicated.

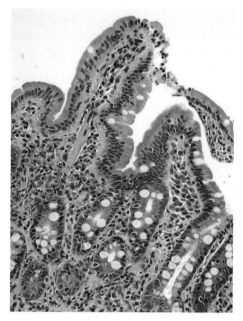

FIGURE 3.34 **Eosinophilic gastroenteritis.** No parasites were found in this patient and this lesion was presumed to be allergic.

Refractory Sprue and Collagenous Sprue

Sadly, there remains a subset of patients that defies current medical management and has a presentation resembling celiac disease. These patients often have negative celiac disease serology. They sometimes respond briefly

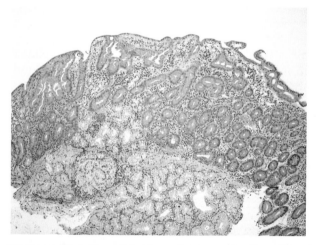

FIGURE 3.35 **Severe malnutrition.** This biopsy from a cachectic patient shows severe atrophy but not intraepithelial lymphocytosis. Presumably the patient has insufficient caloric reserve to manufacture enterocytes.

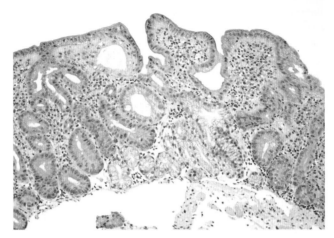

FIGURE 3.36 **Severe malnutrition.** On higher magnification, there is acute inflammation, which suggests a superimposed infection although no organisms are seen in this field.

to a gluten-free diet but then become refractory or they simply never have symptomatic relief from a gluten-free diet. This condition is sometimes descriptively termed "refractory sprue" or "refractory celiac disease" (56) (e-Figs. 3.107–3.109). These patients, like those with classic celiac disease, seem to share the HLA-DQ2 or HLA-DQ8 phenotype (56). Robert et al. (57) reported 10 cases of refractory sprue and found that 5 of 10 refractory patients ultimately developed collagenous sprue as a distinct histologic marker of refractory disease. Additional distinctive findings found in small bowel biopsies in the refractory group were subcryptal chronic inflammation (10 of 10 patients) and marked mucosal thinning in 3 patients. Other nonspecific findings included acute inflammation and gastric metaplasia. One patient with collagenous sprue developed a B-cell lymphoma of the ileum. In general, collagenous sprue was associated with a poor prognosis: 2 of 5 patients died and 2 others required total parenteral nutrition for survival. However, more recently, others have reported relatively good outcomes after gluten-free diet and/or immunomodulatory therapy (58). In our experience, such cases may be clonal by gene rearrangement studies raising the possibility that they may be related to T-cell lymphomas (e-Figs. 3.110–3.112). Two studies by Vakiani et al. (58) and Maguire et al. substantiate our observations of clonality but cast doubt on whether the findings precede the development of lymphoma. The former author documents minor T-cell clones in a polyclonal background in 2 patients (not detected in follow up biopsies) and a dominant T-cell clone in 1 patient out of 15 studied. However, none of the patients in their study developed lymphoma. Similarly, Maguire et al. report clonal T-cell populations in 5 of 6 patients tested. In three of these, clonality was found in sites other than the small bowel, namely colon and peripheral blood. Although one of these patients died from complications of malnutrition, the other four for who follow-up was available improved clinically after treatment (59). Thus, these observations suggest that these clonal T-cell populations may represent short-lived T-cell proliferations. However, these cases are heterogeneous and rare and, as a result, gathering significant numbers of patients to study is a challenging task. Certainly, T-cell lymphoma arising in this setting has been reported and patients with documented T-cell rearrangements benefit from close follow-up (55,60–62). Some patients with collagenous sprue respond to steroids; others are managed with antineoplastic regimens. A diagnostic possibility to ponder when examining biopsies from patients with "refractory sprue" is autoimmune enteropathy, which is further discussed in the following sections.

Refractory sprue can be divided into types (56). In type 1, the IELs mirror the type normally encountered in the small bowel epithelium, whereas those in type 2 have an abnormal (clonal) IEL immunophenotype.

Type 1 refractory sprue: CD3+, CD8+, no clonality on analysis of T-cell receptor gene rearrangements.

Type 2 refractory sprue: CD3+, loss of CD8, clonality on analysis of T-cell receptor gene rearrangements.

Vega et al. (63) have also described a patient with "atypical NK-cell proliferation of the GI tract in a patient with antigliadin antibodies but not celiac disease". T cells in this patient's GI tract expressed CD56, CD7, cytoplasmic CD3 (but not membranous CD3), and TIA-1 but not CD4, CD8, CD10, CD20, CD5, or EBV markers. We suspect this is simply a variant or refractory celiac disease, but the authors' term "NK-cell disease" or a variant may be introduced in the coming years.

IgA Deficiency

The incidence of IgA deficiency ranges from 1:400 to 1:3,000 in healthy blood donors. Most IgA-deficient individuals are healthy, but this condition is associated with protean manifestations (50). A compensatory increase in IgM has been observed in some affected individuals (64). Patients may be asymptomatic or might suffer from recurrent respiratory or GI infections, allergies, or autoimmune disorders (64). For the purposes of GI biopsy interpretation, disorders associated with IgA deficiency include giardiasis, nodular lymphoid hyperplasia, celiac disease (in about 2% of cases), milk intolerance, and inflammatory bowel disease. When reviewing biopsies from IgA-deficient individuals (having serum levels <7 mg per dL with normal IgM and IgG levels), IgA-producing cells may be identified on immunohistochemistry but are usually reduced in number. It may be that, at least in some cases, the secretory component, which mediates endocytosis of IgA into the basolateral aspect of enterocytes, is defective so that IgA-reactive cells are seen, but transport into intestinal secretions is impaired. Since the number of IgA-labeled plasma cells is variable in any population of healthy individuals, the disease can only be suggested by the pathologist when the associated disorders are detected (e-Figs. 3.113–3.118).

Abetalipoproteinemia

This rare, autosomal recessive disorder is characterized by absent apolipoprotein B (apoB), an essential component of chylomicrons, responsible for the transport of dietary fat from the small bowel into the bloodstream. The defect is attributed to defective lipid transfer from the membrane of the endoplasmic reticulum to apoB due to mutations in the gene encoding a microsomal triglyceride transfer protein (MTP) (65,66). As a result, apoB-containing lipoproteins, namely chylomicrons, low density, and very low density lipoproteins, are absent from affected patients' bloodstream. Lipid profile reveals low total cholesterol and triglyceride levels. Patients with this condition usually present during infancy with failure to thrive, diarrhea, and steatorrhea. Malabsorption of fat-soluble vitamins, specifically vitamins E and A, leads to neuromuscular impairment and retinitis pigmentosa later in life (67,68). Lipid membrane defects are evidenced by the presence of acanthotic red blood cells (burr cells) in peripheral smears. Duodenal biopsies show normal villous morphology with lipid-laden, vacuolated or "clear" enterocytes (Fig. 3.37). Similar but less striking findings can be seen in patients who have ingested a fat-containing meal close to the time of endoscopy. Treatment consists of a low-fat diet and administration of fat-soluble vitamins.

Tropical Sprue and Small Bowel Bacterial Overgrowth

Aside from infectious intestinal diseases with known etiology, there is a group of GI disorders mainly affecting the small intestine of individuals predominantly living in and, less often, visiting or returning from the developing world, usually the tropics. These GI disorders range from asymptomatic structural and/or functional abnormalities of the GI mucosa

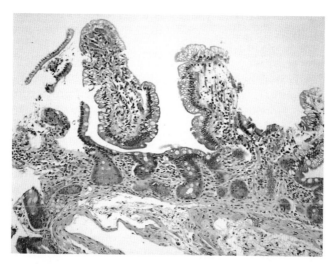

FIGURE 3.37 **Abetalipoproteinemia.** There is abundant lipid retained within enterocytes.

(subclinical enteropathy) to a fully symptomatic condition highlighted by malabsorption of nutrients and associated nutritional deficiencies. These same disorders respond well to folate and broad-spectrum antibiotic treatment (tropical sprue). An infectious etiology is strongly suspected because of (a) the occurrence of tropical sprue in epidemics, particularly in rural areas with poor sanitation; (b) the susceptibility of visitors from developed countries to endemic regions; and (c) the favorable response of these disorders to treatment with antibiotics. In addition, tropical sprue cases have also been associated with bacterial contamination of the small bowel. These patients experience prolonged transit time for digestion through the small intestine, akin to that observed in obstruction (69) and bacterial overgrowth. The appearance of biopsies from these patients is very much like those in patients in Western countries having SBBO. The findings appear similar to the villous attenuation in celiac disease, but with the addition of active inflammation and, at times, features of chronicity, such as gastric mucin cell metaplasia and crypt distortion. These latter conditions also have features that overlap with upper tract Crohn disease. SBBO is relatively common and occurs when small bowel motility is altered and patients present with diarrhea (70–72). This alteration may be the result of underlying medical conditions, such as diabetes, gastroparesis (as a result of diabetes, postsurgical or idiopathic), or scleroderma (which results in sclerosis of the bowel wall), or from surgery (73). An association has been recently reported with use of acid-lowering medications (74). In addition, many patients with so-called irritable bowel syndrome are believed to have this condition. Small bowel aspirate and quantitative cultures have been regarded as the gold standard for diagnosis with more than 10^5 CFU/mL considered the cutoff for SBBO diagnosis. However, the validity of this number is difficult to assess. A systematic review of diagnostic tests for this entity found plenty of diversity regarding definition of SBBO based on culture results with many investigators using values above or below this threshold. Of note, the same review noted that in healthy subjects counts were in the range of 0 to 10^3 CFU/mL (75). Specific antibiotic therapy is determined by sensitivity testing of the cultured agents, which are generally anaerobes (76). A hydrogen breath test has also been used in diagnosing this condition (77), which exploits the hydrogen production from the excess bacteria. However, as with culture, there are multiple definitions in the literature as to what constitutes a positive breath test. Some clinicians rely on response to antibiotics as a means of diagnosing SBBO (75). Sadly, the morphologic features in SBBO range from normal to those like Crohn disease and usually include a component of neutrophilic inflammation (Figs. 3.38 and 3.39, e-Figs. 3.119–3.126). Recent work by Lappinga et al. reiterates the nonspecific histologic features. In their study, the only statistically significant difference between patients with SBBO and controls was a villous:crypt ratio of <3:1 in 24% of the cases of SBBO versus 7% in controls. More than half of the biopsies from patients with SBBO were normal (74). The pathologist reviewing biopsies may be able to raise

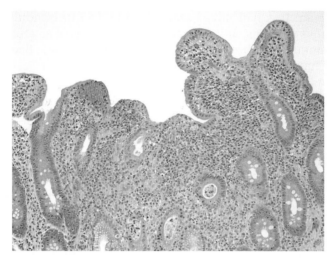

FIGURE 3.38 **Small bowel bacterial overgrowth, biopsy of blind loop.** There is active chronic duodenitis, distortion of the glandular architecture, and villous atrophy. The differential diagnosis is with Crohn disease and tropical sprue.

this possibility and suggest confirmation, but it is difficult to diagnose in isolation of clinical findings.

CROHN DISEASE

Crohn disease is also referred to as regional enteritis, granulomatous enterocolitis, and terminal ileitis. It is a chronic, relapsing, and remitting inflammatory disease of unknown etiology that is often multifocal and can affect any portion of the GI tract. However, the classic disease site is the

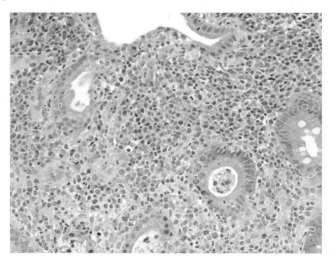

FIGURE 3.39 **Small bowel bacterial overgrowth.** This is a higher magnification image of Figure 3.38.

terminal ileum. It is typically characterized by foci of glandular destruction, aphthous erosions, and serpiginous ulcers, as well as areas of transmural inflammation, fibrosis, and sometimes granulomas. Because of its transmural nature, fissures, sinuses, and fistulas may occur.

Crohn disease affects both sexes about equally and occurs at all ages, with the major peak incidence between 20 and 30 years of age. The initial presentation may be indolent or acute. Symptoms often include cramping pain (typically localized to the right lower quadrant), nonbloody diarrhea, fever, malaise, and anorexia. These findings may mimic acute appendicitis. Hemorrhage and hematochezia are uncommon, but chronic blood loss does occur as a result of erosions and ulcers. Patients with upper GI tract disease may present with dyspepsia, weight loss, hypoalbuminemia, and iron deficiency anemia, which together mimic celiac disease. Fistulas between organs (enterovaginal, enterovesical, and enterocutaneous) may result in the passage of blood, feces, pus, and air from the vagina, urethra, or skin. In some cases, fissuring necrosis with fistula formation is the main complication; in others, stenosis due to fibrosis predominates. Anal and perianal fissures and fistulas are features of many Crohn cases, but rarely of ulcerative colitis. Inflammatory changes can occur in joints, eyes, liver, and skin. There is a familial association: It is estimated that approximately 10% of patients with Crohn disease have another affected family member. Affected patients have a low but documented risk of developing small bowel adenocarcinoma (78), often diagnosed in a postsurgical specimen obtained as a result of obstruction (79,80).

The gross endoscopic appearance of Crohn disease is most consistently characterized as a multifocal process. Aphthous erosions (an "aphtha" is a spot-like small ulcer on a mucous membrane), longitudinal ulcers (train track, tram track, or rake ulcers), and adjacent areas of erythematous or grossly unremarkable mucosa are hallmarks. Additional endoscopic findings include cobblestoning (irregular mucosa due to alternating ulcers and edematous mucosa), strictures, and fissures. The ileum typically shows focal or asymmetric involvement by Crohn disease. This may include erosions, ulcers, and/or strictures. Often, the rectum is not involved (unlike ulcerative colitis). Inflammatory polyps may be present (e-Fig. 3.127–3.129). Rarely, Crohn disease may become confluent, involving the entire bowel, which can be diagnostically difficult for the endoscopist. In both Crohn disease and ulcerative colitis, the normal submucosal vascular network is lost in the involved areas, a feature which assists the endoscopist in the diagnosis of chronic colitis. There is little correlation between the endoscopic appearance and the clinical symptoms of the patient.

Mucosal biopsies, although superficial, can show features that are suggestive of Crohn disease. Discrete foci of inflammation, often associated with neutrophils within crypts (cryptitis) and adjacent to histologically normal crypts, are common (e-Figs. 3.130 and 3.131). Aphthous erosions or ulcers that are characterized by focal surface epithelial necrosis associated with a mixed chronic inflammatory infiltrate–and sometimes

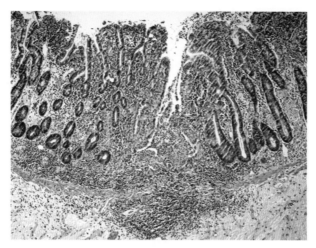

FIGURE 3.40 **Aphthous ulcer, Crohn disease.** This ileal biopsy shows a flat ulcer overlying a lymphoid aggregate.

associated with underlying lymphoid aggregates–are typical early lesions (Fig. 3.40, e-Fig. 3.132). Also typical is variability of inflammation within a single biopsy and among several biopsy fragments from the same anatomic location. The areas of inflammation show architectural changes of chronic crypt-destructive enteritis, while adjacent crypts may appear totally normal. Granulomas are infrequently seen but, when present, are poorly formed and associated with chronic inflammation.

Terminal ileal involvement includes increased lamina propria inflammation, aphthous erosions, and flattened and broad villi. Pyloric metaplasia (mucinous glands, reminiscent of the antral or pyloric mucosa) indicates repeated bouts of inflammation and repair (Figs. 3.41–3.43, e-Figs.

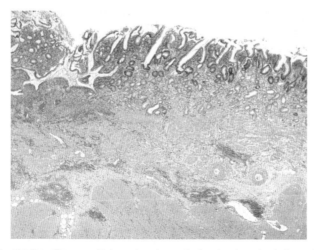

FIGURE 3.41 **Crohn disease.** Note extensive pyloric gland metaplasia and submucosal and muscularis propria lymphoid aggregates.

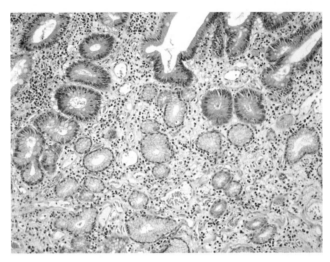

FIGURE 3.42 **Crohn disease.** A higher magnification of Figure 3.41 highlighting pyloric gland metaplasia.

3.133–3.134), and even though this finding is frequently associated with injury as a result of Crohn disease, this type of metaplasia can be encountered in other chronic inflammatory settings (81). One must remember that focal acute ileitis is most commonly caused by medications, particularly NSAID, rather than Crohn disease, and finding the features of chronicity is critical. Medication-induced injury is usually not associated with increased lamina propria inflammation or pyloric metaplasia. Submucosal fibrosis can also be a sequel to NSAID damage. Peyer patches are a normal

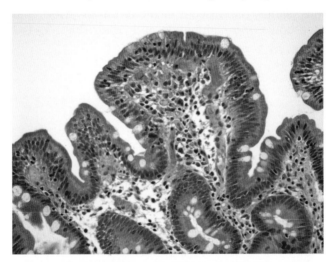

FIGURE 3.43 **Common variable immunodeficiency.** At first glance, the appearances are those of celiac disease, but on closer inspection, there are no plasma cells in the lamina propria. Compare this to Figure 3.36, taken at the same magnification (it appears to be at higher magnification based on severe atrophy) and in which it is easy to recognize plasma cells.

component of the terminal ileum, particularly in young individuals, and should not be diagnosed as chronic inflammation. The mucosa over Peyer patches may be distorted, displaying IELs and flattened villi due to underlying expansion of lymphoid nodules in nonspecific, reactive hyperplasia. Yersiniosis can also result in prominent Peyer patches (e-Fig. 3.135).

Unfortunately, Crohn disease has overlapping features with other inflammatory processes. The endoscopic finding of focal aphthous erosions of early Crohn colitis may be similar to erosions caused by medications and infections. Histologically, the erosions of Crohn disease are associated with a chronic inflammatory infiltrate. Infectious colitis is characterized by a predominance of neutrophils, rather than lymphocytes and plasma cells. Medication-induced erosions (from NSAIDs and other drugs) usually have negligible acute inflammation and only a few neutrophils in the area of erosion. Bowel wall thickening and heaped up masses may be seen in *Yersinia* infection, particularly in the terminal ileum and right colon. The presence of marked inflammation histologically, with numerous granulomas and the clinical information of a mass or stricture, may lead to a diagnosis of Crohn disease in a patient with yersiniosis. Features that suggest *Yersinia* infection over Crohn disease include numerous, well-formed granulomas; granulomas centered in lymphoid follicles; and granulomas with central polymorph-rich suppuration. Histoplasmosis can also mimic Crohn disease both clinically and histologically (e-Figs. 136–138) (82). Any specimen with numerous granulomas should raise suspicion of infection over Crohn disease.

Additionally, some patients with Crohn disease who are given immunomodulatory drugs (such as antitumor necrosis factor-α medications) can become infected with various organisms (acid-fast organisms and histoplasmosis) (e-Figs. 3.136–3.138). Remicade (infliximab) is a monoclonal (IgG) antibody targeting soluble and cellular tumor necrosis factor-α. It has been used to treat a host of inflammatory disorders including psoriasis, rheumatoid arthritis, and Crohn disease. Since it results in immune modulation, reported associated opportunistic infections have included aspergillosis, tuberculosis, and histoplasmosis. In a large Mayo Clinic study of 500 patients treated with Remicade, 8.2% (48 patients) had associated infections. Twenty patients had life-threatening infections, including one with histoplasmosis (83). Other authors have reported about a dozen cases. In general, these patients had severe infections, were undergoing simultaneous treatment with other immune modulators in addition to Remicade, and lived in endemic areas.

BEHÇET DISEASE

Behçet disease is a systemic disorder consisting of oral ulceration, plus any two of the following: Genital ulceration, typical defined eye lesions, typical defined skin lesions, or a positive pathergy test (an exaggerated response to a minor injury of skin) (84–86). The GI tract may be affected anywhere, and deeply penetrating ulcers that lack specific histologic features are found (Fig. 3.43, e-Figs. 3.139–3.144). The most common site is the terminal ileum with ulceration commonly present along the antimesenteric aspect of the bowel in association with Peyer patches (87,88). Confirming the diagnosis requires clinicopathologic correlation, and surgical management is often required.

This syndrome is discussed in more detail in Chapter 4, but diagnosis often requires a resection in order to confirm the characteristic vasculitis.

SMALL INTESTINAL FINDINGS IN ULCERATIVE COLITIS

Generally, the small intestine is unaffected by ulcerative colitis. Unfortunately, there is a subset of patients who have severe pancolitis, which extends a short distance into the ileum as well, and the term "backwash ileitis" has been applied and used with some dissatisfaction by surgeons, gastroenterologists, and pathologists alike. It remains unclear whether such patients have severe ulcerative colitis or something else. In either event, the prevalence of ileal inflammatory changes in patients with ulcerative colitis has been reported at 17% (89). So-called "backwash ileitis" is associated with ileoanal pouch complications in some studies (90), but not others, and is believed by many observers to reflect the severity of the ulcerative colitis. "Backwash ileitis" is sometimes described as "active chronic" or "minimal active (e-Fig. 3.145)"; thus, no real consensus exists. In daily practice, we simply describe what is seen in the ileum. Histologic features are nonspecific and include focal neutrophilic cryptitis and/or crypt microabscesses, partial villous atrophy, and mononuclear lamina propria expansion with or without associated neutrophils; rarely, small, superficial ulceration and pyloric metaplasia may be observed (89). A group of patients with classic ulcerative colitis and severe confluent duodenitis has also been described by Valdez et al. (91). These patients had a good clinical outcome with continent pouches and, therefore, they presumably had a rare form of ulcerative colitis with diffuse duodenal involvement, rather than Crohn disease. Whether these patients had a peculiar SBBO, which complicated their ulcerative colitis, was not clarified in the report. More recently, Hori et al. (92) have reported an association between gastroduodenitis in the setting of ulcerative colitis with pancolitis and low steroid doses.

AMYLOIDOSIS

GI amyloidosis is an almost universal finding in systemic amyloidosis. It consists of extracellular deposition of beta-pleated protein sheets in the mucosa, submucosa, muscularis propria, or serosa.

The older classification divided amyloidosis into "localized" and "generalized," or "primary" and "secondary" amyloidosis. Localized amyloidosis usually does not involve the GI tract. However, systemic amyloidosis almost universally involves the gut. Other common sites of amyloid deposition include the heart, kidneys, liver, and spleen, with restrictive cardiomyopathy, nephrotic syndrome, or hepatosplenomegaly, respectively, depending upon the site of amyloid deposition. As discussed in Chapter 2, the newer classification of amyloidosis is based on the biochemical composition of the amyloid: (a) immunoglobulin light-chain (AL) amyloid, associated with B-cell lymphoma, multiple myeloma, and Waldenstrom macroglobulinemia; (b) amyloid protein A (AA) amyloid, seen in chronic illnesses such as rheumatoid arthritis, tuberculosis, bronchiectasis, Crohn disease, and familial diseases such as familial Mediterranean fever; (c) β-2 microglobulin, associated with renal failure and long-term hemodialysis; (d) β-precursor protein, associated with Alzheimer disease; and (e) transthyretin, which usually involves the heart.

Except for the familial forms, amyloidosis usually affects older adults in their 60s. GI manifestations consist of hemorrhage, nausea and vomiting, weight loss, malabsorption, gastric outlet obstruction, gastroparesis, stasis-related change (such as bacterial overgrowth), or diarrhea. Amyloid deposits in blood vessels cause them to become fragile and leaky, which leads to hemorrhage. Deposits in the muscularis propria and nerve bundles cause impaired motility. Mucosal deposits lead to malabsorption and diarrhea. Rarely, amyloid may present as a tumoral mass and can be mistaken for a carcinoma.

The endoscopic appearance is not specific, consisting of mucosal erosions, ulcers, thickened folds, or even a tumoral mass. Resection specimens with massive amyloid deposition have thick and rigid walls with a waxy appearance. Diagnosis is achieved through tissue biopsy of the GI tract; the rectum and stomach are the preferred sites with a high yield. Biopsy samples must be adequate and deep enough to contain submucosal vessels to increase the diagnostic yield.

Biopsies often show intact and slender villi, and few intramucosal Brunner glands. The lamina propria and muscularis mucosae contain extensive dense, eosinophilic, slightly globular extracellular deposits, which produce the characteristic apple-green birefringence on Congo red stain, consistent with amyloidosis. Amyloid deposits can also be seen in submucosal vessel walls.

The distribution of amyloid in the gut can be patchy or diffuse. Amyloid presents as dense, homogenous, acellular, and eosinophilic extracellular deposits in the lamina propria, submucosa, muscularis propria, nerve trunks, and vascular intima and media. Amyloid deposits often show cracking with slit-like spaces as a result of tissue processing artifact. Amyloid in the lamina propria often appears globular. Massive amyloid accumulation in the muscularis propria and submucosa can occur and is usually associated with AL amyloidosis (e-Figs. 3.146–3.148).

Ultrastructurally, amyloid consists of nonbranching fibrils, 7.5 to 10 nm in diameter. The fibrils are composed of β-pleated sheets of amyloid proteins. Cotton dyes such as Congo red, when polarized, impart a characteristic apple-green birefringence in the presence of amyloid. Other useful stains include Sirius red, Sirius supra scarlet, and thioflavin T (fluorescent dye). Immunolabeling for κ and λ is useful in AL amyloidosis, with the majority showing a λ restriction.

A number of disorders have features that may be mistaken for amyloid. They include (a) arteriosclerosis of vessels, in which resulting hyalinization may be misdiagnosed as amyloid deposits; (b) systemic sclerosis, which can result in fibrosis of muscularis and submucosa that may be mistaken for amyloid; and (c) ischemic injury, which results in lamina propria hyalinization and microcrypts that can resemble amyloid. However, amyloid deposits in the lamina propria appear as globular deposits.

COMMON VARIABLE IMMUNODEFICIENCY

Washington et al. (21) have reported common GI complaints in patients with CVID and related disorders. Daniels et al. (20) documented small bowel biopsy findings in 39 small bowel samples from 19 patients with this condition. Features included a paucity of plasma cells (68%), prominent lymphoid aggregates (47%), increased apoptosis (21%), increased IELs (63%) with or without villous blunting (83% of those with IELs), and granulomas (11%). While these features may suggest celiac disease and/or Crohn disease, both diagnoses can usually be excluded because of the paucity of lamina propria plasma cells (Fig. 3.43) and the likelihood of harboring infectious agents (*Giardia*, Cryptosporidium, microsporidia) (21) (e-Figs. 3.82–3.85). Of course, *Giardia* may be found in immunocompetent hosts as well, but there are often fewer organisms in that setting (e-Figs. 3.78–3.81). It should be stressed that not all patients' biopsies lack plasma cells so clinicopathologic correlation is important.

AUTOIMMUNE ENTEROPATHY

This rare condition is characterized by (a) small intestinal villous atrophy *unresponsive to dietary restrictions*, (b) unrelenting diarrhea, and (c) predisposition to autoimmune disease, as initially proposed by Unsworth and Walker-Smith (93). Though initially thought to affect newborns and young children, adult onset is well-documented in the literature (94–97). Pathophysiology is poorly understood but a proposed mechanism involves loss of self-tolerance and a hyperreactive immune system with inappropriate T-cell activation and cytotoxicity (please see Chapter 2 for a brief discussion of the molecular underpinnings). Increased numbers of mucosal CD4+ and CD8+ T cells have been observed by some (98,99). This activation may be a result of aberrant HLA class II molecule expression in enteric crypt epithelial cells (normally expressed only by mature enterocytes) as documented by Mirakian et al. (100). Certain autoantibodies are associated with this condition, namely antigoblet cell and antienterocyte antibodies. Akram et al. found these antibodies in 13 out of 14 (93%) studied patients. Their presence, however, seems neither necessary nor sufficient for disease development as some patients with the condition have no detectable antibodies (96) and antibodies have been detected in healthy subjects and in patients with celiac disease (101). Additionally, a myriad of other autoantibodies may be present or coexist with the gut-specific antibodies, namely antinuclear, antistriated muscle, antiparietal, anti-SSA, and antiphospholipid antibodies, to name a few. Up to 87% of affected patients suffer from associated autoimmune disorders such as rheumatoid arthritis, myasthenia gravis, psoriatic arthritis, hypothyroidism, autoimmune inflammatory myopathy, idiopathic thrombocytopenic purpura, Raynaud phenomenon, and atrophic gastritis, among others (92,94,102). Two variants of the disorder are described. The first, termed IPEX (immune dysregulation, polyendocrinopathy, enteropathy, X-linked) syndrome, is fatal, X-linked, and characterized by polyendocrinopathy and various autoimmune conditions in association with severe, prolonged diarrhea (103). The second, termed APECED (autoimmune polyendocrinopathy–candidiasis–ectodermal dystrophy) syndrome or APS-1 (autoimmune polyglandular syndrome 1), is autosomal recessive and affected patients suffer from autoimmune enteropathy in association with endocrine abnormalities (hypoparathyroidism, adrenocortical insufficiency, diabetes mellitus, thyroid disease), mucocutaneous candidiasis, and skin manifestations such as alopecia and vitiligo, and nail deformities (104).

The histologic appearance of autoimmune enteropathy varies considerably from case to case. Intestinal biopsies show a picture similar to celiac disease with total or partial villous atrophy, crypt hyperplasia, and expansion of the lamina propria by a lymphoplasmacytic infiltrate. Some cases display intact villous architecture. Active inflammation with or without crypt abscesses may or may not be present (94). Increased IELs may be seen but often to a lesser degree than in celiac disease (94, 96). Crypt apoptosis is striking in some cases. Goblet and/or Paneth cells may be absent (Fig. 3.44, e-Figs. 3.149–3.152). Cases lacking goblet cells and/or Paneth cells are easy to recognize as autoimmune enteropathy if the pathologist is in the habit of assessing for these components in biopsies, whereas the diagnosis can only be listed as part of a differential diagnosis when, e.g., prominent apoptosis is the most salient feature. The diagnosis should be considered when examining biopsies from adult patients labeled as having "refractory sprue" and from babies and children with intractable diarrhea. Treatment consists of nutritional support and immunosuppressive therapy. With treatment, some patients with absent goblet and Paneth cells regain them (Fig. 3.45).

MICROVILLUS INCLUSION DISEASE

Microvillus inclusion disease (or microvillus atrophy) is an uncommon congenital enteropathy, producing intractable secretory diarrhea in early infancy (105–107). It is an inherited disease in an autosomal recessive genetic trait pattern and thus is encountered in populations with prevalent

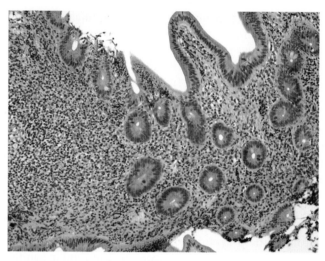

FIGURE 3.44 **Autoimmune enteropathy.** What is absent in a biopsy is as important as what is present. There are no goblet cells or Paneth cells in this biopsy but the architecture is not especially abnormal.

consanguinity. For example, we have encountered both microvillus inclusion disease and the related condition tufting enteropathy in patients from tribal Arab countries. There are several synonyms used for this disease, including Davidson disease (108), familial microvillus atrophy, congenital microvillus atrophy, and intestinal microvillus dystrophy (a variant of microvillus inclusion disease). The outcome is typically poor, with most patients requiring small bowel transplant. Rare cases have resolved.

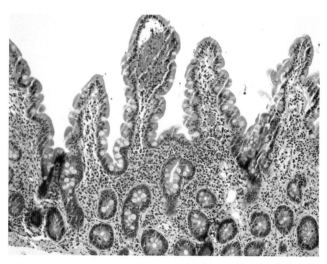

FIGURE 3.45 **Autoimmune enteropathy, treated.** This biopsy was obtained from the same patient as that seen in Figure 3.44 after several months of steroid treatment and improvement of symptoms. Goblet cells and Paneth cells are restored.

The diagnosis criteria for microvillus inclusion disease include

- Intractable watery diarrhea in early infancy
- Diffuse intestinal villous atrophy with no inflammatory reaction
- Apical microvillus inclusions of surface enterocytes identified under electron microscope (definitive diagnosis criterion)
- No evidence of infection, autoimmune disease, or allergy

Biopsies of duodenal mucosa show moderate villous blunting, with no active inflammatory reaction or intraepithelial lymphocytosis. The optimal specimen is a small intestinal biopsy, in which duodenal biopsy is most commonly used. (Rectal biopsy has been proposed as a simple and reliable method for early diagnosis, although the findings may be subtle.) A characteristic feature is architecturally diffuse intestinal villous atrophy with no inflammatory reaction. Due to increased crypt cell apoptosis, either crypt hypoplasia or hyperplasia can be found. Subtle histologic changes in the enterocytes are confined to the villous tips and distal villous lateral borders. Changes are difficult to discern at the base of the villus and in the crypt epithelium; indeed, the enterocytes appear normal in these regions. Cytologically, a bubbly vacuolated appearance of the apical cytoplasm, with extensive or patchy absence of the brush border, is a specific sign for the diagnosis (Fig. 3.46). Typical targetoid cytoplasmic inclusions are occasionally identified in the surface enterocytes (Fig. 3.47).

Instead of a sharp, linear brush border that stains with PAS or alkaline phosphatase histochemically, a bright apical cytoplasmic blush is present and is the most easily recognized change of microvillus inclusion disease (Fig. 3.48). Brush border biomarkers, such as carcinoembryonic antigen (CEA) and CD10, in particular (105,106), are also useful in the

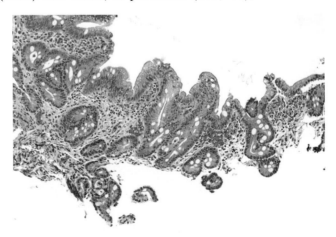

FIGURE 3.46 **Microvillus inclusion disease.** At low magnification, there is villous atrophy but no inflammation. The surface has a peculiar appearance similar to that of gastric mucin cell metaplasia but without a crisply delineated apical mucin cap.

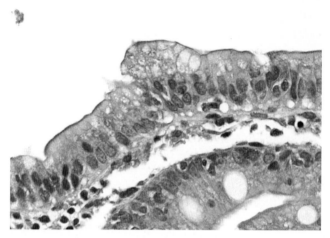

FIGURE 3.47 Microvillus inclusion disease. At high magnification, the brush border focally vanishes and there are targetoid inclusions in the cells.

diagnosis of microvillus inclusion disease. CEA and CD10 stains demonstrate the characteristic, apical cytoplasmic staining pattern in the enterocytes. Ultrastructurally, identification of apical microvillus inclusions in surface enterocytes in intestinal tract biopsies makes a definitive diagnosis, as shown in e-Figures. 3.153–3.156. Tissue orientation, with particular concern to include the apical aspects of the mucosa for electron microscope examination, is crucial for identification of inclusions in apical enterocytes. In addition to electron microscope identification of microvillus inclusions,

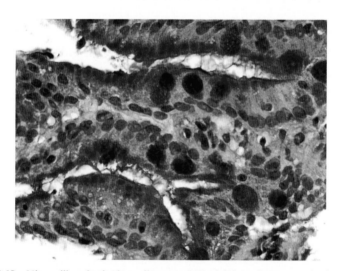

FIGURE 3.48 Microvillus inclusion disease. PAS staining shows a cytoplasmic blush in surface cells. Compare this to Figure 3.12 (gastric mucin cell metaplasia) in which the PAS-positive neutral mucin appears as a crisply demarcated apical mucin cap.

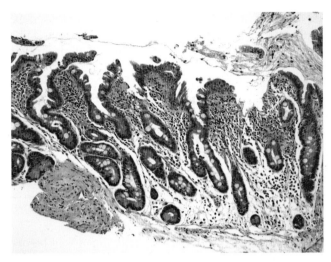

FIGURE 3.49 **Tufting enteropathy.** Presumably as a result of defects in adhesion molecules, the surface enterocytes have disordered nuclei and form tufts.

other unique and diagnostic characteristics of this disease include light microscopic morphologic features, together with biomarker-highlighted apical cytoplasmic blush and inclusions. A variant of this condition (possibly an incomplete form) is called "tufting enteropathy" or "intestinal epithelial dysplasia," and adhesion molecule defects have been implicated (109–111). Histology shows various degree of villous atrophy, with low or without mononuclear cell infiltration of the lamina propria. The epithelium displays disorganization of surface enterocytes with focal crowding, resembling tufts (Figs. 3.49 and 3.50). Deposition of laminin and heparan sulfate

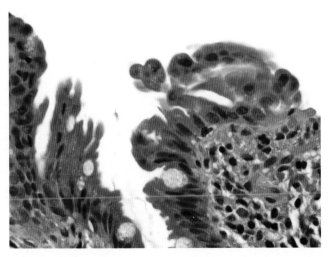

FIGURE 3.50 **Tufting enteropathy.** Higher magnification highlights the so-called tufts.

proteoglycan (HSPG) in the basement membrane, increased expression of desmoglein, ultrastructural changes in the desmosomes, and abnormal distribution of $\alpha2\beta1$ integrin adhesion molecules are all described. An noted above, parental consanguinity and/or affected siblings suggest an autosomal recessive transmission but the causative genes have not been yet identified, making prenatal diagnosis unreliable; EpCAM appears to be the gene at play (110,111). Some infants have a milder phenotype than others, but in most patients, the severity of the intestinal malabsorption even with enteral feeding make them totally dependent on daily long-term parenteral nutrition with a subsequent risk of complications. Intestinal transplantation is often the recommended treatment.

LYMPHANGIECTASIA

Primary intestinal lymphangiectasia is usually diagnosed before 3 years of age (1,2). Most patients have growth retardation. GI complaints vary in severity and consist of diarrhea, vomiting, abdominal pain, and steatorrhea. If large segments of the gut are involved, secondary edema may occur as a result of protein-losing enteropathy and malabsorption. The edema is usually generalized, but asymmetric edema is not uncommon.

Small biopsies taken from these patients may be nondiagnostic, but they simply display multiple dilated lacteals (Figs. 3.51 and 3.52, e-Fig. 3.157), a finding easy to overlook without knowledge of an often dramatic computed tomographic appearance.

The long-term course is variable but usually progresses slowly with intermittent clinical remissions.

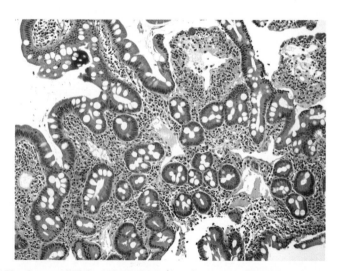

FIGURE 3.51 **Congenital lymphangiectasia.** There are dilated lymphatic spaces. The rather banal appearance of this biopsy belies the dramatic imaging and endoscopic appearances of this condition.

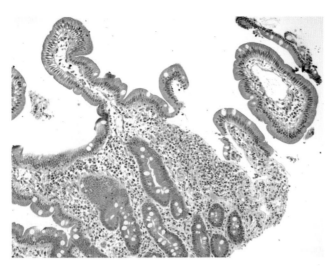

FIGURE 3.52 **Congenital lymphangiectasia.** Higher magnification.

The reported medical treatments for lymphangiectasia are a high-protein, low-fat diet with added medium-chain triglycerides. Also, octreotides have been reported to decrease intestinal protein losses.

REFERENCES

1. Hart MH, Vanderhoof JA, Antonson DL. Failure of blind small bowel biopsy in the diagnosis of intestinal lymphangiectasia. *J Pediatr Gastroenterol Nutr.* 1987;6:803–805.

2. Uguralp S, Mutus M, Kutlu O, et al. Primary intestinal lymphangiectasia: a rare disease in the differential diagnosis of acute abdomen. *J Pediatr Gastroenterol Nutr.* 2001;33:508–510.

3. Dumler JS, Baisden BL, Yardley JH, et al. Immunodetection of *Tropheryma whipplei* in intestinal tissues from Dr. Whipple's 1907 patient. *N Engl J Med.* 2003;348:1411–1412.

4. Brune D. Minor and trace inorganic components of toothpastes. *Scand J Dent Res.* 1980;88:517–520.

5. Marshall BJ, Warren JR. Unidentified curved bacilli in the stomach of patients with gastritis and peptic ulceration. *Lancet.* 1984;1:1311–1315.

6. Martin DF, Montgomery E, Dobek AS, et al. *Campylobacter pylori*, NSAIDS, and smoking: risk factors for peptic ulcer disease. *Am J Gastroenterol.* 1989;84:1268–1272.

7. Riddell RH. Pathobiology of *Helicobacter pylori* infection in children. *Can J Gastroenterol.* 1999;13:599–603.

8. Triadafilopoulos G. Clinical and pathologic features of the nodular duodenum. *Am J Gastroenterol.* 1993;88:1058–1064.

9. Shekitka KM, Helwig EB. Deceptive bizarre stromal cells in polyps and ulcers of the gastrointestinal tract. *Cancer.* 1991;67:2111–2117.

10. Yardley JH, Hendrix TR. Combined electron and light microscopy in Whipple's disease. Demonstration of "bacillary bodies" in the intestine. *Bull Johns Hopkins Hosp.* 1961;109:80–98.

11. Baisden BL, Lepidi H, Raoult D, et al. Diagnosis of Wihipple disease by immunohistochemical analysis: a sensitive and specific method for the detection of *Tropheryma*

whipplei (the Whipple bacillus) in paraffin-embedded tissue. *Am J Clin Pathol.* 2002;118:742–748.

12. Montgomery EA, Popek EJ. Intussusception, adenovirus, and children: a brief reaffirmation. *Hum Pathol.* 1994;25:169–174.

13. Cano MV, Hajjeh RA. The epidemiology of histoplasmosis: a review. *Semin Respir Infect.* 2001;16:109–118.

14. Allendoerfer R, Deepe GS Jr. Blockade of endogenous TNF-alpha exacerbates primary and secondary pulmonary histoplasmosis by differential mechanisms. *J Immunol.* 1998;160:6072–6082.

15. Lamps LW, Molina CP, West AB, et al. The pathologic spectrum of gastrointestinal and hepatic histoplasmosis. *Am J Clin Pathol.* 2000;113:64–72.

16. Lamps LW, Madhusudhan KT, Greenson JK, et al. The role of *Yersinia enterocolitica* and *Yersinia pseudotuberculosis* in granulomatous appendicitis: a histologic and molecular study. *Am J Surg Pathol.* 2001;25:508–515.

17. Lamps LW, Madhusudhan KT, Havens JM, et al. Pathogenic *Yersinia* DNA is detected in bowel and mesenteric lymph nodes from patients with Crohn's disease. *Am J Surg Pathol.* 2003;27:220–227.

18. Marciano BE, Rosenzweig SD, Kleiner DE, et al. Gastrointestinal involvement in chronic granulomatous disease. *Pediatrics.* 2004;114:462–468.

19. Levine S, Smith VV, Malone M, et al. Histopathological features of chronic granulomatous disease (CGD) in childhood. *Histopathology.* 2005;47:508–516.

20. Daniels JA, Lederman HM, Maitra A, et al. Gastrointestinal tract pathology in patients with common variable immunodeficiency (CVID): a clinicopathologic study and review. *Am J Surg Pathol.* 2007;31:1800–1812.

21. Washington K, Stenzel TT, Buckley RH, et al. Gastrointestinal pathology in patients with common variable immunodeficiency and X-linked agammaglobulinemia. *Am J Surg Pathol.* 1996;20:1240–1252.

22. Plutzer J, Ongerth J, Karanis P. Giardia taxonomy, phylogeny and epidemiology: facts and open questions. *Int J Hyg Environ Health.* 2010;213:321–333.

23. Szyszko T, Al-Nahhas A, Tait P, et al. Management and prevention of adverse effects related to treatment of liver tumours with 90Y microspheres. *Nucl Med Commun.* 2007;28:21–24.

24. Cortina G, Wren S, Armstrong B, et al. Clinical and pathologic overlap in nonsteroidal anti-inflammatory drug-related small bowel diaphragm disease and the neuromuscular and vascular hamartoma of the small bowel. *Am J Surg Pathol.* 1999;23:1414–1417.

25. Lang J, Price AB, Levi AJ, et al. Diaphragm disease: pathology of disease of the small intestine induced by non-steroidal anti-inflammatory drugs. *J Clin Pathol.* 1988;41:516–526.

26. Smith JA, Pineau BC. Endoscopic therapy of NSAID-induced colonic diaphragm disease: two cases and a review of published reports. *Gastrointest Endosc.* 2000;52:120–125.

27. Roy J, Snover D, Weisdorf S, et al. Simultaneous upper and lower endoscopic biopsy in the diagnosis of intestinal graft-versus-host disease. *Transplantation.* 1991;51:642–646.

28. Snover DC, Weisdorf SA, Vercellotti GM, et al. A histopathologic study of gastric and small intestinal graft-versus-host disease following allogeneic bone marrow transplantation. *Hum Pathol.* 1985;16:387–392.

29. Weisdorf DJ, Snover DC, Haake R, et al. Acute upper gastrointestinal graft-versus-host disease: clinical significance and response to immunosuppressive therapy. *Blood.* 1990;76:624–629.

30. Cruz-Correa M, Poonawala A, Abraham SC, et al. Endoscopic findings predict the histologic diagnosis in gastrointestinal graft-versus-host disease. *Endoscopy.* 2002;34:808–813.

31. Papadimitriou JC, Cangro CB, Lustberg A, et al. Histologic features of mycophenolate mofetil-related colitis: a graft-versus-host disease-like pattern. *Int J Surg Pathol.* 2003;11:295–302.

32. Nguyen T, Park JY, Scudiere JR, et al. Mycophenolic acid (CellCept and Myofortic) induced injury of the upper GI tract. *Am J Surg Pathol.* 2009;33:1355–1363.

33. Parfitt JR, Jayakumar S, Driman DK. Mycophenolate mofetil-related gastrointestinal mucosal injury: variable injury patterns, including graft-versus-host disease-like changes. *Am J Surg Pathol.* 2008;32:1367–1372.

34. Talmon GA, Saigh QM, Dimaio D, et al. Characterization of epithelial apoptosis in biopsies of small-bowel allografts using cleaved caspase 3 immunostaining. *Int J Surg Pathol.* 2010.

35. Oble DA, Mino-Kenudson M, Goldsmith J, et al. Alpha-CTLA-4 mAb-associated panenteritis: a histologic and immunohistochemical analysis. *Am J Surg Pathol.* 2008;32:1130–1137.

36. Iacobuzio-Donahue CA, Lee EL, Abraham SC, et al. Colchicine toxicity: distinct morphologic findings in gastrointestinal biopsies. *Am J Surg Pathol.* 2001;25:1067–1073.

37. Johnson TC, Diamond B, Memeo L, et al. Relationship of HLA-DQ8 and severity of celiac disease: comparison of New York and Parisian cohorts. *Clin Gastroenterol Hepatol.* 2004;2:888–894.

38. Carlsson A, Axelsson I, Borulf S, et al. Prevalence of IgA-antigliadin antibodies and IgA-antiendomysium antibodies related to celiac disease in children with Down syndrome. *Pediatrics.* 1998;101:272–275.

39. Maki M, Mustalahti K, Kokkonen J, et al. Prevalence of Celiac disease among children in Finland. *N Engl J Med.* 2003;348:2517–2524.

40. Fasano A, Berti I, Gerarduzzi T, et al. Prevalence of celiac disease in at-risk and not-at-risk groups in the United States: a large multicenter study. *Arch Intern Med.* 2003;163:286–292.

41. Fasano A. European and North American populations should be screened for coeliac disease. *Gut.* 2003;52:168–169.

42. Catassi C, Ratsch IM, Gandolfi L, et al. Why is coeliac disease endemic in the people of the Sahara? *Lancet.* 1999;354:647–648.

43. Rostami K, Malekzadeh R, Shahbazkhani B, et al. Coeliac disease in Middle Eastern countries: a challenge for the evolutionary history of this complex disorder? *Dig Liver Dis.* 2004;36:694–697.

44. Catassi C, Fasano A. Celiac disease as a cause of growth retardation in childhood. *Curr Opin Pediatr.* 2004;16:445–449.

45. Dickey W, Hughes D. Prevalence of celiac disease and its endoscopic markers among patients having routine upper gastrointestinal endoscopy. *Am J Gastroenterol.* 1999;94:2182–2186.

46. Prasad KK, Thapa BR, Nain CK, et al. The frequency of histologic lesion variability of the duodenal mucosa in children with celiac disease. *World J Pediatr.* 2010;6:60–64.

47. Weir DC, Glickman JN, Roiff T, et al. Variability of histopathological changes in childhood celiac disease. *Am J Gastroenterol.* 2010;105:207–212.

48. Marsh MN. Gluten, major histocompatibility complex, and the small intestine. A molecular and immunobiologic approach to the spectrum of gluten sensitivity ('celiac sprue'). *Gastroenterology.* 1992;102:330–354.

49. Rostami K, Kerckhaert J, Tiemessen R, et al. Sensitivity of antiendomysium and antigliadin antibodies in untreated celiac disease: disappointing in clinical practice. *Am J Gastroenterol.* 1999;94:888–894.

50. Goldstein NS, Underhill J. Morphologic features suggestive of gluten sensitivity in architecturally normal duodenal biopsy specimens. *Am J Clin Pathol.* 2001;116:63–71.

51. Mino M, Lauwers GY. Role of lymphocytic immunophenotyping in the diagnosis of gluten-sensitive enteropathy with preserved villous architecture. *Am J Surg Pathol.* 2003;27:1237–1242.

52. Goldstein NS. Non-gluten sensitivity-related small bowel villous flattening with increased intraepithelial lymphocytes: not all that flattens is celiac sprue. *Am J Clin Pathol.* 2004;121:546–550.

53. Goldstein NS. Proximal small-bowel mucosal villous intraepithelial lymphocytes. *Histopathology.* 2004;44:199–205.

54. Kurppa K, Collin P, Viljamaa M, et al. Diagnosing mild enteropathy celiac disease: a randomized, controlled clinical study. *Gastroenterology.* 2009;136:816–823.

55. Wahab PJ, Meijer JW, Mulder CJ. Histologic follow-up of people with celiac disease on a gluten-free diet: slow and incomplete recovery. *Am J Clin Pathol.* 2002;118:459–463.

56. Rubio-Tapia A, Murray JA. Classification and management of refractory coeliac disease. *Gut.* 2010;59:547–557.

57. Robert ME, Ament ME, Weinstein WM. The histologic spectrum and clinical outcome of refractory and unclassified sprue. *Am J Surg Pathol.* 2000;24:676–687.

58. Vakiani E, Arguelles-Grande C, Mansukhani MM, et al. Collagenous sprue is not always associated with dismal outcomes: a clinicopathological study of 19 patients. *Mod Pathol.* 2010;23:12–26.

59. Maguire AA, Greenson JK, Lauwers GY, et al. Collagenous sprue: a clinicopathologic study of 12 cases. *Am J Surg Pathol.* 2009;33:1440–1449.

60. Cellier C, Delabesse E, Helmer C, et al. Refractory sprue, coeliac disease, and enteropathy-associated T-cell lymphoma. French Coeliac Disease Study Group. *Lancet.* 2000;356:203–208.

61. Daum S, Hummel M, Weiss D, et al. Refractory sprue syndrome with clonal intraepithelial lymphocytes evolving into overt enteropathy-type intestinal T-cell lymphoma. *Digestion.* 2000;62:60–65.

62. Daum S, Weiss D, Hummel M, et al. Frequency of clonal intraepithelial T lymphocyte proliferations in enteropathy-type intestinal T cell lymphoma, coeliac disease, and refractory sprue. *Gut.* 2001;49:804–812.

63. Vega F, Chang CC, Schwartz MR, et al. Atypical NK-cell proliferation of the gastrointestinal tract in a patient with antigliadin antibodies but not celiac disease. *Am J Surg Pathol.* 2006;30:539–544.

64. Aghamohammadi A, Cheraghi T, Gharagozlou M, et al. IgA deficiency: correlation between clinical and immunological phenotypes. *J Clin Immunol.* 2009;29:130–136.

65. Shoulders CC, Brett DJ, Bayliss JD, et al. Abetalipoproteinemia is caused by defects of the gene encoding the 97 kDa subunit of a microsomal triglyceride transfer protein. *Hum Mol Genet.* 1993;2:2109–2116.

66. Wetterau JR, Aggerbeck LP, Bouma ME, et al. Absence of microsomal triglyceride transfer protein in individuals with abetalipoproteinemia. *Science.* 1992;258:999–1001.

67. Sperling MA, Hengstenberg F, Yunis E, et al. Abetalipoproteinemia: metabolic, endocrine, and electron-microscopic investigations. *Pediatrics.* 1971;48:91–102.

68. Triantafillidis JK, Kottaras G, Sgourous S, et al. A-beta-lipoproteinemia: clinical and laboratory features, therapeutic manipulations, and follow-up study of three members of a Greek family. *J Clin Gastroenterol.* 1998;26:207–211.

69. Ghoshal UC, Ghoshal U, Ayyagari A, et al. Tropical sprue is associated with contamination of small bowel with aerobic bacteria and reversible prolongation of orocecal transit time. *J Gastroenterol Hepatol.* 2003;18:540–547.

70. Castiglione F, Rispo A, Di Girolamo E, et al. Antibiotic treatment of small bowel bacterial overgrowth in patients with Crohn's disease. *Aliment Pharmacol Ther.* 2003;18:1107–1112.

71. King T. Small intestinal bacterial overgrowth and irritable bowel syndrome. *JAMA.* 2004;292:2213; author reply 2213–2214.

72. Teo M, Chung S, Chitti L, et al. Small bowel bacterial overgrowth is a common cause of chronic diarrhea. *J Gastroenterol Hepatol.* 2004;19:904–909.

73. Reddymasu SC, McCallum RW. Small intestinal bacterial overgrowth in gastroparesis: are there any predictors? *J Clin Gastroenterol.* 2010;44:e8–13.

74. Lappinga PJ, Abraham SC, Murray JA, et al. Small intestinal bacterial overgrowth: histopathologic features and clinical correlates in an underrecognized entity. *Arch Pathol Lab Med.* 2010;134:264–270.

75. Khoshini R, Dai SC, Lezcano S, et al. A systematic review of diagnostic tests for small intestinal bacterial overgrowth. *Dig Dis Sci.* 2008;53:1443–1454.

76. Stotzer PO, Brandberg A, Kilander AF. Diagnosis of small intestinal bacterial overgrowth in clinical praxis: a comparison of the culture of small bowel aspirate, duodenal biopsies and gastric aspirate. *Hepatogastroenterology.* 1998;45:1018–1022.

77. Corazza GR, Menozzi MG, Strocchi A, et al. The diagnosis of small bowel bacterial overgrowth. Reliability of jejunal culture and inadequacy of breath hydrogen testing. *Gastroenterology.* 1990;98:302–309.

78. Jess T, Winther KV, Munkholm P, et al. Intestinal and extra-intestinal cancer in Crohn's disease: follow-up of a population-based cohort in Copenhagen County, Denmark. *Aliment Pharmacol Ther.* 2004;19:287–293.

79. Palascak-Juif V, Bouvier AM, Cosnes J, et al. Small bowel adenocarcinoma in patients with Crohn's disease compared with small bowel adenocarcinoma de novo. *Inflamm Bowel Dis.* 2005;11:828–832.

80. Tougeron D, Lefebure B, Savoye G, et al. Small-bowel adenocarcinoma in patient with Crohn's disease: report of a series of three cases. *Scand J Gastroenterol.* 2008; 43:1397–1400.

81. Drut R, Altamirano E. Small bowel gastric metaplasia: a report of three cases in children. *J Clin Pathol.* 2008;61:382–384.

82. Steiner SJ, Kleiman MB, Corkins MR, et al. Ileocecal histoplasmosis simulating Crohn disease in a patient with hyperimmunoglobulin E syndrome. *Pediatr Infect Dis J.* 2009;28:744–746.

83. Colombel JF, Loftus EV Jr, Tremaine WJ, et al. The safety profile of infliximab in patients with Crohn's disease: the Mayo clinic experience in 500 patients. *Gastroenterology.* 2004;126:19–31.

84. Criteria for diagnosis of Behcet's disease. International Study Group for Behcet's Disease. *Lancet.* 1990;335:1078–1080.

85. O'Neill TW, Rigby AS, Silman AJ, et al. Validation of the International Study Group criteria for Behcet's disease. *Br J Rheumatol.* 1994;33:115–117.

86. Ergun T, Gurbuz O, Harvell J, et al. The histopathology of pathergy: a chronologic study of skin hyperreactivity in Behcet's disease. *Int J Dermatol.* 1998;37:929–933.

87. Isomoto H, Shikuwa S, Suematsu T, et al. Ileal lesions in Behcet's disease originate in Peyer patches: findings on magnifying endoscopy. *Scand J Gastroenterol.* 2008;43:249–250.

88. Takada Y, Fujita Y, Igarashi M, et al. Intestinal Behcet disease–pathognomonic changes in intramucosal lymphoid tissues and effect of a "rest cure" on intestinal lesions. *J Gastroenterol.* 1997;32:598–604.

89. Haskell H, Andrews CW Jr, Reddy SI, et al. Pathologic features and clinical significance of "backwash" ileitis in ulcerative colitis. *Am J Surg Pathol.* 2005;29:1472–1481.

90. Schmidt CM, Lazenby AJ, Hendrickson RJ, et al. Preoperative terminal ileal and colonic resection histopathology predicts risk of pouchitis in patients after ileoanal pull-through procedure. *Ann Surg.* 1998;227:654–662; discussion 663–655.

91. Valdez R, Appelman HD, Bronner MP, et al. Diffuse duodenitis associated with ulcerative colitis. *Am J Surg Pathol.* 2000;24:1407–1413.

92. Hori K, Ikeuchi H, Nakano H, et al. Gastroduodenitis associated with ulcerative colitis. *J Gastroenterol.* 2008;43:193–201.

93. Unsworth DJ, Walker-Smith JA. Autoimmunity in diarrhoeal disease. *J Pediatr Gastroenterol Nutr.* 1985;4:375–380.

94. Akram S, Murray JA, Pardi DS, et al. Adult autoimmune enteropathy: Mayo Clinic Rochester experience. *Clin Gastroenterol Hepatol.* 2007;5:1282–1290; quiz 1245.

95. Carroccio A, Volta U, Di Prima L, et al. Autoimmune enteropathy and colitis in an adult patient. *Dig Dis Sci.* 2003;48:1600–1606.

96. Casis B, Fernandez-Vazquez I, Barnardos E, et al. Autoimmune enteropathy in an adult with autoimmune multisystemic involvement. *Scand J Gastroenterol.* 2002;37:1012–1016.

97. Volta U, De Angelis GL, Granito A, et al. Autoimmune enteropathy and rheumatoid arthritis: a new association in the field of autoimmunity. *Dig Liver Dis.* 2006;38:926–929.

98. Lachaux A, Loras-Duclaux I, Bouvier R. Autoimmune enteropathy in infants. Pathological study of the disease in two familial cases. *Virchows Arch.* 1998;433:481–485.

99. Moore L, Xu X, Davidson G, et al. Autoimmune enteropathy with anti-goblet cell antibodies. *Hum Pathol.* 1995;26:1162–1168.

100. Mirakian R, Hill S, Richardson A, et al. HLA product expression and lymphocyte subpopulations in jejunum biopsies of children with idiopathic protracted diarrhoea and enterocyte autoantibodies. *J Autoimmun.* 1988;1:263–277.

101. Biagi F, Bianchi PI, Trotta L, et al. Anti-goblet cell antibodies for the diagnosis of autoimmune enteropathy? *Am J Gastroenterol.* 2009;104:3112.

102. Mitomi H, Tanabe S, Igarashi M, et al. Autoimmune enteropathy with severe atrophic gastritis and colitis in an adult: proposal of a generalized autoimmune disorder of the alimentary tract. *Scand J Gastroenterol.* 1998;33:716–720.

103. Powell BR, Buist NR, Stenzel P. An X-linked syndrome of diarrhea, polyendocrinopathy, and fatal infection in infancy. *J Pediatr.* 1982;100:731–737.

104. Perheentupa J. APS-I/APECED: the clinical disease and therapy. *Endocrinol Metab Clin North Am.* 2002;31:295–320, vi.

105. Groisman GM, Amar M, Livne E. CD10: a valuable tool for the light microscopic diagnosis of microvillous inclusion disease (familial microvillous atrophy). *Am J Surg Pathol.* 2002;26:902–907.

106. Groisman GM, Ben-Izhak O, Schwersenz A, et al. The value of polyclonal carcinoembryonic antigen immunostaining in the diagnosis of microvillous inclusion disease. *Hum Pathol.* 1993;24:1232–1237.

107. Groisman GM, Sabo E, Meir A, et al. Enterocyte apoptosis and proliferation are increased in microvillous inclusion disease (familial microvillous atrophy). *Hum Pathol.* 2000;31:1404–1410.

108. Davidson GP, Cutz E, Hamilton JR, et al. Familial enteropathy: a syndrome of protracted diarrhea from birth, failure to thrive, and hypoplastic villus atrophy. *Gastroenterology.* 1978;75:783–790.

109. Goulet O, Salomon J, Ruemmele F, et al. Intestinal epithelial dysplasia (tufting enteropathy). *Orphanet J Rare Dis.* 2007;2:20.

110. Sivagnanam M, Mueller JL, Lee H, et al. Identification of EpCAM as the gene for congenital tufting enteropathy. *Gastroenterology.* 2008;135:429–437.

111. Sivagnanam M, Schaible T, Szigeti R, et al. Further evidence for EpCAM as the gene for congenital tufting enteropathy. *Am J Med Genet A.* 2010;152A:222–224.

4

COLON

Review of nonneoplastic colon biopsies requires a check of each compartment, namely, the epithelium, lamina propria, muscularis mucosae, and submucosa (if present). A few "tips" on what to look for include

a. If muscularis propria is present on biopsy samples, communication with the endoscopist to address the possibility that the patient has an iatrogenic perforation is advised (Fig. 4.1, e-Fig 4.1). On rare occasion, one might encounter tissue foreign to the gut admixed with colonic tissue, and this might be the only clue to an iatrogenic perforation (see e-Figs. 4.2 and 4.3).

b. Surface epithelium should be scanned for microorganisms (i.e., *Cryptosporidium*, spirochetosis), and the presence of an exudate should prompt a search for other organisms, especially *Amebae*.

c. It is useful to know if the patient has diverticular disease because this can result in inflammatory changes that mimic inflammatory bowel disease (IBD), as well as mucosal prolapse changes.

d. The constituents of an expanded lamina propria should be examined at high magnification as some diagnostic findings that involve exclusively this compartment can be subtle. For example, mast cells in the setting of mastocytosis can be difficult to discern as mast cell contents attract numerous eosinophils; neoplasms may only expand the lamina propria, barely affecting the glandular architecture; and granulomas tend to have the same tinctorial quality as the lamina propria, at times causing only slight expansion of this compartment.

Like the rest of the gastrointestinal (GI) tract, the colonic mucosa has a limited repertoire of responses to many injuries. The purpose of diagnostic biopsies in inflammatory disorders of the intestine is to (a) establish the presence of colitis, (b) differentiate idiopathic IBD from other inflammatory conditions, (c) attempt to distinguish ulcerative from Crohn colitis, (d) document extent of disease, (e) detect dysplasia and carcinoma, and (f) identify (when feasible) infectious agents (i.e., viral cytopathic changes). A large number of disorders can result in intestinal inflammation; these are partially listed in Table 4.1. In a certain percentage of cases, neither etiology nor characteristic features of a known entity can be identified, and such cases are diagnosed as "nonspecific colitis."

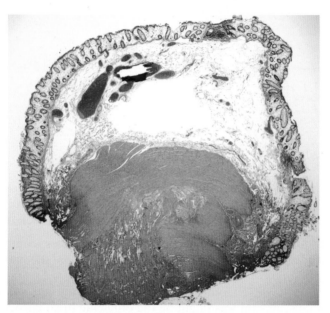

FIGURE 4.1 **Iatrogenic perforation.** This specimen comes from an endoscopic attempt to resect a polyp following infiltration of the submucosa to elevate the mucosa, which resulted in perforation of the bowel wall. There is muscularis propria on the biopsy, a finding that should prompt contacting the endoscopist.

It should be noted that the diagnosis of colitis requires evidence of injury to the epithelium, and not simply a mild increase in the amount of chronic inflammatory infiltrate within the lamina propria. In fact, it is entirely normal to find more lymphoplasmacytic cells in the lamina propria of the cecum than the distal colon, and practicing pathologists need to be aware of this (Figs. 4.2 and 4.3). Unless further specified, the histopathologic diagnosis of inflammation in colorectal biopsies is of limited value. Fortunately, in a review by Tsang and Rotterdam of biopsies from 100 patients having colon biopsies for nonneoplastic diseases, only 17 were interpreted as having "nonspecific inflammation" (1). Among the cases with inflammation, a specific diagnosis was rendered in 75% (51 cases had features of a specific diagnosis, 17 were "nonspecific," and 32 were normal). The study was retrospective and the reviewers' diagnoses were compared to the diagnoses rendered at original review: 30 of the 51 cases (59%), which had a specific diagnosis initially, had been diagnosed as "nonspecific" colitis. Thus, it would appear that improved familiarity with diagnostic criteria might strongly reduce the incidence of "nonspecific" colitis.

Tsang and Rotterdam defined "nonspecific inflammation" as the increase in inflammatory cells beyond what one would expect physiologically in the corresponding anatomic sites. Crypts may show reactive changes, such as an increase in mitoses or slight irregularity in shape. The lack of either sufficient clinical data or distinctive histopathologic features often precludes further classification.

TABLE 4.1 Inflammatory Intestinal Disorders	
Idiopathic Inflammatory Bowel Disease	**Iatrogenic Inflammation**
Ulcerative colitis	Enemas and laxatives
Crohn colitis	Drug-induced colitis
"Indeterminate" colitis	Therapeutic radiation colitis
Inflammation secondary to infectious agents	GVHD
Inflammation associated with motor disorders	Diversion colitis
Diverticulitis	**Associated with specific diseases**
Solitary rectal ulcer syndrome (and other mucosal prolapse disorders)	Chronic granulomatous disease
Inflammation secondary to vascular hypoperfusion	Immunodeficiency syndromes
Ischemic colitis	Hemolytic uremic syndrome
Vasculitis	Behçet disease
Necrotizing enterocolitis	**Miscellaneous**
Colitis complicating intestinal obstruction	Collagenous and lymphocytic colitis
	Neutropenic enterocolitis (typhlitis)
	Eosinophilic colitis
	Uremic colitis/Mycophenolate injury

In this chapter, an attempt is made to present features that allow some diagnostic specificity, with the caveat that nonneoplastic GI biopsies require correlation with the clinical and endoscopic findings. Also, it is important to inform colleagues when biopsies are normal, since this may

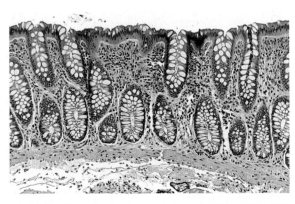

FIGURE 4.2 **Normal right colon.** The lamina propria contains lymphocytes, plasma cells, and scattered eosinophils.

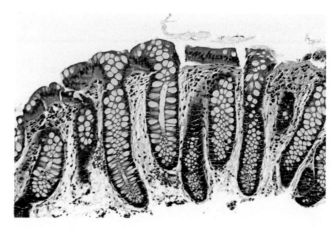

FIGURE 4.3 **Normal left colon.** This is from the same patient as depicted in Figure 4.2. There are fewer normal lamina propria constituents.

reflect functional disorders of motility as an etiology for the patient's symptoms (e.g., irritable bowel syndrome [IBS]) (2).

COLON HISTOLOGY

Normal histology in the colon reflects function of the specific site. Liquid stool from the small intestine enters the cecum, where water is progressively absorbed until it has the consistency of feces by the time it reaches the descending colon. The colonic mucosa produces abundant mucus that lubricates the surface and facilitates the passage of fecal material. The differences in the normal histology of the right and left colonic mucosa reflect these functions of absorption and lubrication. In the crypts of the right and transverse colon, absorptive cells predominate, although the larger goblet cells are more conspicuous.

The lamina propria in these proximal segments of the colon is more cellular than that of the distal colon and rectum and includes abundant plasma cells (involving the full thickness of the mucosa), lymphocytes, and eosinophils. Paneth cells may be found in the cecum and right colon. In contrast, goblet cells increase sharply in number in the left colon, and absorptive cells are fewer in the left colon and rectum. The lamina propria is much less cellular, with fewer eosinophils. Plasma cells are present only beneath the surface epithelium more distally.

If κ and λ immunostaining are performed on colon biopsies, there are normally more κ- than λ-reactive plasma cells so somewhat more prominent κ than λ immunolabeling can be disregarded (e-Figs. 4.4 and 4.5).

Lymphoid aggregates are normal and can be a prominent feature, at times providing the only explanation for the endoscopic appearance of a "polyp." Intraepithelial lymphocytes are normally found in increased numbers over lymphoid aggregates (Fig. 4.4) and should not generate concern for lymphocytic colitis, especially in the absence of other features, such as lymphoplasmacytic expansion of the lamina propria or surface epithelial damage. Macrophages are normally present and play a role in the

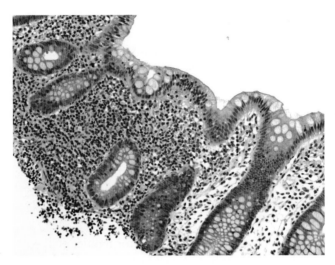

FIGURE 4.4 **Normal colon histology.** Intraepithelial lymphocytes are normally found in increased numbers over lymphoid aggregates and should not generate concern for lymphocytic colitis. Notice few intraepithelial lymphocytes away from the lymphoid aggregate (right side of the field).

processing and presentation of antigens. They aggregate in the superficial lamina propria where they form a rind just under the epithelium, where they phagocytose cellular debris from the normal apoptosis of surface epithelial cells (e-Figs. 4.6 and 4.7). Surface apoptosis is more prominent in the left colon and rectum than in the proximal colon.

Although eosinophils are present in the lamina propria of nearly all right colonic biopsies, their numbers vary greatly, particularly in patients from diverse geographic regions. In fact, eosinophils are generally more numerous in patients living in warmer areas of the United States (3). Paneth cells are abnormal outside of the right colon (although we accept them up to the splenic flexure); their presence in the left colon is metaplastic, usually in response to chronic inflammation or injury (e-Fig. 4.8). It is not uncommon for the untrained eye to mistake enterochromaffin cells (also known as Kulchitsky cells) for Paneth cells in the left (e-Fig. 4.9). The giveaway rests on the location of the eosinophilic granules: Paneth cell granules are exposed to the luminal surface, while neuroendocrine cell granules are located toward the basement membrane. Prior mucosal injury from any source can result in scattered intramucosal ganglion cells (e-Figs. 4.10 and 4.11); atypical reactive stromal cells can be found in ulcer beds in the colon, as well as in the remainder of the GI tract (e-Fig. 4.12).

IRRITABLE BOWEL SYNDROME

In the United States, the most common cause of chronic diarrhea is IBS, a condition with a prevalence of between 6% and 20% of cases, depending on inclusion criteria. Diagnosis is based on criteria that include continuous or recurrent abdominal discomfort, bloating or distention, and sometimes a change in stool frequency or appearance. The American Gastroenterological Association advocates colonoscopy as part of the evaluation of patients with presumed IBS who are >50 years old, or in whom there are symptoms (e.g., diarrhea predominance and/or weight loss) that might suggest another disease (2). Thus, most of the colonic biopsies that we review as part of the evaluation for chronic diarrhea can be expected to have essentially normal histology, and they should be reported as such. This requires an understanding of the histologic features of normal mucosa from all parts of the colon and rectum, as well as the ability to recognize histologic "abnormalities" that can be ignored.

EFFECTS OF BOWEL PREPARATION AND OTHER ARTIFACTS

There are a number of common, trivial abnormalities that we must recognize (and usually disregard) to report a biopsy as normal.

Bowel preparation for sigmoidoscopy and colonoscopy may induce a number of mucosal injuries that must be recognized, lest they be misinterpreted as pathologic. Hypertonic enemas, generally used before sigmoidoscopy, may injure the mucosal surface and result in flattened or absent surface epithelium, loss of epithelial mucin, or slight neutrophilic inflammation. The lamina propria may be edematous or hemorrhagic (4).

The two most commonly used preparations for full colonoscopy are sodium phosphate and balanced electrolyte solutions containing polyethylene glycol (PEG). Sodium phosphate bowel preparations (e.g., Fleet's enema) are preferred by many patients and thus are a commonly used bowel preparation in adult patients, except for those who cannot tolerate the potential fluid and electrolyte shifts. Oral sodium phosphate preparations are strong osmotic laxatives that induce a number of endoscopic and histologic changes. The most common endoscopic change is the presence of what appears to be small aphthous (spot-like) lesions—small foci of pale mucosa surrounded by erythematous rings that look like shallow erosions. These aphthous-like lesions have been described in up to one quarter of patients after sodium phosphate bowel preparation. Histologically, these are usually large lymphoid aggregates, although some authors have described edema, hemorrhage, or acute inflammation (5). The lesions disappear when colonoscopy is repeated with an alternate bowel preparation and therefore are clinically unimportant. Oral sodium phosphate bowel preparation is also believed to induce foci of neutrophilic cryptitis—focal active colitis (FAC)—in about 3% of patients (e-Figs. 4.13 and 4.14). Whereas apoptosis is normal in the surface epithelium, scattered apoptotic bodies at the bases of crypts are found after sodium phosphate bowel preparation. These apoptotic bodies have been counted at about 1 per 10 well-oriented crypts in contrast to about 1 per 20 crypts in controls (5). However, since these preparations create alterations that overlap with the findings in various diseases and have some patient tolerance issues, more recently, many gastroenterologists have encouraged patients to use various preparations that contain PEG with electrolytes (miralax, glycolax, colyte, golytely, nulytely); these preparations seem to produce fewer histologic artifacts.

OTHER ENDOSCOPIC AND BIOPSY-RELATED ARTIFACTS

During the course of colonoscopy, gas is introduced to insufflate the bowel for better visualization of the mucosa. Small amounts of this gas may infiltrate tissue and appear as small, clear, bubble-like spaces in the mucosa or superficial submucosa, often in or near lymphoid aggregates. Because these spaces resemble adipocytes, this phenomenon has been termed "pseudolipomatosis" (6) (Fig. 4.5, e-Figs. 4.15 and 4.16). It lacks clinical importance and need not be reported, except perhaps in the uncommon event that it has created an endoscopic finding—a whitish, poorly demarcated, slightly raised plaque. Biopsy forceps can also induce tissue trauma, resulting in mucosal hemorrhage, crushing of epithelium that may resemble dysplasia, and an artifact in which the epithelium is squeezed entirely out of crypts leaving empty crypts. This "squeeze" artifact (e-Fig. 4.17) is common on the edges of mucosal biopsies and is usually readily recognized. However, when a large area is involved, it may be mistaken for ischemic injury. A common giveaway to this artifact is that the glands that have been "squeezed out" of their crypts are frequently seen detached but adjacent to the main tissue fragment with no significant signs of injury; additionally, the lamina propria around the missing glands is undamaged.

FOCAL ACTIVE COLITIS

FAC is the term used to describe focal neutrophilic infiltration of colonic crypts (e-Fig. 4.18). It may consist of one focus in a single biopsy, or multiple foci. Because focal inflammation is a feature of Crohn disease, studies

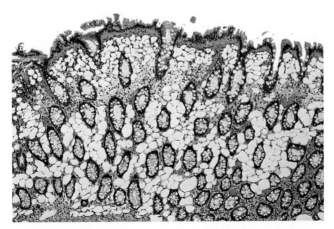

FIGURE 4.5 **Pseudolipomatosis.** Gas used to insufflate the bowel may penetrate the tissue and appear as clear, round spaces in the lamina propria resembling adipocytes.

of FAC have examined whether it antedates subsequent development or diagnosis of Crohn disease. In studies of adult patients with FAC in colon biopsies, very few have developed Crohn disease (7,8). Many seem to have a clinical course that resembles infectious diarrhea and about 20% have been shown to harbor *Campylobacter jejuni* by PCR (9), although this may have no relationship to the FAC and simply may reflect a common indication for endoscopy. In contrast, in a group of pediatric patients with FAC, a higher proportion (27.6%) went on to develop Crohn disease (10). In Greenson's studies, no adult patient with FAC developed Crohn disease (7,10), and the only endoscopic abnormalities were aphthous or aphthous-like ulcers, possibly artifacts of bowel preparation. In contrast, in the pediatric group, 2 of 17 patients with normal colonoscopy developed Crohn disease, compared with 6 of 11 with abnormal colonoscopy. Thus, it seems that in adult patients without history or the endoscopic features suggestive of Crohn disease, FAC can be safely ignored. However, it should be noted when reporting pediatric biopsies.

LAMINA PROPRIA MACROPHAGES

Macrophages are a normal constituent of the colonic lamina propria, where they serve roles in antigen processing and phagocytosis of surface epithelial cells that have undergone apoptosis. CD68 immunostaining highlights a gradient in their distribution, with more macrophages in the upper lamina propria and fewer in deeper areas (11). When pigmented macrophages are found, this is referred to as melanosis coli (Fig. 4.6). Macrophages containing mucin are called muciphages (e-Fig. 4.19).

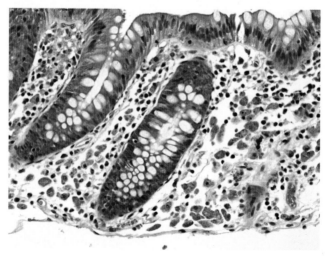

FIGURE 4.6 **Melanosis coli.** These pigmented macrophages in the lamina propria contain lipofuscin, not melanin.

When muciphages are present in otherwise normal biopsies, the usual gradient is reversed as they tend to accumulate in the lower part of the mucosa (e-Fig. 4.19). Muciphage aggregates are found associated with crypt rupture from any cause and are therefore seen in many settings (11), including in asymptomatic patients. Ultrastructural study supports degenerated epithelial cells as the source of the mucin (12). Muciphages must be distinguished from the macrophages of Whipple disease, mycobacterial infection, and carcinoma, but it is not usually necessary to perform a full workup in any given case because aggregates of muciphages are very common in colorectal mucosa; they are present in 40% of otherwise normal rectal biopsies (13). They are presumed to reflect occult and clinically unimportant epithelial injury, such as trauma related to stool passage, or subclinical infection. There is no need to note them in reports of otherwise normal colorectal mucosa. Sometimes macrophages contain barium from imaging studies (e-Figs. 4.20 and 4.21), which has a golden brown-to-yellow color and does not polarize strikingly.

The term melanosis coli is a misnomer. The brown pigment that accumulates in lamina propria macrophages in this condition is lipofuscin, not melanin (Fig. 4.6). Although it is most often seen in the cecum and rectum, it can be found throughout the colorectum, appendix, and terminal ileum. It is extremely common and is detected in the majority of elderly individuals. In one study of 200 patients, among men and women in the age group of 20 to 54 years, 32% of the men and 44% of the women were affected. For patients >75 years of age, 76% of the men and 67% of the women were affected (14). Lipofuscin accumulates by phagocytosis of apoptotic epithelial cells (15–17). There is a strong association with anthraquinone and other laxatives because they induce apoptosis (18–20). While many patients with melanosis do not report use of laxatives (15), some may be ingesting them inadvertently. One such example has been reported associated with ingestion of aloe-vera (which contains anthraquinones) as a "wellness drink" (21). Melanosis may result from any process associated with apoptosis, such as nonsteroidal anti-inflammatory drug (NSAID) use and has been described in patients with ulcerative colitis and Crohn colitis (22). In our practice, we typically mention melanosis coli if the finding is striking, or if the endoscopist reports seeing pigmented mucosa, but we ignore it otherwise.

Another type of lesion consists of nodules of lipid-laden macrophages that resemble xanthomas but appear in crops. These lesions have been likened to chicken skin and are called "chicken skin mucosa" by endoscopists (23–25) and were initially described in association with colonic polyps and neoplasms (23–25) (Figs. 4.7 and 4.8, e-Figs. 4.22–4.26). That notwithstanding, there is no evidence to suggest premalignant potential and "chicken skin mucosa" may only serve as a marker of local injury as this finding tends to be localized to the vicinity of large-volume polyps (23). We do mention the presence of lipid-laden macrophages in reports since it provides a histologic correlate for the endoscopic finding. Similarly, sometimes hemosiderin-laden macrophages are seen and should also be reported because they reflect resolving GI tract hemorrhage (e-Figs. 4.27 and 4.28).

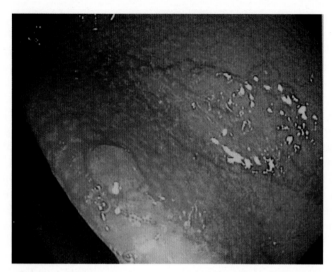

FIGURE 4.7 **Chicken skin mucosa.** These are nodules of lipid-laden macrophages.

REACTIVE CHANGES THAT CAN MIMIC NEOPLASIA

Signet Cell Change

Signet cell change describes a finding often seen in association with pseudomembranous colitis in which epithelium in damaged columnar mucosa becomes detached and begins to slough. As the cells detach from the basement membrane to be sloughed into the lumen, they round up and intracytoplasmic mucin can compress the nuclei, imparting an appearance like the cells in signet ring cell carcinomas. This phenomenon has been reported in

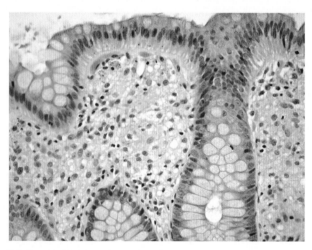

FIGURE 4.8 **Chicken skin mucosa.** Notice aggregates of lipid-laden macrophages within the lamina propria. These are a marker of local injury.

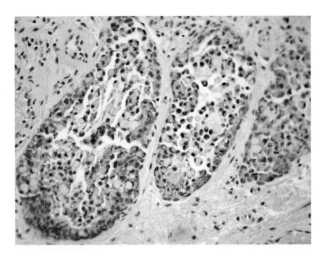

FIGURE 4.9 **Signet cell change.** The signet cells are contained within the basement membrane of damaged glands.

the upper GI tract as well as in the colon (26–29). Signet ring cell change is seen in cells contained within the basement membrane of damaged glands but can be quite striking at times (Fig. 4.9, e-Figs. 4.29 and 4.30). Since the cells in question tend to also feature reparative changes, they can appear especially alarming. In doubtful cases, an e-cadherin stain can be performed and will demonstrate intact membranous labeling (in contrast to many true signet cell carcinomas, which lose their labeling) (e-Fig. 4.30).

Atypical Stromal Cells

These cells can be encountered in polyps and ulcers anywhere in the GI tract (30,31) and the colon is not an exception. They are encountered in a rind at the interface where hypoxic necroinflammatory debris meets viable underlying granulation tissue. They have an alarming histologic appearance with features similar to those of pleomorphic sarcomas but differ by being encountered in a monolayer in an ulcer or polyp rather than by forming a mass themselves. They may be mitotically active with occasional atypical mitoses (Figs. 4.10 and 4.11, e-Fig. 4.31). If immunolabeling is performed, these cells are "vimentin only" fibroblasts (i.e., negative for keratins, S100 protein, CD117, desmin and usually negative with actins). In any doubtful case, resampling can be requested of the gastroenterologist, but most examples of atypical stromal cells in polyps and ulcers can be readily recognized as benign.

IDIOPATHIC INFLAMMATORY BOWEL DISEASE

Idiopathic IBD primarily includes chronic ulcerative colitis and Crohn disease. These differ in natural history, clinical, and pathologic associations; effective therapies; and response to treatment. These differences

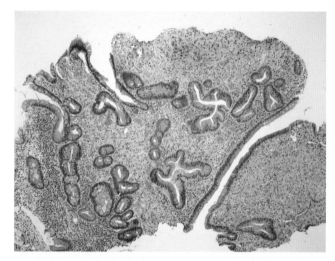

FIGURE 4.10 Atypical stromal cells. Notice atypical spindle cells within the lamina propria. These are often encountered in a rind at the interface where hypoxic necroinflammatory debris meets viable underlying granulation tissue.

underscore the importance of distinguishing between the two diseases. While classic cases can be separated, there may be gross, clinical, and histologic overlap of features—not only between ulcerative colitis and Crohn disease, but also with other inflammatory conditions of the colon. This results in an initial diagnosis of indeterminate colitis in up to 20% of cases of idiopathic IBD (32,33).

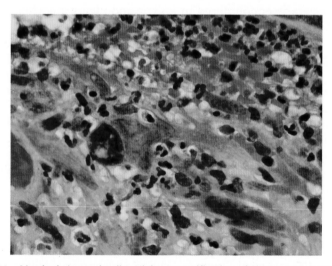

FIGURE 4.11 Atypical stromal cells. Higher magnification of Figure 4.10. Cytologic atypia can be alarming. These cells are seen in a monolayer in an ulcer or polyp without forming a mass.

ULCERATIVE COLITIS

Ulcerative colitis is a chronic crypt-destructive, inflammatory process of unknown cause, characterized by a predominantly mucosal-based disease and clinically associated with exacerbations and remissions of bloody diarrhea (1). There is no gender predilection. Disease presents at all ages with the major peak incidence in the 15- to 25-year age range and a minor peak in the 7th decade. There is a familial association: Up to 25% of patients have another affected family member. Ulcerative colitis is characterized by recurrent episodes of bloody diarrhea that can undergo spontaneous or therapy-induced remission. The initial presentation may be indolent in onset or may be a severe and acute presentation with toxic hemorrhagic colitis. In children, initial biopsies may be nondiagnostic because children are often brought for medical attention before histologic features of chronicity are evident (whereas adults wait until they have been symptomatic for months to years before seeking evaluation) (10,34,35).

The gross endoscopic appearance of ulcerative colitis varies with the degree of activity, duration of disease, and response to therapy (36). It is characterized by diffuse disease with rectal involvement extending proximally. In the more active phases, the mucosa is typically erythematous, bloody, friable, and has a granular appearance. Quiescent disease may appear granular with areas of punctuate erythema (e-Fig. 4.32). Pseudopolyps (mucosal remnants) and inflammatory polyps (e-Fig. 4.33) may be seen in active disease; postinflammatory (filiform) polyps (e-Fig. 4.34) may be seen in active or quiescent disease. In all cases, the normal submucosal vascular network is lost, and this is an important clue to the endoscopist, indicating chronic colitis. In patients who have had repeated bouts of colitis, the normal haustral folds may be absent. The transition between normal and abnormal mucosa is generally gradual but may be abrupt. Except for the occasional presence of focal cecal or periappendiceal ("cecal patch") involvement as "skip areas," (e-Fig. 4.35) there is no loss of disease continuity in untreated disease.

On biopsies, crypt architectural distortion and increased mucosal chronic inflammation are the two characteristic histologic findings. Neutrophils, the hallmark of active disease, are located within crypt epithelium (cryptitis) and crypt lumina (crypt abscesses), with fewer within the lamina propria around the crypts (Figs. 4.12 and 4.13, e-Figs. 4.8, 4.36–4.40). Architectural distortion results from prior mucosal destruction and imperfect repair, resulting in decreased numbers of crypts and shortened, branched, malformed, regenerated crypts. ("Crypt-destructive colitis" refers to the distortion of regenerated crypts, rather than acute injury of crypts due to cryptitis.) The chronic inflammatory components consist of variable numbers of plasma cells, eosinophils, and lymphocytes. Eosinophils may predominate. Lymphoid aggregates are commonly seen at the mucosal–submucosal interface. The regenerating epithelium is immature and, as such, does not contain mucin typical of a mature goblet cell (and thus

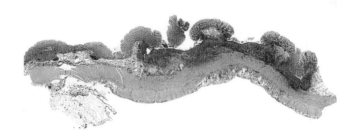

FIGURE 4.12 Ulcerative colitis. Notice lymphoid aggregates at the mucosal–submucosal interface. Mucosal remnants between ulcerated areas appear as polyps (pseudopolyps) to the endoscopist.

indicates mucin depletion). Biopsy fragments from the same topographic area typically show similar findings with the same degree of inflammation and injury (e-Fig. 4.41). Inflammation is usually more severe distally. Of course, granulomas are lacking, but occasionally, a foreign body response to a ruptured crypt may be found, which is in some respects a granuloma but reporting it as such will result in confusion with Crohn disease. Usually, the offending crypt can be found on serial sections and mucin associates with a foreign body–type giant cell, rather than a classic epithelioid granuloma (Fig. 4.14). Although Paneth cell metaplasia is common (e-Fig. 4.8), pyloric metaplasia is occasionally encountered in ulcerative colitis (e-Fig. 4.39 and 4.40), but it is more typical of Crohn disease. Of course, knowledge of upper tract findings is important because ulcerative colitis theoretically

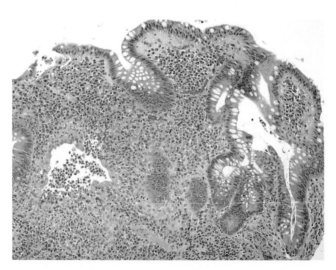

FIGURE 4.13 Ulcerative colitis. Crypt architectural distortion, lymphoplasmacytic expansion of the lamina propria, cryptitis, and crypt abscesses are all seen in this example. Notice immature regenerating epithelium devoid of mucin.

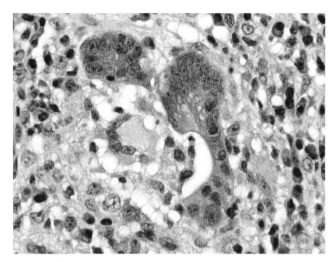

FIGURE 4.14 **Ulcerative colitis.** The center of the field shows a damaged crypt with a foreign body giant cell response. It is probably best to report such findings as "damaged crypts with foreign body responses" (if at all) since reporting such foci as "granulomas" may result in concern that a patient with well-established ulcerative colitis instead has Crohn disease.

involves only the colon and not the upper tract. However, some observers have reported diffuse duodenitis in patients who they otherwise would believe to have classic ulcerative colitis (37,38). Overall, however, most ulcerative colitis patients have no upper GI inflammation in biopsies, and most of the inflammatory lesions they have are not specific (39). The most common upper GI inflammatory pattern in patients with ulcerative colitis is focal gastritis, which is highly nonspecific, followed by gastric basal mixed inflammation and superficial plasmacytosis (e-Fig. 4.42, 4.43). The diffuse chronic duodenitis associated with ulcerative colitis seems to be a strong predictor of pouchitis (39).

When specimens are resected, the inflammatory process is confined predominantly to the mucosal surface, with an abrupt interface with the submucosa. At low magnification, the mucosa is cellular, often congested, has decreased numbers of crypts, and shows loss of the normal perpendicular or "test tube" arrangement of crypts. There may be lymphoid aggregates at the mucosal interface, which can be numerous. In areas of significant activity, ulcers can be adjacent to preserved mucosa. These mounds of residual mucosa, surrounded by ulcers, are termed "pseudopolyps." With time, as the adjacent mucosa regenerates, the mound may protrude and form an inflammatory polyp (Fig. 4.15, e-Fig. 4.44). The submucosa typically lacks significant inflammation and fibrosis. There is often edema and congestion. Transmural chronic inflammation and lymphoid aggregates are not present, except in areas of deep ulceration associated with toxic megacolon.

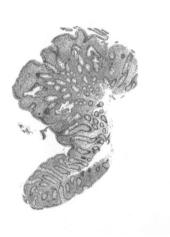

FIGURE 4.15 **Colonic inflammatory pseudopolyp.** The lower portion of the field shows essentially normal mucosa, whereas the upper portion of the field shows an inflammatory polyp.

No specific tests for ulcerative colitis are available, and genetic susceptibility tests are not currently suitable for clinical use, despite interesting advances (40). Initially, patients should be tested for infectious causes that are associated with long-standing and toxic colitis, to exclude *Shigella, Salmonella,* and *Campylobacter jejuni,* in particular. Patients who have a flare of ulcerative colitis, while being treated with immunosuppressives, may also benefit from testing for cytomegalovirus (CMV) infection, which can present with deep ulcers in the background of ulcerative colitis. Serologic tests for perinuclear antineutrophil cytoplasmic antibody (p-ANCA) are often reactive in patients with ulcerative colitis (but not Crohn disease).

Patients with IBD have, as their central defect, alterations in their gut immune surveillance, which causes them to have antibodies to various bacteria. Some observers have suggested a role for serology for antibodies to certain bacteria in diagnosis of IBD with inconsistent reported results for various markers. One commercial laboratory (Prometheus Laboratories) offers a panel consisting of the following:

Anti-*Saccharomyces cerevisiae* (ASCA) (both IgG and IgA based) by ELISA
Anti-*Escherichia coli* outer membrane porin (OmpC) by ELISA
Pseudomonas fluorescens–associated sequence 12 by ELISA
Flagellin CBIR1 by ELISA
p-ANCA by ELISA (see above)
p-ANCA by direct immunofluorescence
DNAse-sensitive p-ANCA by direct immunofluorescence

The company suggests that their panel will allow serology to separate out subtypes of IBD and distinguish it from IBS. Since each marker by itself lacks sufficient sensitivity and specificity to establish an accurate diagnosis, the panel approach is offered. In one pediatric study, however, the authors found the panel (about $450) less effective than routine CBC and ESR (about $100) in screening for IBD (41) but, once a diagnosis of inflammatory disease is established, it can sometimes help separate Crohn disease from ulcerative colitis (42,43). In general, ulcerative colitis correlates with p-ANCA and Crohn disease with ASCA.

Ulcerative colitis must be distinguished from infectious colitis, medication-induced colitis, ischemic colitis, and Crohn disease. Long-standing infectious colitis may display the features of ulcerative colitis, including increased chronic inflammation, neutrophils, basal plasmacytosis, and diffuse colonic involvement. A predominance of neutrophils within the lamina propria (rather than within the crypt epithelium), and overall architectural preservation, supports infectious over ulcerative colitis. The initial episode of ulcerative colitis may histologically appear similar to infectious colitis; therefore, infectious etiologies should be excluded prior to confirming a diagnosis of ulcerative colitis. Medications, particularly NSAIDs, may be associated with focal acute colitis or ulcers throughout the colon. Histologically, NSAID ulcers are typically abrupt, with no significant inflammation in the adjacent mucosa and with minimal chronic inflammation. Chronic ischemic colitis can be mistaken for ulcerative colitis, particularly because ischemia—due to low vascular flow—often affects the left colon and may be intermittent. As such, abrupt episodes of ischemia can result in mucosal ulceration which, following reperfusion, may become inflamed and show all of the architectural features of ulcerative colitis. Features that support ischemia include the age of the patient, location of the ulceration, involvement of the muscularis propria, and importantly, the lack of neutrophils destroying crypt epithelium. Crohn lesions characterized by crypt destruction are typically patchy, with areas that appear involved and others that appear uninvolved, within single biopsies and among different fragments from one area. Crohn colitis typically lacks the diffuse crypt destruction that is characteristic of ulcerative colitis.

There is no curative therapy for ulcerative colitis. Treatment goals include inducing and maintaining remission, minimizing side effects, and improving the quality of life. Standard therapy includes anti-inflammatory drugs, specifically the 5-ASA compounds (sulfasalazine and other salicylates), which are effective in preventing exacerbations in patients in remission. Steroids, either topical (enemas) or systemic, are effective in treating acute exacerbations. Once a patient is treated, the characteristic distribution of ulcerative colitis may become altered. Thus, a patient may display iatrogenic rectal sparing, something that should be remembered by pathologists interpreting biopsies from treated patients (the usual case). Most patients have mild-to-moderately active disease, which does not require colectomy. Although uncommon, if mortality does occur, it is usually in the first 2 years of the disease and results from severe fulminant disease (toxic colitis). Mortality may also result from disease-associated complications, including colorectal carcinoma, primary sclerosing cholangitis, therapeutic complications, and thromboembolic disease. Colectomy is required in up to 20% of patients, usually within the first 2 years for fulminant disease. Colectomy is also performed following the detection of dysplasia or adenocarcinoma.

Long-standing ulcerative colitis is associated with an increased risk of dysplasia and adenocarcinoma, even in patients with well-controlled, quiescent disease. Periodic colonoscopic exams are used to survey for dysplasia and adenocarcinoma. Routine surveillance with biopsies is recommended annually for patients with extensive disease of >8 years' duration because there is an increasing annual incidence of adenocarcinoma. Biopsies are generally taken from the cecum, ascending, splenic flexure, transverse, hepatic flexure, descending, and sigmoid colon; and rectum. The pathologist records evidence of colitis, inflammatory activity, and the presence or absence of dysplasia. As noted above, these surveillance biopsies often lack the typical distribution of ulcerative colitis because it has been altered by treatment. But, this should not prompt a diagnosis of Crohn disease, but of treated ulcerative colitis instead (44,45). Dysplasia and carcinoma in this setting are further addressed in Volume 2. The clinicopathologic features of ulcerative colitis are summarized in Table 4.2.

CROHN DISEASE

Crohn disease (regional enteritis, granulomatous enterocolitis, and terminal ileitis) is a chronic, relapsing, and remitting inflammatory disease of unknown etiology that is often multifocal and can affect any portion of the GI tract. Its hallmarks include focally distributed glandular destruction, aphthous erosions, and serpiginous ulcers, as well as transmural inflammation, fibrosis, and sometimes granulomas. Because of its transmural nature, fissures, sinuses, and fistulas may develop. Crohn disease has an equal gender incidence and occurs at all ages, with the major peak incidence between 20 and 30 years of age. The initial presentation may be indolent, or acute and severe. The symptoms are variable but often include cramping pain, typically localized to the right lower quadrant; nonbloody diarrhea; fever; malaise; and anorexia. These findings may mimic acute appendicitis. Although the appendix may be involved with Crohn disease, appendicitis as a presenting feature is extremely rare. Hemorrhage and hematochezia are uncommon, but chronic blood loss can result from erosions and ulcers. Patients with upper intestinal disease may present with dyspepsia, weight loss, hypoalbuminemia, and iron deficiency anemia, mimicking celiac disease. Fistulas (enterovaginal, enterovesical, and enterocutaneous) may result in the passage of blood, feces, pus, and air from the vagina, urethra, or skin. In some cases, fissuring necrosis with fistula formation is the main complication; in others, stenosis predominates. Anal and perianal

TABLE 4.2 Features of Ulcerative Colitis

Definition

A chronic idiopathic IBD with episodes of bloody diarrhea, and histologically characterized by mucosal-based, chronic crypt-destructive colitis with continuous involvement from the rectum extending proximally

Incidence

Uncommon (4 to 20 people out of 100,000 annually)

Higher incidence in North America, Western Europe, South Africa

Demographics

Equal female-to-male ratio

Caucasians > other ethnic groups

Jewish > other religious groups

Rare in first decade of life

Major peak at 15–25 years of age

Minor peak at 60–70 years of age

Familial association: Up to 25% have affected relative

Clinical

Recurrent episodes of bloody diarrhea

Endoscopic

Active phase: Mucosa erythematous, bloody, friable, and granular

Quiescent phase: Mucosa granular with punctuate erythema; loss of haustral folds (tube-like appearance)

Polyps: Pseudopolyps (mucosal remnants) and inflammatory polyps in active disease; postinflammatory polyps in active or quiescent disease

All phases: Normal submucosal vascular network is lost

Biopsy findings

Crypt architectural distortion

Increased mucosal chronic inflammation

Neutrophils, the hallmark of active disease, are located within crypt epithelium (cryptitis) and crypt lumens (crypt abscesses)

Lymphoid aggregates commonly seen at mucosal–submucosal interface

Regenerating epithelium is immature and does not contain mucin (mucin depletion)

Biopsy fragments from the same topographic area typically show similar findings

Inflammation is usually more severe distally

Differential diagnosis

Infectious colitis

Medication-induced colitis (especially NSAIDs)

Ischemic colitis

Crohn disease

NSAIDs, nonsteroidal anti-inflammatory drugs.

fissures and fistulas are often a component of Crohn disease, but rarely of ulcerative colitis. Inflammatory changes can occur in joints, eyes, liver, and skin. Approximately 10% of patients have an affected family member.

There is little correlation between the endoscopic appearance and the clinical symptoms. The endoscopic appearance of Crohn disease is most consistently a multifocal process. Aphthous erosions, longitudinal ulcers (tram track or rake ulcers), and adjacent areas of erythematous or grossly unremarkable mucosa are the key features. Additional endoscopic findings include cobblestoning (alternating ulcers and edematous mucosa), strictures, and fissures. The ileum typically shows focal or asymmetric involvement by Crohn disease. This may include erosions, ulcers, and/or strictures. The rectum is often spared (unlike in untreated ulcerative colitis). Inflammatory polyps may be present. Rarely, Crohn disease may become confluent, involving the entire bowel, which can be diagnostically misleading for both the endoscopist and the pathologist. In both Crohn disease and ulcerative colitis, the normal submucosal vascular network is lost in the involved areas.

Resection is typically reserved for patients with severe complications, such as obstruction due to strictures, fistulas, perforation, severe chronic anemia, or hemorrhage (Fig. 4.16, e-Figs. 4.45 and 4.46). Since milder disease is not resected, the gross pathologic findings are usually striking when resection is performed. The subserosal fat (so-called "creeping fat") is often firm and contracted over areas of involvement. Longitudinal opening of the bowel may reveal areas of normal bowel wall thickness and other areas of the bowel that are firm, thickened, and pipe-like. The mucosa may show aphthous erosions, longitudinal "rake" ulcers, cobblestoning, polyps, fissures, and fistulas. The process is usually multifocal, often with rectal sparing but may become confluent. When confluent, the firm, pipe-like nature of the bowel may help to distinguish Crohn disease from ulcerative colitis, in which fibrosis is unusual.

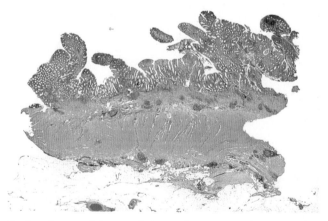

FIGURE 4.16 **Crohn disease.** Microscopic image from a resection. Note the transmural lymphoid aggregates arranged in a pattern reminiscent of a string of pearls.

Mucosal biopsies, although superficial, can show features that are suggestive of Crohn disease. For example, when several biopsies from the same general site are received in a single container, often, even at low magnification, it is clear that each of the fragments has a different degree of inflammation and some might be completely uninflamed (e-Fig. 4.47). Discrete foci of inflammation, often associated with neutrophils within crypts (cryptitis) adjacent to histologically normal crypts, are common. Aphthous erosions or ulcers, characterized by focal surface epithelial necrosis associated with a mixed chronic inflammatory infiltrate and sometimes associated with underlying lymphoid aggregates, are typical early lesions (e-Fig. 4.48). As above, variability of inflammation within a single biopsy, and among several biopsy fragments from the same anatomic location, is also typical. The areas of inflammation show architectural changes of chronic crypt-destructive colitis, while adjacent crypts may appear normal (Fig. 4.17, e-Fig. 4.49). Fissures may be apparent even on mucosal biopsies (Fig. 4.18, e-Fig. 4.50). Granulomas are infrequent but, when present, are usually poorly formed and associated with chronic inflammation (Fig. 4.19, e-Figs. 4.51–4.54). Finding necrotizing or particularly exuberant granulomas should prompt a diligent search for organisms (Fig. 4.20, e-Fig. 4.55–4.61).

If submucosa is present in the biopsy, there may be significant submucosal chronic inflammation, while the overlying mucosa may only be slightly expanded by chronic inflammatory cells, a feature absent in infectious or ulcerative colitis. Terminal ileal involvement includes increased lamina propria inflammation, aphthous erosions, and flattened and broad villi. Pyloric metaplasia (mucinous glands, reminiscent of the antral or pyloric mucosa) indicates repeated bouts of inflammation and repair

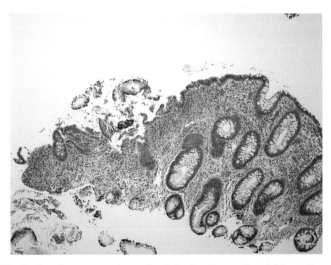

FIGURE 4.17 Crohn disease, early and subtle findings. The right portion of the field appears essentially normal, whereas there is a suggestion of erosion in the left portion of the field.

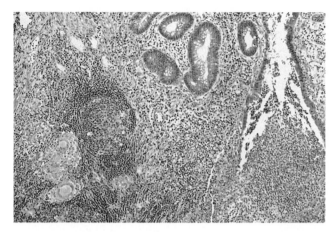

FIGURE 4.18 **Crohn disease.** This image shows a fissure on the right and granulomatous inflammation on the left.

(Fig. 4.21). Unfortunately, focal acute ileitis is most commonly caused by medications, particularly NSAIDs, rather than Crohn disease. Medication-induced injury is usually not associated with increased lamina propria inflammation or pyloric metaplasia. Submucosal fibrosis can also follow NSAID damage. Peyer patches are a normal component of the terminal ileum, particularly in young individuals, and should not be diagnosed as chronic inflammation. The mucosa over Peyer patches may be distorted, showing flattened villi due to underlying expansion of lymphoid nodules in nonspecific reactive hyperplasia or from infections (e.g., yersiniosis).

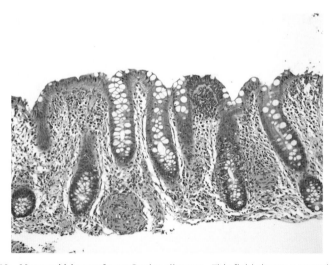

FIGURE 4.19 **Mucosal biopsy from Crohn disease.** This field shows a granuloma on the left and cryptitis on the right.

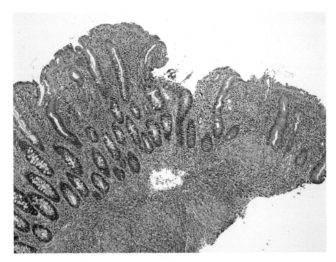

FIGURE 4.20 **Crohn disease complicated by histoplasmosis.** Exuberant or necrotizing granulomatous inflammation should prompt a search for microorganisms, as granulomas in the setting of Crohn disease are nonnecrotizing, poorly formed, and not prominent.

No specific tests for Crohn colitis are available. However, as with ulcerative colitis, exclusion of infectious etiologies is important, particularly *Yersinia* infection (Fig. 4.22). As above, serologic testing for ASCA can be helpful; approximately 70% of Crohn patients are positive, and usually ulcerative colitis patients are negative. In cases where there is difficulty distinguishing between ulcerative colitis and Crohn colitis, performance of both ASCA and p-ANCA may help in the differential diagnosis since

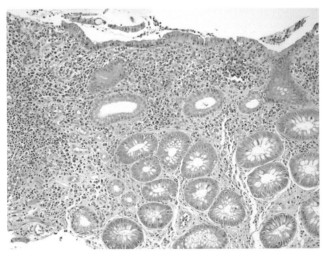

FIGURE 4.21 **Crohn disease.** Pyloric metaplasia can be seen in the setting of Crohn disease and indicates repeated bouts of ulceration and repair.

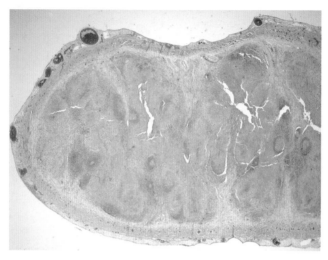

FIGURE 4.22 **Yersinia enterocolitis/appendicitis.** Necrotizing granulomas should suggest an infectious etiology rather than Crohn disease.

p-ANCA is positive in approximately 70% of ulcerative colitis patients and in 10% to 30% of Crohn patients. However, there is overlap in the results between Crohn and ulcerative colitis, and adding additional markers can sometimes refine the testing, something that has been exploited in the so-called Prometheus test, outlined in the section above on ulcerative colitis. As noted above, despite promising information concerning the *NOD2/CARD15* gene and other colitis-associated genes, it remains premature to offer genetic screening on patients.

Crohn colitis must be distinguished from infectious colitis, medication-associated colitis, and ulcerative colitis. The endoscopic finding of focal aphthous erosions of early Crohn colitis may be similar to erosions caused by medications, bowel preparation, and infections. Erosions of Crohn disease are associated with a chronic inflammatory infiltrate. Infectious colitis is characterized by a predominance of neutrophils, rather than lymphocytes and plasma cells. Medication-induced erosions (from NSAIDs and others) usually have negligible acute inflammation; typically, only a few neutrophils appear in the area of erosion. The more advanced changes of Crohn colitis, particularly discrete ulcers and masses seen endoscopically, must also be distinguished from medications and infection. NSAID ulcers may be multiple and deep. They tend to be on the top of mucosal folds and are circumferential, rather than longitudinal. Biopsies often show fibrosis with only minimal inflammation. NSAID strictures may form; when these are circumferential, they are termed "diaphragms", especially in the small bowel. Bowel wall thickening and heaped up masses may be seen in *Yersinia* infection, particularly in the terminal ileum and right colon. The presence of marked inflammation histologically, with numerous granulomas and the clinical information of a mass or stricture, may lead to a diagnosis of Crohn disease in a patient with yersiniosis or histoplasmosis. Features that suggest infection over Crohn disease include numerous granulomas, granulomas centered in lymphoid follicles, and granulomas with central necrosis. Any specimen with numerous granulomas should suggest infection over Crohn disease.

Fulminant Crohn colitis is difficult or impossible to distinguish from ulcerative colitis in a mucosal biopsy specimen because many of the distinguishing features are deep to the mucosa. Furthermore, in fulminant (toxic) ulcerative colitis, inflammation may become transmural. In resection specimens, the most important features are the presence of transmural lymphoid aggregates and the presence of occasional poorly formed granulomas at all levels of the bowel wall. The effects of treatment can also cause diagnostic difficulty, as treated ulcerative colitis may show areas of involved and uninvolved mucosa, and variable degrees of disease activity. It is important to review original pretreatment material, if possible, to help distinguish between ulcerative colitis and Crohn disease because patients with ulcerative colitis are candidates for ileal pouch anal anastomosis (IPAA). Those with Crohn disease, however, are poor candidates for IPAA because of the high risk of pouch failure due to anastomotic breakdown.

Since Crohn disease is incurable, treatment goals focus on inducing and maintaining remission, minimizing side effects, and improving the quality of life. Standard therapy includes anti-inflammatory drugs, specifically the 5-ASA compounds (sulfasalazine and other salicylates), and steroids. Infliximab (Remicade) and related drugs (adalimumab/Humira, etanercept/Enbrel), monoclonal antibodies (mAbs) against tumor necrosis factor-α (TNF-α), have been helpful in treating acute episodes of Crohn colitis, particularly fistulas and other complications (46). Budesonide (Entocort), a topical steroid that is taken orally, has also been shown to be very effective in treating ileal Crohn disease (47). It is locally absorbed and metabolized in the liver, thereby reducing the systemic side effects associated with other steroids. Surgery is reserved for patients who are unresponsive to medical therapy. Patients who have undergone surgical intervention are at an increased risk of requiring additional surgery for anastomotic complications (strictures, anastomotic leaks, and fistulas).

Recent improvements in therapy have markedly decreased the mortality and morbidity of Crohn disease. The most significant complications are seen in the first few years of the disease; younger patients tend to have more active disease, perhaps due to an active immune system, which diminishes with age. The most common complications include perianal fistulas, toxic colitis, anemia, arthritis, and drug-associated problems. Patients who have strictures tend not to have fistulas and vice versa. Key features of Crohn disease are summarized in Table 4.3.

Granulomatous inflammation may be a manifestation of Crohn disease in extraintestinal sites such as lymph nodes, lungs, and skin (e-Figs. 4.62 and 4.63 [lung], e-Figs. 4.64 and 4.65 [skin]). Diagnosis requires a high index of

TABLE 4.3 Crohn Colitis

Definition

A chronic multifocal, relapsing and remitting, progressive inflammatory disease that can affect any portion of the GI tract, it is typically characterized by foci of epithelial destruction, aphthous erosions, and serpiginous ulcers, as well as transmural inflammation, fibrosis, and granulomas in the small and large bowel

Incidence

Uncommon (5–20 people of 100,000 annually)

Higher incidence in North America, Northern Europe

Demographics

Equal female-to-male distribution

Caucasians > other ethnic groups

Ashkenazi Jews > other religious groups

Major peak at 20–30 years of age

Minor peak at 60–70 years of age

Familial association: approximately 10% have affected relative

Clinical

Cramping pain, nonbloody diarrhea, fever, malaise, and anorexia

Hemorrhage and hematochezia are uncommon

Upper intestinal disease: dyspepsia, weight loss, hypoalbuminemia, and iron deficiency anemia

Fistulas, stenosis

Anal and perianal fissures, and fistulas

Inflammatory changes can occur in joints, eyes, liver, and skin

Endoscopic

Aphthous erosions

Longitudinal ulcers (tram track or rake ulcers) and adjacent unremarkable mucosa

Cobblestoning

Strictures

Fissures and fistulas

Terminal ileal involvement

Submucosal vascular network lost

Frequent rectal sparing

Biopsy features

Discrete foci of inflammation and architectural changes adjacent to histologically normal crypts

Aphthous erosions often associated with underlying lymphoid aggregates

(continued)

TABLE 4.3 **Crohn Colitis** (*Continued*)
Variability of inflammation within a single biopsy and among several biopsy fragments from the same anatomic location
Granulomas uncommon and, if present, are poorly formed and associated with chronic inflammation
Submucosal chronic inflammation disproportionate to that in the overlying mucosa
Terminal ileal involvement: Aphthous erosions; distorted, flattened villi; pyloric metaplasia
Differential diagnosis
Infectious colitis
Medication-associated colitis (especially NSAIDs)
Ulcerative colitis

GI, gastrointestinal; NSAIDs, nonsteroidal anti-inflammatory drugs.

suspicion, correlation with clinical history, and exclusion of infectious etiologies. This is occasionally referred to as "metastatic" Crohn disease.

POUCHITIS

Although, technically, pouchitis is a topic for the nonneoplastic small bowel (Chapter 3), it is included here because the continent pouch plays the role of a rectum. When Kock described the creation of a continent ileoanal operation to create a continent pouch that could function as a rectum, he described an inflammatory lesion that followed, and it has been referred to as "pouchitis" (48–50). Pouchitis is different from "diversion colitis" found in blind pouches (Hartmann pouches), in contrast to continent ones such as Kock pouches or IPAA. In a nutshell, the problem in pouchitis is that there really are no absolute histologic criteria to determine whether the inflammation in a pouch is a reflection of the response of the ileal mucosa to serving as a rectum, or a manifestation of recurrent inflammatory disease. When the pouch has been created after a colectomy for a neoplasm or familial adenomatous polyposis (FAP), rather than for inflammatory disease, it is easier to dismiss the possibility of recurrent inflammatory disease. But, this is the minority of cases. In one study, pathologic features that were associated with the subsequent development of pouchitis included the presence of severe colitis that extended into the cecum (severe pancolitis), early fissuring ulcers, active inflammation of the appendix, and appendiceal ulceration (51). No significant differences in patient gender or age, depth or extent of ulceration, or the presence or absence of "backwash ileitis" were identified in patients with pouchitis versus those without it. However, other observers have found an association between "backwash ileitis" and subsequent pouchitis (52). As noted above, the diffuse chronic duodenitis associated with ulcerative colitis seems to be a strong predictor of pouchitis (39). The incidence of pouchitis has a wide range; about half of patients have at least one episode (53), but it is not usually sufficiently severe to merit revision of the pouch. The cause of pouchitis remains unclear, but factors cited include stasis, immunologic alterations, and epithelial damage (53).

The classic histologic description includes neutrophilic inflammation in acute pouchitis and classic features of chronicity with villous atrophy in the chronic setting, all features that are identical to those of ulcerative colitis or Crohn disease (54,55) (e-Figs. 4.66–4.70). In fact, pyloric metaplasia is even seen in some examples and appears identical to that in the ileum in Crohn disease (56) (Fig. 4.21). Some observers have offered criteria that they believe establish the diagnosis of pouchitis in the presence of diarrhea and inflammation visible on sigmoidoscopy, which include a moderate-to-severe polymorphonuclear infiltrate in >25% of a low-power field (57). But, these criteria certainly do not exclude infection or that the presumed ulcerative colitis patient actually has Crohn disease. In some studies, pouchitis is classified as type A, B, or C, as follows. Type A is defined as normal mucosa or mild villous atrophy with no or mild inflammation. Type B mucosa shows transient atrophy with temporary, moderate inflammation followed by normalization of architecture. Type C mucosa is defined as a pattern of persistent atrophy with severe inflammation (58). Some patients (type C) experience striking villous atrophy, and this may be the precursor to the small number of patients who develop dysplasia in their pouches (58–60). In daily practice, we do not list response types as above. We do make some attempt to report the degree of inflammation and the presence of extensive atrophy, and we allow our clinical colleagues to form the correlation with the endoscopic findings. A pouchitis activity disease index has been developed that combines clinical, endoscopic, and microscopic findings (61). Initial treatment is usually with metronidazole or other combinations of antibiotics.

A more distressing concern in interpreting biopsies, from patients believed to have ulcerative colitis at the time of resection, revolves around the occasional patient who develops pouch complications that are indistinguishable from Crohn disease. The conclusion of surgical and endoscopic colleagues is generally that the pathologist has misdiagnosed the resection specimen with ulcerative colitis when the patient, in fact, has Crohn disease. In some instances, this may be the case because patients with Crohn disease, in whom a continent pouch is attempted, have terrible complications about half the time. Most surgeons avoid creating continent pouches in individuals for whom there is no clear diagnosis. (In patients with "indeterminate colitis," severe pouch complications are documented about 20% of the time; in ulcerative colitis, complications occur in about 8% to 10% of cases.) However, there is a small set of patients with classic ulcerative colitis who develop an idiosyncratic, Crohn-like disease in their continent pouch, which requires revision. Being aware of this phenomenon can be occasionally useful (62).

"CUFFITIS"

Often, when pouches are created in patients with ulcerative colitis, a slender ring of the original rectal mucosa is present at the anastomosis between the small bowel (pouch) and upper anus (squamous-line) (e-Figs. 4.71–4.74). This short zone is termed the rectal cuff. As such, it remains diseased and thus can be inflamed and encountered on biopsies that are performed for surveillance of the patient's pouch. The pathologist may encounter relatively uninflamed small bowel mucosa (e-Figs. 4.71 and 4.72) and highly damaged residual rectal mucosa with "cuffitis" (e-Figs 4.73 and 4.74). The risk of neoplasia is low (about 1%) in this residual pocket of rectal mucosa, but, not surprisingly, most likely to be encountered in patients whose resections were performed for neoplasia complicating their ulcerative colitis (63). Based on the concern for neoplasia in the residual rectal cuff, mucosal stripping has been advocated by some, but this can lead to pouch complications and is probably not justified in all patients with ulcerative colitis but is probably worth performing in individuals with ulcerative colitis-associated dysplasia/carcinoma who undergo proctocolectomy with ileoanal pullthrough (64).

EOSINOPHILIC COLITIS

Attempting to diagnose eosinophilic colitis is frustrating since there are no references that allow clear diagnostic criteria. In contrast to the esophagus, which displays a monolayer of epithelium and minimal lamina propria on biopsies such that it is easy to perform counts of eosinophils per high-power field (and thus for which there are suggested cutoffs for abnormal numbers of intraepithelial eosinophils in various conditions), colon biopsies display minimal epithelium compared to lamina propria and eosinophils in the lamina propria of the colon are a normal finding. The number of eosinophils in the lamina propria of the colons of healthy individuals is highly variable and is influenced by geography (3,65), season (66), and location in the colon (there are more eosinophils in the right colon) (66). In a formal study of counts of normal persons, occasional (1 to 4 eosinophils/4 consecutive crypts) were seen in approximately half of mucosal biopsy samples from the ascending colon; eosinophils were always present singly in the crypt epithelium and were virtually absent from the epithelium of the descending colon (66). The lamina propria in 4 consecutive intercrypt spaces contained 30 to 45 eosinophils in the right colon and 7 to 22 eosinophils in the left colon (66). Thus, we typically ignore a few intraepithelial eosinophils in colon biopsies and also do not bother to count eosinophils in the lamina propria. However, if there are numerous intraepithelial eosinophils and eosinophils

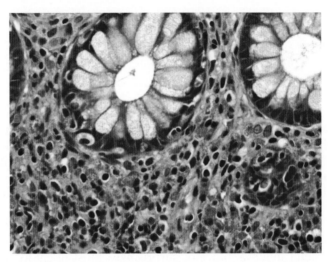

FIGURE 4.23 **Eosinophilic colitis pattern.** Finding numerous intraepithelial and lamina propria eosinophils is an abnormal but nonspecific finding that requires clinical correlation.

in the muscularis mucosae (Fig. 4.23, e-Fig. 4.75–4.77), we regard this as an abnormal finding and report it with a note that the eosinophilia should be correlated with peripheral blood eosinophilia and other allergic manifestations such as atopy and asthma. In infants, finding rectal intraepithelial eosinophils can correlate with milk allergy and atopy (67), but in older children, there seems to be little correlation between biopsies reported with eosinophilic colitis and other stigmata of allergic disease (68). Of course, prominent colonic eosinophils can be encountered in patients with IBD, medication allergies, parasitic infections, mastocytosis, and Langerhans cell histiocytosis (LCH), so their presence is hardly specific.

INFECTIOUS COLITIS

Acute self-limited colitis is used here to invoke the features of colitis secondary to various bacteriologic etiologies, with the exception of enterohemorrhagic *Escherichia coli* (mentioned below), since it produces an ischemic colitis appearance. Such cases display neutrophils with crypt abscesses that tend to appear in the upper half of the mucosa and prominent neutrophils in the lamina propria (69) (Figs. 4.24–4.26, e-Figs. 4.78–4.80). The basal plasmacytosis seen in ulcerative colitis and Crohn colitis is lacking (70) (e-Fig. 4.80). Glandular architecture is preserved. Erosions and lamina propria edema may be seen. The course is self-limited and correlates with pertinent stool cultures. As acute self-limiting colitis heals (which has often occurred by the time biopsies are taken), there are reactive epithelial changes, but crypt architecture remains intact.

As for specific infectious agents affecting the colon, bacterial colitis is often a result of *Campylobacter sp.* or *Aeromonas sp.*, but culture is

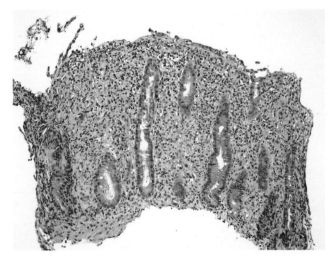

FIGURE 4.24 **Acute colitis.** Biopsies of patients with infectious colitis tend to show a neutrophilic infiltrate that predominates superficially within the crypts and lamina propria. There is no basal plasmacytosis or significant architectural distortion.

required for precise typing. Of course, CMV infection, and various parasites, may be encountered in many settings in which patients are immuno-suppressed (Fig. 4.27, e-Figs. 4.81–4.87). The ova of schistosomes can be encountered and *Strongyloides* is occasionally found on colon biopsies. Sometimes human immunodeficiency virus (HIV) patients have a peculiar giant cell colitis (e-Fig. 4.88) (71), apparent on colon biopsies.

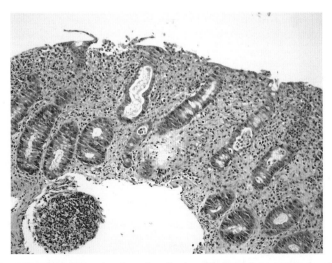

FIGURE 4.25 **Acute colitis.** Biopsies of patients with infectious colitis tend to show a neutrophilic infiltrate that predominates superficially within the crypts and lamina propria. There is no basal plasmacytosis or significant architectural distortion.

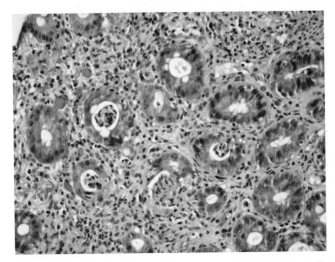

FIGURE 4.26 **Acute colitis.** This higher magnification of figure 4.25 better illustrates reactive epithelial changes often seen in association with infectious colitis.

Colonic spirochetosis is a peculiar condition in which numerous, unusual Warthin-Starry reactive organisms carpet the colon surface (Figs. 4.28 and 4.29, e-Figs. 4.89–4.92). It has been associated with abdominal pain, appendicitis, chronic diarrhea, and rectal bleeding in some cases. But in the majority of cases, spirochetosis is an incidental finding with no clear clinical correlates. The mucosa may appear entirely normal to the endoscopist or may show areas of ulceration, erosion, edema, and/ or erythema (72–74). The anaerobic intestinal spirochetes *Brachyspira*

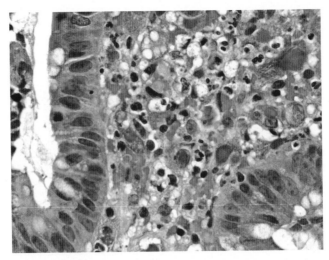

FIGURE 4.27 **Cytomegalovirus (CMV) colitis.** The cell in the center shows the classic intranuclear inclusion associated with CMV, while the cell on the right shows a smudged chromatin pattern and intracytoplasmic inclusions.

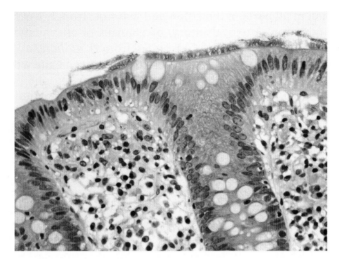

FIGURE 4.28 **Intestinal spirochetosis.** Anaerobic intestinal spirochetes carpet the epithelial surface in this case of colonic spirochetosis.

aalborgi and *Brachyspira pilosicoli* seem to be responsible for most cases of spirochetosis. *B. pilosicoli* colonizes the intestinal tract of many animal species, especially pigs, and can be found in approximately 30% of feces from persons in developing countries. Koteish et al. have reported a retrospective analysis of colonic spirochetosis in 14 cases, including 4 children and 10 adults seen at our hospital (75). Two men had HIV infections. All children and both HIV-infected men had abdominal complaints, diarrhea, or both. Most other adults underwent colonoscopy for polyp screening (four) and follow-up of Crohn disease (one). Histologically, spirochetosis

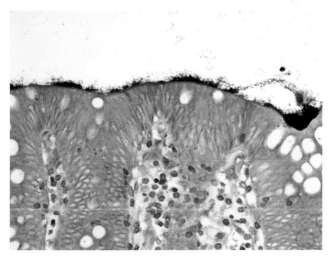

FIGURE 4.29 **Intestinal spirochetosis.** This Warthin-Starry stain highlights the surface spirochetes.

was identified in all parts of the colon and was not strongly associated with active inflammation, mucosal injury, or changes of chronicity. Genotype analysis of 13 cases showed that 11 resulted from *B. aalborgi* and 2 from *B. pilosicoli* infections. Only 2 patients were treated specifically with antibiotics, with complete resolution of abdominal symptoms in one patient with follow-up. Follow-up biopsy results were available for 2 patients who did not receive treatment; one showed persistent spirochetosis, and the other was negative. Spirochetosis in this series had a male predominance, was generally caused by *B. aalborgi*, and occurred in two distinct clinical settings: Children who often have abdominal symptoms and adults who are typically asymptomatic. A Spanish group identified the organism in 0.7% of patients with chronic watery diarrhea (76). The same authors noticed mild lamina propria expansion by inflammatory cells in 7 of 10 affected patients. Symptomatic patients are typically treated with metronidazole, while antibiotics are not typically administered to asymptomatic individuals.

It is well-known that a large number of infectious processes can mimic idiopathic inflammatory disease. Generally, the features of *Campylobacter*, *Salmonella*, and *Shigella* are distinguished from IBD by the proclivity of responding neutrophils to involve the lamina propria (more than the glands), and the lack of architectural distortion and basal plasmacytosis. But overlapping features do occur. Necrotizing epithelioid granulomatous inflammation may accompany *Yersinia pseudotuberculosis*, and aggregates of macrophages may accompany *Yersinia enterocolitica* (Fig. 4.22, e-Figs. 4.93 and 4.94). Although granulomas may raise the possibility of Crohn disease, these tend to be bigger and more prominent in the setting of *Yersinia* infection. To the extent that the morphologic features of pseudomembranous colitis (Figs. 4.30 and 4.31, e-Figs. 4.95 and 4.96) and

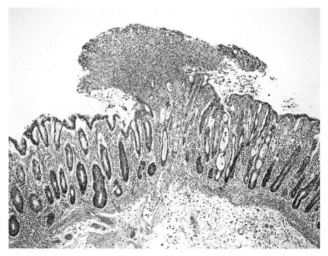

FIGURE 4.30 **Pseudomembranous colitis.** Note the exudative appearance of the pseudomembrane and the relative preservation of crypt architecture.

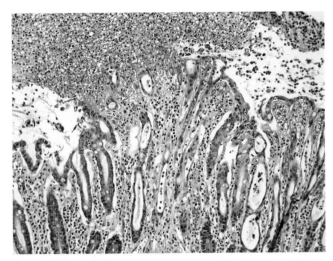

FIGURE 4.31 Pseudomembranous colitis, higher magnification of figure 4.30. Note the predominance of neutrophils with little expansion of the lamina propria by chronic inflammatory cells.

enterohemorrhagic *E. coli* colitis mimic IBD, these must also be considered (although these mimic ischemic effects more than they mimic IBD). The proclivity for GI histoplasmosis to mimic IBD has been emphasized by Lamps et al. (77). The presentation of IBD and GI histoplasmosis can be identical (fever, malaise, GI bleeding, diarrhea, nausea and vomiting, ulcers, fissures, perforation, and colitis), and the histologic presence of granulomas and full-thickness inflammation can lead to an interpretation of Crohn colitis (e-Figs. 4.97–4.99). The disease may be seen in nonendemic areas and in immunocompetent hosts. Ulcerated areas should always be screened for *E. histolytica* (amebic colitis) (Fig. 4.32, e-Figs. 4.100–4.103) and CMV. The former tends to appear in the exudate itself, whereas the latter is found frequently in endothelial and, less frequently, epithelial cells. The classic, targetoid CMV intranuclear inclusion is often not evident and, instead, the only histologic clue to the diagnosis is a large nucleus with smudged chromatin pattern. CMV-infected cells may also show intracytoplasmic inclusions. Adenovirus may involve the bowel in immunocompetent individuals, in which it invokes an impressive lymphoid response (particularly in the terminal ileum), and is accompanied by loss of nuclear polarity and subtle basophilic intranuclear inclusions without cytoplasmic counterparts (61) (e-Figs. 4.104 and 4.105). The virus typically infects goblet cells, which may appear aberrant with the characteristic mucin vacuole located underneath, instead of above the nucleus (78). The necrotizing granulomas associated with *Yersinia sp.* are lacking in adenovirus infection. Adenovirus proctocolitis is often overlooked on biopsy material and has been reported to coinfect with CMV about one third of the time (78). Immunohistochemical staining for adenovirus may be of value in doubtful cases. *Mycobacterium avium*

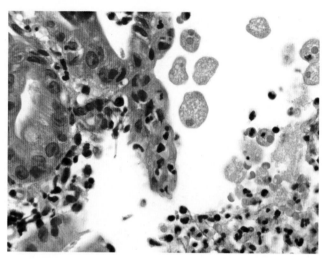

FIGURE 4.32 **Amebic colitis.** These organisms are often found within ulcer-associated exudates.

complex (e-Figs. 4.106–4.108), other Mycobacteria (e-Fig. 4.109–4.112), *Cryptosporidium,* and *Microsporidium* (Fig. 4.33, e-Figs. 4.113–4.114) can be found in immunosuppressed hosts. We sometimes have noted prominent lymphoid aggregates in biopsies from patients with a course that is clinically in keeping with viral gastroenteritis (e-Fig. 4.115).

Of course, malakoplakia, while usually in the genitourinary tract, can also be found in the GI tract and reflects a curious response to degenerating bacteria, which assume a targetoid appearance when ingested by macrophages (Michaelis-Gutmann bodies) (e-Figs. 4.116–4.120).

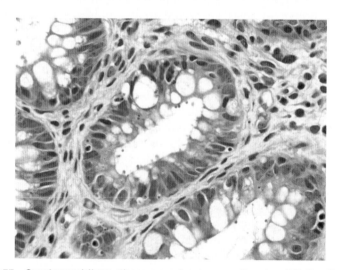

FIGURE 4.33 *Cryptosporidium.* These organisms are easily missed if the tissue is not examined at high magnification.

Sexually transmitted diseases (STDs) affecting the rectum are not commonly encountered by pathologists but must be kept in mind when examining biopsies from at-risk patients (HIV infected, men who have sex with men [MSM]). The etiology of sexually transmitted proctitis is varied. A retrospective chart review of MSM who presented with rectal symptoms identified *Neisseria gonorrhoeae* (30%) as the most common causative organism, followed by *Chlamydia trachomatis* (19%), *Herpes simplex* (2%), and *Treponema pallidum* (2%) (79). Symptoms may mimic IBD and include anorectal pain with or without a purulent, mucoid, or bloody discharge, tenesmus, and urgency to defecate. Although pathologists are seldom provided with pertinent clinical history, there are histologic clues that allow us to raise some of these diagnostic possibilities. Unfortunately, the histologic changes seen with gonorrheal infection are nonspecific and consist predominantly of an acute proctitis. Lymphogranuloma venereum (LV) can be histologically similar to Crohn disease. The former shows a predominance of follicular lymphohistiocytic and plasma cell infiltrates in the submucosa, muscularis propria, and serosa with neural hyperplasia in the submucosal and myenteric plexuses. A superficial biopsy may show nonspecific findings. Similar to Crohn disease, there may be extensive thickening and fibrosis of the bowel wall but lesion distribution tends to be limited to the rectum in LV (80).

Treponema pallidum is the causative agent of syphilis, an STD characterized by primary, secondary, and tertiary stages. Briefly, the primary stage presents with a chancre, a painless firm, red lesion at the site of inoculation, which heals after 3 to 6 weeks. The secondary stage, characterized by a maculopapular rash, is the result of spirochete multiplication within the skin and mucous membranes and occurs 2 to 10 weeks after the initial stage. Condyloma lata (raised, broad-based plaques) may be seen during this stage and may provoke concern for HPV infection. The tertiary stage is rare in this day and age when antibiotics are readily available but is characterized by aortitis, tabes dorsalis, and gummas (rubbery nodules composed of a necrotic center with surrounding macrophages, fibroblasts, lymphocytes, and plasma cells). Endoscopically, syphilitic proctitis may present granular, friable, erythematous, thick, or ulcerated mucosa (81–83). On histologic exam, one sees a neutrophilic cryptitis with ulceration, granulation tissue, and massive associated mucosal and submucosal lymphoplasmacytic infiltration that tends to be angiocentric (Fig. 4.34, e-Fig. 4.121–4.123). Poorly formed granulomas may be seen. Although a silver stain may be employed to highlight the spirochetes, these are frequently not identified. Definitive diagnosis requires serologic confirmation with rapid plasma reagin (RPR) and fluorescent treponemal antibody–absorption test (FTA).

The large intestine can also harbor protozoan organisms such as *Blastocystis hominis* and *Entamoeba histolytica* in both immunocompetent and immunosuppressed hosts. Protozoal infection is prevalent among patients with IBD and has been proposed as a potential cause for disease exacerbation and persistent activity by some observers. Although

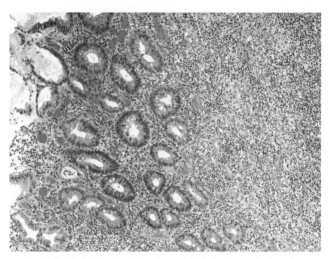

FIGURE 4.34 Syphilis proctitis. The findings in syphilitic proctitis are nonspecific and include a neutrophilic cryptitis with ulceration and massive associated mucosal and submucosal lymphoplasmacytic infiltration. The predominance of plasma cells should trigger this diagnostic possibility.

documented cases of *B. hominis*–associated colitis exist, its role as a definite cause of GI injury is unclear as the organism can be found in well-formed stool from asymptomatic patients (albeit in low numbers), and infection does not seem to alter intestinal permeability. Symptomatic patients with such organisms on stool examination lacking other proven pathogens may benefit from treatment with metronidazole. *E. histolytica* is the only member of the *Entamoeba* genus that is associated with intestinal injury. Histologic exam shows grey, round to oval organisms with a round nucleus, intracytoplasmic red blood cells, and associated active inflammation (Fig. 4.32, e-Figs. 4.100–4.103). Infection may result in formation of an ameboma mimicking colonic malignancy endoscopically and on imaging studies. Though organisms are usually found in association with surface exudate, rarely ameba may invade deep into the bowel wall with subsequent perforation and need for surgical intervention (84,85). Though amebiasis is a health concern predominantly in developing countries, cases in the United States may be encountered in travelers returning from such areas. Similarly, *Paracoccidioides brasiliensis* colitis is occasionally encountered in South American patients but not in the North American population (e-Figs. 4.124 and 4.125).

Helminths can be directly visualized endoscopically. Infection is rare outside of endemic areas (tropical and subtropical countries) where they pose a significant health burden leading to impair in growth, physical fitness, cognition, and reduction in school attendance and performance (86). *Trichuris trichiura* (whipworm), *Enterobius vermicularis* (pinworm), *Ascaris lumbricoides* (roundworm), and *Schistosoma* spp. are some examples of the most clinically significant pathogens. Patients may be asymptomatic or may report nonspecific symptoms such as abdominal pain, discomfort, constipation, rectal bleeding, or diarrhea. Some patients with *T. trichiura* (whipworm) infection may present with iron deficiency anemia, and a heavy organism burden is associated with a dysentery-like syndrome (87,88). Stool examination is frequently negative and the diagnosis is frequently made endoscopically (89). Since organisms are usually directly visualized through the endoscope, tissue biopsies are not necessary to establish the diagnosis. If taken, however, one sees a prominent eosinophilic mucosal infiltrate with or without associated worms. *T. trichiura* worms have a thick outer cuticle; females display a posterior gravid uterus filled with barrel-shaped eggs, while males show a copulatory organ (e-Figs. 4.41–4.44 in Chapter 3.). Patients with *E. vermicularis* infection can be completely asymptomatic or may present with the classic symptom of pruritus ani. It is the most common helminth found in appendectomies and has been associated with symptoms of acute appendicitis, in many cases without histologic evidence of inflammation (90,91). Cross sections of the organism show lateral ala with centrally located internal organs (e-Figs. 4.126–4.129) (91).

Colonic schistosomiasis is also rare in the United States but is common in endemic tropical and subtropical areas. Although the rectosigmoid area is preferentially affected, the entire colon may show endoscopic abnormalities. The mucosa may appear granular, erythematous, ulcerated, friable, or edematous in the acute setting. Long-standing infections may present a pale, nodular or polypoid mucosa with loss of vascular pattern (92–95). Biopsies show *Schistosoma* ova within a lamina propria rich in inflammatory cells, particularly eosinophils with or without an associated foreign body giant cell reaction (e-Figs. 4.130–4.132). A lateral spine serves to identify eggs from *S. mansoni*, while a terminal spine is characteristic of *S. hematobium*. The former is associated with intestinal infections, while the latter affects the genitourinary system. Some cases lack a significant inflammatory response (93). Infection-associated bowel perforation has been reported (94,96) and some cases are associated with development of colonic adenocarcinoma (92,95,97). Whether infection represents a definite risk factor for malignancy as it does for squamous cell carcinoma of the urinary bladder is unclear.

Although strongyloidiasis is typically encountered in the small bowel, it can occasionally be seen in the colon (e-Fig. 4.133).

ISCHEMIC COLITIS

The biopsy features that are classically associated with ischemic colitis include marked surface injury, mucin loss in crypts, "atrophic microcrypts", and the hyalinization of the lamina propria, such that the normal loose connective tissue (punctuated with plasma cells, lymphocytes, and eosinophils) is replaced with a dense eosinophilic matrix, and the residual glands become more closely spaced (lamina propria "collapse") (98) (Fig. 4.35 and 4.36, e-Figs. 4.134–4.138). Cytologic atypia in the form of

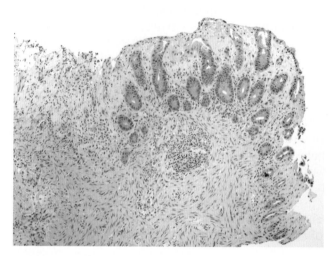

FIGURE 4.35 **Ischemic colitis.** This image shows surface injury, mucin loss, and hyalinization of the lamina propria. Residual glands appear more closely spaced (lamina propria "collapse").

hyperchromatic, enlarged nuclei is a frequent finding and atypical mitoses can even be encountered (Fig. 4.138). In older patients, ischemic disease is typically attributable to atherosclerotic mesenteric vascular disease. In the setting of global hypoperfusion or splanchnic constriction, the "watershed" zones are prone to vascular disease. The classic "watershed zone" is at the splenic flexure, an area supplied by the distal-most reaches of both the superior mesenteric artery and the inferior mesenteric artery, but not by more proximal branches of either source. As such, any vascular

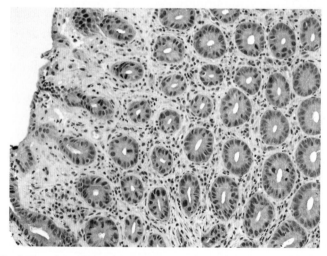

FIGURE 4.36 **Ischemic colitis.** This case shows hyalinization of the lamina propria and cytologic atypia in the form of hyperchromatic, enlarged nuclei.

compromise—from hypovolemia to splanchnic shunting during exercise or global hypotension (such as after trauma)—can affect this zone (the Griffith point) more substantially than other areas in the colon. A similar "watershed zone" is present in the ileocecal region (the Sudeck point) (99).

There are many etiologies for ischemic colitis and the condition is associated with a myriad of diseases and drugs (prescribed and "over-the-counter") (100). Associated risk factors include hypertension, diabetes, chronic obstructive pulmonary disease, coronary artery disease, abdominal surgery, use of opioids, antihypertensives, hormone replacement therapy, performance-enhancing supplements, and immunomodulators, to name a few (100–102). Distance running is known to be associated with varying degrees of colonic ischemia. As an indication of this, it is known that about one quarter of both male and female runners who previously lacked ischemic colitis have occult blood in their stool following participation in a marathon (103). More extensively documented colonic ischemia has also been reported in such athletes; this generally resolves uneventfully (104–106). In contrast to the effect of splanchnic constriction in athletic settings, however, ischemic colitis due to hypovolemia in young trauma patients is unusual (107).

Certain infectious agents are also known to produce an ischemic picture, classically enterohemorrhagic (verotoxin-producing) *E. coli* and *Clostridium difficile*. The prototype infectious agent for producing ischemic colitis is *E. coli* O157:H7 (e-Figs. 4.139 and 4.140), which first came to attention in the early 1980s (108,109). It is a primary cause of severe hemorrhagic diarrhea and one of its complications—hemolytic uremic syndrome, which develops in up to 20% of cases—is a serious consequence. Ground beef and other bovine products have been implicated as sources. The largest outbreak of this organism occurred in upstate New York in association with an agricultural fair (110). Since *E. coli* is ubiquitous in stool, enterohemorrhagic strains must be specifically sought by stool cultures using sorbitol-MacConkey medium, from which sorbitol non-fermenting colonies are selected and assayed for the specific organism, with either an enzyme immunoassay or a latex agglutination assay (111). Unfortunately, about 3% to 18% of toxin-producing *E. coli* are able to ferment sorbitol (and thus appear as "ordinary" *E. coli* on culture plates). This bacterium may also be responsible for outbreaks that are not detected by routine screening protocols for these organisms (112).

The key pathogenetic mechanism underlying the manifestations of enterohemorrhagic *E. coli* is the direct effect of its cytotoxicity on endothelium (113). This direct effect results in GI manifestations if the process is limited or in hemolytic uremic syndrome if the process becomes systemic. Endoscopic biopsies taken from infected patients may display ischemic colitis features with prominent fibrin thrombi, findings that allow the pathologist to suggest pertinent laboratory evaluation (114) but which are by no means specific. An immunohistochemical test has been developed, although there is limited experience with it in tissue diagnosis (115).

In younger patients with ischemic colitis, a variety of drug associations can be invoked, including illegal drugs (cocaine) (116–121) (e-Figs. 4.141 and 4.142), over-the-counter decongestant medications (122–124), oral contraceptives (125,126), NSAIDs (127,128), Kayexalate (given for hyperkalemia in renal patients and suspended in a sorbitol solution that induces osmotic ischemia) (e-Figs. 4.143 and 4.144) (129), and the migraine headache medication, sumatriptan (130,131). The introduction, withdrawal, and reintroduction of the drug alosetron hydrochloride (Lotronex) have been associated with cases, some fatal, of ischemic colitis (132,135). Lotronex, a potent selective 5-hydroxytryptamine receptor antagonist, was approved in February of 2000 in the United States for the treatment of diarrhea-predominant IBS in women. Marketing was suspended in November of 2000, after reports of colonic ischemia and serious complications of constipation. After public outcry from patients and their advocates, the drug was reintroduced in 2002 and its use is now restricted to patients with severe disease with a high benefit:risk ratio. Follow-up studies of the reintroduced drug have not demonstrated untoward ischemic events (136,137).

Other causes of ischemic intestinal disease in young adults include coagulopathies, anorexic behavior, and vasculitides such as lymphocytic phlebitis and giant cell arteritis, among others (138,139) (see below). A 2001 report from the Mayo Clinic of 39 young adults with ischemic bowel disease included 13 (of 25) women taking oral contraceptives, 4 patients with vascular thrombi, 4 taking vasoactive drugs, 4 with hypovolemia, and 2 with vasculitis. No etiology was demonstrated in the remaining 19 patients (140). Genetic predisposition may also play a role in younger patients as some patients younger than 55 with ischemic colitis are more prone to harbor factor V and plasminogen activator inhibitor gene polymorphisms when compared with healthy controls (141).

In older patients, the differential diagnosis is often between pseudomembranous and ischemic colitis. The diagnosis of ischemic colitis often requires careful clinicopathologic correlation. The process may resolve spontaneously. Involvement is segmental, and the splenic flexure area is particularly vulnerable. In early cases, there is desquamation and necrosis of the mucosa, particularly the superficial mucosa. Pseudomembranes are often seen microscopically, although the endoscopic appearances of ischemia and pseudomembranous colitis differ (compare e-Fig. 4.134 to e-Fig. 4.95). Hemorrhage and hemosiderin-laden macrophages are seen in the lamina propria. Fibrin thrombi may be seen as the process progresses. Chronicity is evidenced by crypt atrophy and hyalinized lamina propria. Dignan and Greenson have published helpful criteria to distinguish ischemic colitis from pseudomembranous colitis (Table 4.4) (98). These criteria allow distinction of most cases, but not all, in which this differential diagnosis arises. *C. difficile* is often the etiologic agent in pseudomembranous colitis, but not all pseudomembranes are caused by this bacterium, and not all infestations with *C. difficile* result in pseudomembranes. Cases are typically associated with antibiotics.

TABLE 4.4 Features for Distinguishing Pseudomembranous from Ischemic Colitis

	Pseudomembranous Colitis (*Clostridium difficile*)	Ischemic Colitis
Endoscopic Appearance	Diffusely distributed discrete, 0.2 to 0.3 cm pseudomembranes throughout colon	Localized process with expansive pseudomembrane or mass ("thumbprinting" radiographically)
Hyalinized lamina propria	No	Yes
Atrophic microcrypts	+	+++
Full-thickness mucosal necrosis	+	+++
Diffuse microscopic distribution of pseudomembranes	+	+++

+, occasionally; +++, commonly.
Adapted from Dignan CR, Greenson JK. Can ischemic colitis be differentiated from *C. difficile* colitis in biopsy specimens? *Am J Surg Pathol.* 1997;21(6):706–710.

FINDINGS IN SYSTEMIC DISEASES

Scleroderma

GI involvement is seen in the majority of patients with scleroderma and can be a significant source of morbidity. Although upper GI tract complaints are more common, approximately 30% experience lower GI tract symptoms (142). This connective tissue disorder can result in hypomotility and intestinal pseudo-obstruction resulting in constipation and bacterial overgrowth (143). There are no specific biopsy changes as the muscularis propria is the involved layer, typically showing sclerosis of the inner circular muscle (144) (e-Figs. 4.145 and 4.146).

Vasculitis

It is treacherous to attempt diagnosis of vasculitis on colonic biopsies; if ischemic ulcers are present, any inflammation in walls of small vessels may be secondary rather than primary. The systemic vasculitides are clinically diverse, multisystem diseases, and their unifying pathologic feature is inflammation of blood vessel walls. Vasculitis may be categorized according to vessel size. Small vessel vasculitis includes systemic lupus erythematosus (SLE) (Fig. 4.37, e-Figs. 4.147 and 4.148), microscopic

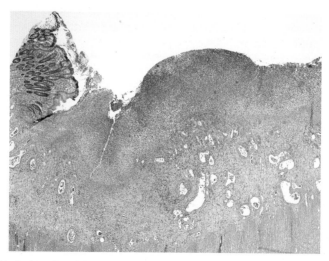

FIGURE 4.37 Ischemic colitis. This image is from a patient with mucosal ischemic necrosis as a result of lupus vasculitis.

polyangiitis, Wegener granulomatosis (WG), Churg-Strauss syndrome, Henoch-Schönlein syndrome, Adamantiades-Behçet disease, and rheumatoid vasculitis. Medium-sized vessel vasculitis includes SLE, polyarteritis nodosa (PAN), thromboangiitis obliterans, and Kawasaki disease. Large vessel vasculitis refers to Takayasu arteritis and giant cell arteritis. However, there may be considerable overlap among the various syndromes. In addition, both Crohn disease and ulcerative colitis, itself, may result in vasculitis. The type of IBD most often associated with vasculitis is Crohn disease, which usually affects the arteries.

Intestinal vasculitis may accompany a variety of systemic vasculitides, such as PAN, Churg-Strauss syndrome, Henoch-Schönlein purpura, lupus, and rheumatoid arthritis (145–150). PAN, SLE, and Henoch-Schönlein are the angiitides most commonly accompanied by GI complications (147). Key features of the vasculitides affecting the GI tract are tabulated in Table 4.5. Isolated venulitis of the GI tract has been reported under a variety of terms (lymphocytic phlebitis, necrotizing and giant cell granulomatous phlebitis, idiopathic myointimal hyperplasia of mesenteric veins, mesenteric inflammatory veno-occlusive disease, intramural mesenteric venulitis, and idiopathic colonic phlebitis) (e-Figs. 4.149–4.155) (138,148,151). The trouble with this entity, as is frequently the case in GI tract lesions, is that it describes a pattern of injury, but the etiology remains unknown.

Behçet disease (BD) refers to a systemic inflammatory disorder of uncertain etiology characterized by oral and genital ulcers, ocular inflammation, and pustular/ulcerating skin lesions. GI tract disease manifests with well-defined, "punched-out" or "geographic" mucosal ulceration, which may be deep into the wall with subsequent perforation (152–154). Ulcers can be single or multiple with skip lesions, raising clinical suspicion

TABLE 4.5 Summary: Vasculitis Affecting the GI Tract

Type	Definition	Vessel Size Typically Affected	Microscopic Features
Henoch-Schönlein syndrome (also called anaphylactoid purpura, Schönlein-Henoch syndrome)	Most common vasculitis in children characterized by purpuric skin eruption, fever, arthralgia, and visceral symptoms; seasonal incidence (peaks in winter); renal involvement in up to half of cases; patients present with skin purpura, and hemorrhage of bowel, kidney, or lung	Small	Small vessel necrotizing vasculitis, histologically indistinguishable from small vessel forms of polyarteritis; IgA immune deposits in affected vessel walls
PAN (periarteritis nodosa, polyarteritis)	Necrotizing vasculitis of medium- and small-sized arteries; involvement of the aorta is unknown; patients present with involvement of any organ; in descending order: Kidneys, muscles, nerves, viscera, and heart; in children, the heart is the most common site	Medium (arteries)	Focal segmental necrotizing arteritis with fibrinoid necrosis is hallmark of acute lesions, which have a proclivity for microaneurysm formation; healing lesions have vessel wall sclerosis; the characteristic feature is the presence of coexisting acute and healing lesions, with intervening segments of unaffected artery
Lupus vasculitis	Vasculitis affecting patients known to have lupus	Medium	Variable and nonspecific histology
Wegener vasculitis	A necrotizing granulomatous vasculitis that, in classic form, affects the lungs and kidneys; most affected (75%) are c-ANCA-positive	Small	The lesions have geographic necrosis, granuloma formation, and vasculitis; all three components are of extrapulmonary cases, so diagnosis requires clinicopathologic correlation

(Continued)

TABLE 4.5 Summary: Vasculitis Affecting the GI Tract (*Continued*)

Type	Definition	Vessel Size Typically Affected	Microscopic Features
Churg-Strauss vasculitis (allergic granulomatosis and angiitis)	A subset or "overlap syndrome" of polyarteritis nodosa; the pathologic diagnostic criteria require systemic and pulmonary necrotizing vasculitis, with an eosinophilic infiltrate and extravascular granulomas; clinical diagnostic triad: History of asthma or allergy, peripheral blood eosinophilia, and pulmonary and systemic vasculitis with eosinophilic infiltrate	Medium	Like PAN with an eosinophilic infiltrate; when changes are limited to an isolated organ system, the condition is known as limited or isolated Churg-Strauss syndrome
Buerger disease (thromboangiitis obliterans)	Nonarteriosclerotic segmental inflammatory occlusive disease of medium-sized and small arteries and veins, usually affecting limbs, with occasional visceral involvement; strong association with smoking; male predilection (9:1); usually in young men (<40 years); begins with the Raynaud phenomenon	Medium	Diagnostic only in its early stages with clinically evident thrombophlebitis; there are inflammatory thrombi of arteries and veins with "endovascular" microabscesses with scattered giant cells; the later stages are less diagnostic and organizing thrombi are seen; the end stage is nondiagnostic with fibrotic occluded vessels

GI, gastrointestinal; IgA, immunoglobulin A; c-ANCA, c-antineutrophil cytoplasmic antibody; PAN, polyarteritis nodosa.

for Crohn disease (155). The ileum, cecum, and ascending colon are the more commonly affected areas (155,156). Upper tract lesions are uncommon. As with any vasculitis, findings on superficial biopsies are nonspecific showing chronic active mucosal inflammation, and architectural distortion with or without ulceration, reminiscent of IBD (e-Fig. 4.156–4.158). Biopsies are typically too superficial for identification of a vasculitis, which usually involves submucosal and serosal venules. Massive hemorrhage as a result of extensive ulceration is a rare but documented phenomenon (157).

On biopsies, vasculitis involving the GI tract vessels results in ischemic changes that cannot be distinguished from other causes of ischemia. This is a setting in which clinical correlation is critical and working closely with the endoscopist is key. For example, the angiographic features of PAN are characteristic, and the diagnosis can be made prospectively by noting ischemic features on a mucosal biopsy. If steroid therapy is promptly initiated, surgery can be avoided. Exclusive involvement of the GI tract by vasculitis is uncommon (158) and correlation with other pertinent clinical and imaging findings can be extremely valuable.

Autoimmune Enterocolopathy

Patients with autoimmune enteropathy may have accompanying colonic inflammation with grossly abnormal, friable, erythematous mucosa with loss of vascular pattern. Histologic changes range from only mild expansion of the lamina propria by a lymphohistiocytic, neutrophilic, and eosinophilic infiltrate to goblet cell depletion, architectural distortion, and crypt abscess formation (Fig. 4.38, e-Fig. 4.159). As is the case in the small bowel, aberrant HLA II expression has been detected on surface and crypt epithelial cells (159,160). Autoimmune enteropathy is further discussed in Chapter 3.

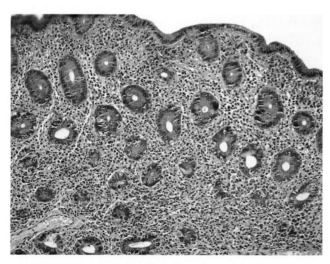

FIGURE 4.38 **Autoimmune enterocolopathy.** Notice the absence of goblet cells.

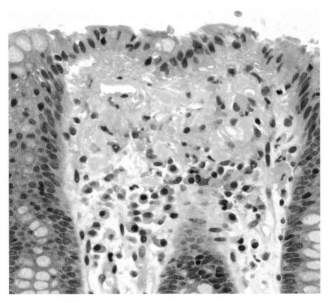

FIGURE 4.39 **Amyloidosis.** In this subtle example, the basement membrane, which is laden with amyloid, appears damaged and friable.

Amyloidosis

Amyloidosis can affect the colon just as it can affect the remainder of the GI tract (Fig. 4.39, e-Figs. 4.160–4.165). GI tract disease may occur as part of systemic amyloidosis or, rarely, it can be localized to the gut. This distinction is clinically important as patients with localized amyloidosis have a good prognosis with no need for medical intervention, while those with systemic amyloidosis have a worse prognosis and commonly require treatment with alkylating agents (161). Patients may be asymptomatic or present with rectal bleeding and/or abdominal pain. The endoscopist may report areas of petechiae, erythema, nodularity, ulceration, or friability. The characteristic acellular, eosinophilic material can be seen within the lamina propria, muscularis mucosae, submucosa, or thickened vessel walls. The process may be transmural with potential for perforation (162,163). Occasionally, because it imparts a thickened basement membrane, it may have overlapping features with collagenous colitis. In contrast to the collagen in the latter, which is punctuated with nuclei of fibroblasts and entrapped endothelial cells, the thick basement membrane in amyloidosis contains no nuclei.

Mastocytosis

Normally, the gut has scattered lamina propria and submucosal mast cells, usually not easily identified unless they are specifically searched for or highlighted with immunohistochemical stains (mast cell tryptase or CD117). Increased numbers of mast cells in the GI tract can be seen in a

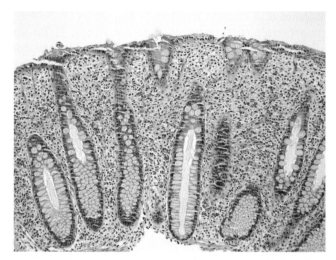

FIGURE 4.40 **Mastocytosis.** Notice the predominance of eosinophils at low power.

number of inflammatory disorders including patients with allergic disease, parasitic infections, and eosinophilic colitis.

While rarely encountered, neoplastic mast cell infiltration of the GI tract can occur in the setting of systemic mastocytosis (SM). The GI symptoms in SM are often attributable to the histamines and other compounds produced by the mast cells, rather than to their presence in the GI tract (164–169). Clinical and endoscopic features may overlap with those of IBD (168,170). Mast cells are CD117-reactive and can be identified with CD117/c-kit stains (Figs. 4.40 and 4.41 e-Figs. 4.166–4.175). Although correlation

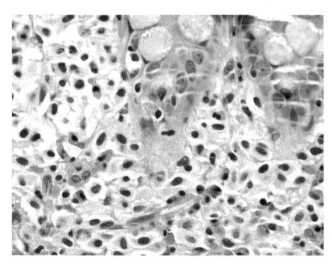

FIGURE 4.41 **Mastocytosis.** Higher magnification of Figure 4.40 showing prominent eosinophils and associated mast cells with ovoid, deeply basophilic nuclei and abundant cytoplasm.

with skin biopsies and clinical features is helpful in elucidating the etiology for their presence (neoplastic vs. inflammatory), Hahn and Hornick (166) reported histologic clues that are useful in this regard, namely, mast cell density and CD25 expression. In their study, biopsies from patients with SM showed significantly higher mast cell density (>100/hpf) when compared with biopsies from patients with cutaneous mastocytosis or GI inflammatory conditions. In addition, immunostaining with CD25 (IL-2 receptor expressed by neoplastic mast cells) is specific for SM and is not expressed in GI tract mast cells from patients with cutaneous mastocytosis or GI inflammatory processes (166). The classic D816V *KIT* mutation associated with SM is also seen in cases with GI involvement (168). Unfortunately, mastocytosis is not as responsive to imatinib as the CD117 expression would suggest (169).

In contrast to SM, so-called "mastocytic enterocolitis" refers to a condition in which patients have chronic protracted diarrhea and demonstrate increased numbers of normal mast cells in their GI biopsies (more than 20/hpf) (e-Figs 4.176 and 4.177). Sixty-seven percent of those affected respond to treatment with H_1 and H_2 receptor antagonists and cromolyn sodium (mast cell mediator release inhibitor) (171). This observation has led to requests for performing mast cell stains on biopsies from patients with diarrhea but without features of typical inflammatory disease; in some respects, this is a request to perform mast cell stains on patients with IBS and the meaning of so-called "mastocytic enterocolitis" is unclear. We do not perform such stains routinely and hesitate to perform them when asked since similar treatment is often offered empirically for such patients.

Langerhans Cell Histiocytosis

Colonic involvement in Langerhans cell histiocytosis (LCH, previously known as histiocytosis X) has been reported in 3.3% of pediatric patients with multisystemic disease and is even less common in children with single organ system involvement (172). A poorly understood and potentially fatal disease, LCH occurs in both children and adults and results from uncontrolled proliferation or augmented survival of macrophage-like cells, which are histologically and immunohistochemically similar to epidermal, antigen-presenting Langerhans cells. Pediatric patients with GI involvement present with nonspecific symptoms such as diarrhea, abdominal pain, lower GI bleeding, and failure to thrive (172,173). The colon may appear endoscopically normal or show edema, erythema, or ulceration (172,174,175). In most adult patients, LCH seems to be an isolated finding typically (but not invariably) associated with an indolent course (176). The condition is characterized histologically by the presence of numerous macrophages with a "kidney bean"–shaped nucleus in the lamina propria and/or submucosa in the background of variable numbers of T lymphocytes, eosinophils, and giant cells. Classical Birbeck granules can be identified on electron microscopy, but the diagnosis is more easily confirmed by positive immunohistochemical staining for S100 and CD1a (e-Figs. 4.178–4.182).

Prominence of eosinophils may be the first clue to the diagnosis. Some cases, however, display a paucity of eosinophils and diagnosis requires a high index of suspicion.

Common Variable Immunodeficiency

Common variable immunodeficiency (CVID) presents colonic findings that are similar to those in the small bowel (Chapter 3) (177). CVID syndrome is the second most common immunodeficiency syndrome after select IgA deficiency. The hallmark of CVID presentation is persistent sinonasal infections, but many such patients have GI tract complaints attributable to small intestinal atrophy, chronic giardiasis, pernicious anemia, and colitis. Such patients are at risk for development of small bowel lymphoma and gastric carcinoma. Because CVID is a chronic disease, injury to the colon in patients with this condition is lifelong. As such, although these patients have decreased number of lamina propria plasma cells (Fig. 4.42), other features of their disease mimic "quiescent" or active IBD, such as marked crypt distortion (e-Figs. 4.183–4.189) and/or intraepithelial neutrophils. Apoptosis is often a prominent feature of CVID, mimicking graft versus host disease (GVHD), and these patients are prone to a host of infections (e-Figs. 4.190 and 4.191). CVID is also associated with lymphocytic and collagenous colitis (e-Figs. 4.183–4.187, 4.192). Granulomas and lymphoid aggregates can also be encountered in this setting (177). The diagnosis can be difficult in isolation of the clinical findings. Although the possibility of CVID can be suggested when plasma cells are decreased, this finding is seen in approximately 66% of the patients and about a third of biopsies from CVID patients have (hypofunctional) plasma cells (177).

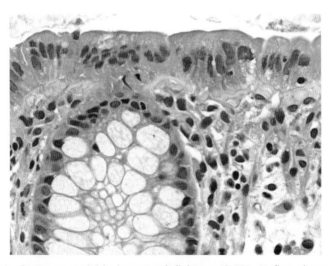

FIGURE 4.42 **Common variable immunodeficiency (CVID).** At first glance, this colon biopsy appears normal, but on closer inspection, plasma cells, usually abundant, are absent from the lamina propria, a finding seen in about two thirds of GI tract samples from patients with CVID.

Chronic Granulomatous Disease

Chronic granulomatous disease is an inherited disorder manifesting as immune deficiency caused by mutations in any of the genes that encode the various subunits of the superoxide-generating phagocyte NADPH oxidase system responsible for the respiratory burst involved in organism killing. This disease affects around 1 in 250 000 children and is associated with significant morbidity and mortality, with the predicted life expectancy reduced to around 25 to 30 years of age, with recurrent severe bacterial and fungal infections with granuloma formation. Treatment usually involves the use of prophylactic and therapeutic antibiotics, and newer therapies have been developed such as interferon-γ (IFN)-γ, bone marrow transplantation, and gene therapy. Chronic granulomatous disease can affect the colon in about a third of patients and displays prominent macrophages and eosinophils (178). Granulomas, if present, are often poorly formed. Macrophages are often pigmented (Fig. 4.43, e-Fig. 4.193–4.195). Occasional cases of CVID also show granuloma formation (177,179), but of course, the hallmark is the absence of lamina propria plasma cells and apoptosis.

IATROGENIC INJURY

Radiation Colitis/Proctitis

Radiation colitis may be acute or chronic. The acute phase occurs hours to days following irradiation and shows an edematous, dusky pattern with loss of the vascular pattern at endoscopy. On biopsy, nuclear pyknosis, karyorrhexis, and enlarged nuclei are seen with diminished mitotic activity and mucin (e-Figs. 4.196–4.199). These changes are reversible over a 1- to 2-month period of time. Chronic radiation colitis develops weeks to

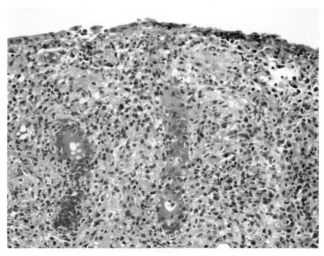

FIGURE 4.43 **Chronic granulomatous disease.** The lamina propria is replaced by poorly formed granulomas.

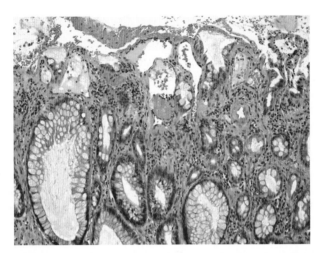

FIGURE 4.44 **Radiation injury.** Notice hyalinized vessels aligned parallel to the surface epithelial basement membrane.

years following therapy. Hyalinized connective tissue is seen in any of the bowel wall layers accompanied by atypical fibroblasts, telangiectasia, vessel wall hyalinization, phlebosclerosis, and atrophy of the muscularis propria (e-Figs. 4.200–4.203). The changes may be seen best in the submucosa and not detected by mucosal biopsy. Of course, stromal changes may be striking and, occasionally, epithelial changes may as well (180). We have noted a pattern in which hyalinized vessels are aligned parallel to the surface epithelial basement membrane, a finding that is very common in rectal biopsies from men who have had irradiation for prostate cancer (Figs. 4.44 and 4.45).

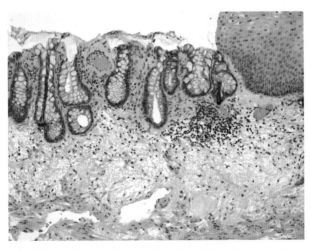

FIGURE 4.45 **Radiation injury.** Notice hyalinized vessels aligned parallel to the surface epithelial basement membrane and atrophic glands that fail to reach the basement membrane.

Mycophenolate (Cellcept)-Associated Colonic Injury

Probably referred to in the past as "uremic colitis" (e-Fig. 4.204), mycophenolate-associated colonic injury is similar to that encountered elsewhere in the GI tract and characterized by changes that mimic those of GVHD (181). As noted in prior chapters, mycophenolate is an immunosuppressive drug used mainly in patients with solid organ transplants (kidney, liver, heart, lung) to maintain their grafts, but this medication is also administered to patients with a wide range of other conditions. In the United States, there are two available preparations for this compound: mycophenolate mofetil (MMF; Cellcept; Roche Pharmaceuticals) and mycophenolate sodium (Myfortic, Novartis Inc.). The difference between the two preparations is that Myfortic is an enteric-coated drug, while MMF is not. Myfortic is therefore absorbed in the intestine, while MMF is absorbed in the stomach. Their efficacy and toxicity profiles are similar.

Mycophenolic acid (MPA) functions by inhibiting the *de novo* pathway of purine synthesis. In general, almost 100% of B and T lymphocytes depend on the *de novo* pathway for purine synthesis, while this dependency is lower for enterocytes (about 50%). Therefore, by inhibiting guanosine synthesis in lymphocytes, cytotoxic T lymphocytes responsible for cellular rejection and antibody production by B lymphocytes are suppressed in transplanted patients. Although the dependency of enterocytes on the *de novo* pathway for purine genesis is lower than that of lymphocytes, MPA can inhibit the proliferation of enterocytes, leading to epithelial injury.

The side effects of MPA predominantly involve the GI tract and hematopoiesis and include diarrhea, nausea, vomiting, gastritis, ulcers, opportunistic infections, and anemia. Changes in the lower GI tract were initially studied, consisting of GVHD-like findings. Finding apoptosis is not specific for mycophenolate-associated injury. The findings are essentially identical to those of GVHD such that clinical correlation is always required—if the patient has had a bone marrow rather than solid organ transplant then prominent apoptosis is generally a reflection of GVHD. CMV infection (and other viral infections) is also associated with apoptosis. If a patient taking mycophenolate has CMV gastritis as well, there is no way to determine the cause of any apoptotic bodies that may be encountered.

Ipilimumab-Associated Injury

Monoclonal antibodies (mAbs) against the cytotoxic T lymphocyte antigen-4 (CTLA-4) molecule have been used as an adjuvant to experimental tumor immunization protocols in the treatment of malignant melanomas and various cancers. One of the side effects includes severe gastroenteritis (182). In symptomatic patients taking this medication, endoscopic findings are variable, ranging from normal to diffusely erythematous and ulcerated mucosa. The constant histologic findings include a lymphoplasmacytic expansion of the lamina propria with increase in intraepithelial

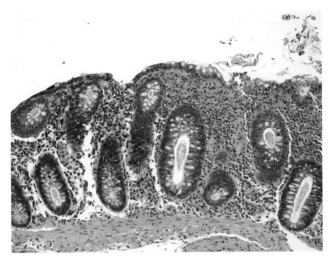

FIGURE 4.46 **Ipilimumab-associated injury.** This example shows mild lymphoplasmacytic expansion of the lamina propria with increased intraepithelial lymphocytes and apoptotic bodies.

lymphocytes. Increased epithelial apoptosis is also a distinctive feature. Cryptitis and glandular inflammation are observed in the colon (Fig. 4.46, e-Figs. 4.205–4.207). The responsible immune cells are T-cell subsets (CD3+, CD4+, and CD8+) and CD4CD25 regulatory T cells. The features are similar to those encountered in autoimmune enterocolopathy (see Chapter 4). The pathogenesis may relate to increased numbers of regulatory T cells in the GI mucosa.

Kayexalate (Sodium Polystyrene Sulfonate)-Associated Injury

Kayexalate-associated injury is discussed in some detail in Chapter 1, although the severe ischemic hyperosmotic injury that has been associated with this medication was initially reported in the colon (129). As noted in Chapter 1, Kayexalate is a cation-exchange resin. When administered orally, by nasogastric tube, or by enema, sodium cations are released from the resin and exchanged for hydrogen ions. As the resin then passes through the intestines, hydrogen is exchanged for potassium, which is then eliminated in the feces along with the remainder of the altered resin, thereby lowering the serum potassium concentration.

In the early use of Kayexalate, the resin was suspended in water and then administered. Although it was generally well tolerated, some patients were reported to develop gastric and bowel opacifications as a result of concretions of crystalline resin. Therefore, it became increasingly popular to administer Kayexalate in a suspension with hypertonic sorbitol. This solution reduces both the frequency of Kayexalate bezoar formation and the colonic impaction by promoting an osmotic diarrhea. However, this hyperosmotic effect results in mucosal injury in a subset of patients, as

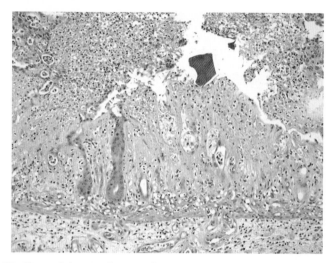

FIGURE 4.47 Kayexalate (sodium polystyrene sulfonate)-associated injury. The histologic appearance is the same regardless of where it is encountered (upper or lower tract). Kayexalate crystals appear purplish on H&E stain and display a cracked appearance resembling fish scales. Compare to cholestyramine crystals in Figure 4.48.

discussed in Chapter 1. The hallmark is the presence of ischemic pattern injury, with mucosal necrosis, and hyalinized lamina propria exactly like ischemic injury from other causes. However, the appearance of the sodium polystyrene sulfonate crystals associated with the injury is the same regardless of where they are encountered. They appear purplish on hematoxylin and eosin (H&E) stains and display a cracked appearance resembling fish scales (Fig. 4.47, e-Figs 4.208–4.210) although they may be bile-stained (and thus greenish to grey black) in patients in whom the preparation has been administered orally. The differential diagnosis is with cholestyramine, the crystals of which lack cracks and are usually red in color on H&E stains (Fig. 4.48, e-Fig. 4.211). These are seen as "innocent bystanders," usually in normal mucosa.

Graft Versus Host Disease

The features of GVHD of the colon are similar to those elsewhere, with varying degrees of apoptosis and crypt dropout. It can be graded as a construct to compare to prior biopsies (grade 1, increased crypt apoptosis; grade 2, apoptosis with crypt abscess; grade 3, individual crypt necrosis [Fig. 4.49, e-Fig. 4.212]; and grade 4, total denudation of areas of mucosa). Like GVHD elsewhere, it can have a chronic phase in which crypt distortion appears but lacks the active inflammation and prominent basal plasmacytosis that characterize ulcerative and Crohn colitis. Of course, it typically accompanies bone marrow rather than solid organ transplant. In addition, GVHD is always diagnosed in the proper clinical setting, so correlation with the clinical impression is critical. The differential diagnosis is with entities resulting in apoptosis, such as viral infection (always check

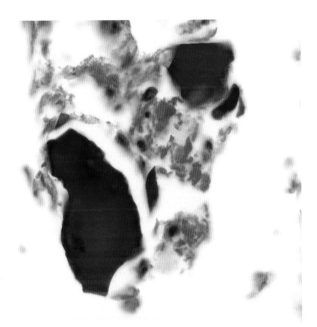

FIGURE 4.48 **Cholestyramine crystals.** These crystals lack cracks and are usually red on H&E stain. They are seen as "innocent bystanders," usually in normal mucosa. Compare with Kayexalate crystals in Figure 4.47.

biopsies for CMV on routine stains and obtain immunohistochemical ones at low threshold), autoimmune disease, NSAID use, and medications. For example, mycophenolate mofetil (Cellcept) administered to solid organ transplant patients can result in colon biopsy findings that are identical

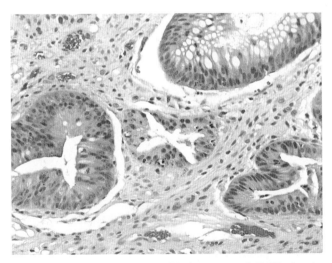

FIGURE 4.49 **Graft-versus-host-disease.** This is a case of GVHD showing prominent apoptosis.

to those of GVHD (181) (e-Fig. 4.204), and chemotherapy or other prolonged injury can produce similar features (e-Fig. 4.213).

Diversion Colitis

Sometimes, when a segment of bowel is resected, the surgeon is forced to create an ileostomy or colostomy because there is simply too much inflammation (or tumor) to reanastomose the remaining bowel without clinical compromise. In this case, the remaining bowel (often the rectum) has no passing fecal stream. If the rectum is left as a blind opening, continuous with the anus, it is called a "Hartmann pouch," and the pathologist should consider that there might be diversion colitis. Colitis following diversion of the fecal sream is usually mild (Fig. 4.50, e-Figs. 4.214 and 4.215). However, in severe cases, the features may perfectly mimic both ulcerative colitis and Crohn colitis. Regression of the colitis generally follows restoration of the normal continuity of the fecal stream. Diversion colitis is common, occurring as subclinical disease in about 70% of diverted patients. Some authors have reported that lymphoid follicle hyperplasia is a typical finding, although others have reported variable histology (183). If the diverted colon is reconstructed into another anatomic structure (such as a neovagina), it is still prone to diversion colitis (184–186). The hypothesis is that the condition results from the absence of luminal, short-chain fatty acids (the preferred metabolic substrate of colonic epithelium) and is secondary to a change in the bacterial milieu, based on the finding that the condition can be reversed in many cases, with the instillation of these compounds into the diverted segment (187). An ischemic etiology has also been proposed as short-chain fatty acids may play a role in vascular smooth muscle relaxation (183).

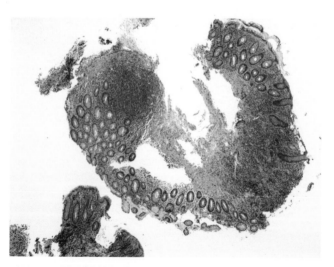

FIGURE 4.50 **Diversion colitis.** This particular case shows prominent lymphoid aggregates.

MICROSCOPIC COLITIS

The term "microscopic colitis" has been applied to biopsies of patients with symptomatic colitis in whom there are no endoscopic (gross) anomalies, but in which specific microscopic features are found. Coined by Read in 1980, the term was used to describe patients who each had chronic diarrhea, a normal colonoscopy, a normal barium enema, and mucosal inflammation in their colonic biopsies (188). There are two types of microscopic colitis that account for most such patients—collagenous and lymphocytic colitis. Both entities feature an inflamed lamina propria and surface injury but seem to be distinct entities that differ in their demographics, disease associations, and clinical course. Neither seems to confer an increased risk for development of malignancy or IBD (189).

Collagenous colitis was first described in 1976 (190). Patients have chronic watery diarrhea that may have an insidious onset or develop abruptly. In addition to diarrhea, many patients report abdominal pain, fatigue, or weight loss. Rare patients may complain of constipation. While in most cases the mucosa appears endoscopically normal, some cases of collagenous colitis may feature linear mucosal tears or defects (e-Figs. 4.216–4.218), especially in cases associated with the use of the proton pump inhibitor lansoprazole (191–193). Patients with lansoprazole-associated collagenous colitis experience symptom resolution upon discontinuation of the medication (192). There may also be an association with the use of NSAIDs (194,195) and there is evidence that some ulcers in collagenous colitis relate to use of this medication (196). Collagenous colitis is more common in women, with a female-to-male ratio of 6 to 8:1 and a median age at diagnosis of 55 years. However, the age range is broad, and many cases are diagnosed in patients under the age of 45 years. Forty percent of patients have an associated disease (Table 4.6). The most common of these associated diseases are rheumatoid arthritis, thyroid disorders, celiac disease, and diabetes mellitus. Rare cases associated with perforation, either during or after colonoscopy, are documented (197).

Lymphocytic colitis was separated as a specific form of microscopic colitis by Lazenby et al. in 1989 (198). Patients with lymphocytic colitis have chronic watery diarrhea and normal colonoscopy (199). There is a broad age range at diagnosis, ranging from young adults to elderly patients, with a mean in the 6th to 7th decade. In sharp contrast to collagenous colitis, men and women are equally affected. Some patients report abdominal pain and/or weight loss. Also, lymphocytic colitis has a stronger association with celiac disease than collagenous colitis. Among patients with celiac disease, about one third have histologic features of lymphocytic colitis on biopsy. Of patients with lymphocytic colitis, as many as one quarter may have celiac disease (199). As with collagenous colitis, there may be an association with NSAID use.

These two microscopic colitides share many histologic features, including increased lamina propria cellularity, which is primarily attributable to

TABLE 4.6 Conditions Associated with the Watery Diarrhea–Colitis Syndrome	
Extraintestinal	Gastrointestinal
Rheumatoid arthritis	Sprue/celiac disease
Seronegative arthritis	Lymphocytic gastritis
Hypothyroidism	Chronic atrophic gastritis
Hyperthyroidism	Ulcerative colitis
Juvenile diabetes	Crohn disease
Uveitis	Ileal carcinoid
Idiopathic pulmonary fibrosis	Colon carcinoma
Alopecia areata	Bacterial overgrowth
Asthma	IBS
Scleroderma	
Giant cell arteritis	
Rheumatic fever	
Raynaud syndrome	
Idiopathic thrombocytopenic purpura	
Primary biliary cirrhosis	
Chronic hepatitis	
NSAID use	
Drug allergies	
Hodgkin disease	
Non-Hodgkin lymphoma	

plasma cells, but also lymphocytes and eosinophils. The crypts are nondistorted or minimally distorted. There is surface epithelial injury associated with infiltration by lymphocytes and degenerative features such as cytoplasmic vacuoles, loss of mucin, nuclear irregularity, pyknosis, and flattening. Thus, lymphocytic colitis shows increased intraepithelial lymphocytes, surface mucin loss, and an expanded lamina propria. Scattered eosinophils are not uncommon but are a more prominent feature of collagenous colitis. (Figs. 4.51 and 4.52, e-Figs. 4.219–4.226). Increased intraepithelial lymphocytes are a normal finding in surface epithelium overlying lymphoid aggregates and should not be misinterpreted as lymphocytic colitis (Fig. 4.4).

The key diagnostic distinction between collagenous colitis and lymphocytic colitis is that the former has the deposition of an abnormal layer of collagen between the surface epithelium (Figs. 4.53 and 4.54). This can vary and tends to be more pronounced in the proximal colon and less so in the rectosigmoid. When compared to normal (e-Fig. 4.227) the lower border is irregular, with strands of collagen extending into the underlying

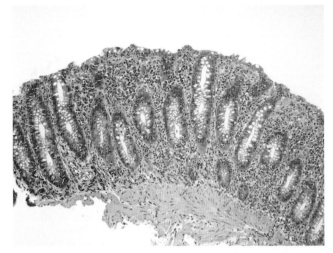

FIGURE 4.51 **Lymphocytic colitis.** At low power, one sees expansion of the lamina propria by a chronic inflammatory infiltrate and superficial injury with loss of surface mucin.

lamina propria and incorporating dilated capillaries and fibroblast nuclei (e-Fig. 4.228–4.233). Eosinophils are quite often prominent in collagenous colitis, both in the lamina propria and within surface and crypt epithelium (e-Fig. 4.234). Scattered neutrophils are often found in collagenous colitis but are not a feature of lymphocytic colitis. When neutrophils are prominent, it suggests superimposed infectious colitis. In collagenous colitis, the surface epithelium tends to separate from the basement membrane beneath, leaving stretches in which abnormal collagen is exposed on the

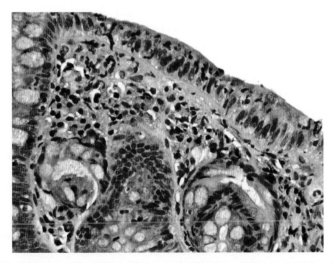

FIGURE 4.52 **Lymphocytic colitis.** Higher magnification of Figure 4.51 showing marked increase in intraepithelial lymphocytes and prominent eosinophils.

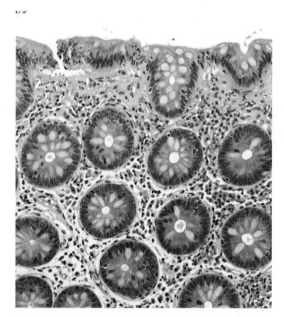

FIGURE 4.53 **Collagenous colitis**. These cases show an irregular collagen table underlying the surface epithelium with entrapped capillaries and eosinophils. Not uncommonly, the tissue is friable and the surface epithelium strips away from the collagen table.

surface. In lymphocytic colitis, the surface lymphocytosis is usually more prominent, eosinophils are less common, and prominent crypt-epithelial lymphocytosis is often a feature. There is no need to count lymphocytes; most pathologists have a good idea of what is "too many" (e-Fig. 4.235 and 4.236) from reviewing adjoining tissue next to adenomas and knowing the normal amount. Since surface intraepithelial lymphocytosis is only one of several features for a diagnosis, counts are really not necessary. There should be intraepithelial lymphocytosis in crypts as well as on the surface of the biopsy (e-Fig. 4.219).

Most cases of lymphocytic and collagenous colitis appear as above, but problems may arise when cases do not fit the usual pattern or lack some of the expected findings.

The abnormal subsurface collagen that is typical of collagenous colitis is not always thick enough to be appreciated on routine H&E staining. There is no minimal thickness required for the diagnosis of collagenous colitis. In normal colonic mucosa, the trichrome stain marks the basement membrane lying at the base of the surface epithelium, forming a smooth, thin line (e-Fig. 4.227). When collagen is deposited beneath this epithelium, the trichrome stain has an irregular lower border, with strands

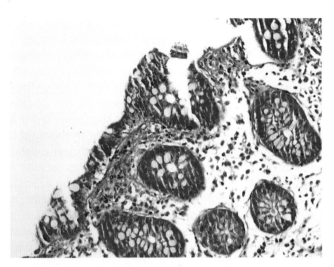

FIGURE 4.54 **Collagenous colitis.** A thick and irregular basement membrane can be highlighted with a trichrome stain.

of collagen extending into the adjacent lamina propria and trapping capillaries (Fig. 4.55). It is this abnormal pattern, rather than the absolute thickness of the collagen, that is the key feature in collagenous colitis. There is no reason to measure the deposited collagen to diagnose collagenous colitis. The abnormal collagen deposition is not always evident on routine stains, and we generally order a trichrome stain when we plan to diagnose lymphocytic colitis to detect subtle collagenous colitis. An abnormal collagen band alone is insufficient for the diagnosis of collagenous colitis but must be present in the appropriate context (200). In addition, obtaining

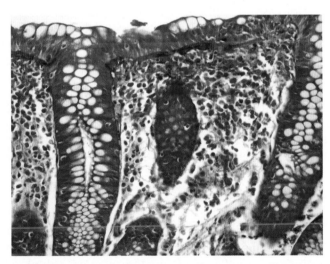

FIGURE 4.55 **Collagenous colitis.** The basal collagen entraps nuclei. It is the quality rather than the quantity of the collagen that is abnormal.

such measurement is problematic as the lowermost border of this irregular collagen table is difficult to define. Occasionally, thick bands of collagen may be seen in the colonic mucosa as a result of healed ischemia, radiation injury, ulcerative colitis, or mucosal prolapse (201).

Just as collagen deposition is not the only feature of collagenous colitis, surface lymphocytosis, alone, is not sufficient for the diagnosis of lymphocytic colitis. It must be present along with the increased inflammatory component of the lamina propria and must appear in the right clinical setting, since there are other situations in which lymphocytic colitis–like histology has been described. Some of these other settings include drugs (such as ticlopidine), infectious colitis (Brainerd diarrhea), the presence of other immune diseases (such as Hashimoto thyroiditis), and inconsistent GI symptoms, such as hematochezia or constipation (201). In addition, patchy collagenous or lymphocytic colitis has been reported as a harbinger for Crohn disease (202). Pathologists are often faced with biopsies obtained with a suspicion of microscopic colitis, which show mild intraepithelial lymphocytosis with no other accompanying abnormalities. When faced with this situation, we render a descriptive diagnosis and provide a differential diagnosis that includes early lymphocytic colitis, NSAID-associated changes, or resolving colitis. Intraepithelial lymphocytosis in pediatric patients has similar associations as in the adult setting with autoimmune enteropathy representing an additional association in the former group (203).

The classic descriptions of collagenous and lymphocytic colitis do not stress neutrophilic inflammation, cryptitis, or foci of crypt distortion, but these may be present in some examples (204). Cryptitis might raise concern for another disorder, but if the histologic and clinical evidence are otherwise consistent with a microscopic colitis, such foci do not preclude the diagnosis.

A subset of cases of collagenous and lymphocytic colitis cases present superficial lamina propria giant cells (without granuloma formation) (e-Figs. 4.237–4.240), and this rare variant has been termed "microscopic colitis with giant cells". The finding is a mere curiosity and is of no clinical significance (205). As an aside, similar giant cells may be encountered in the lamina propria of patients infected with HIV in association with hyperplasia of mucosa-associated lymphoid tissue (e-Fig. 4.88) (71). Foreign-body–type giant cells may rarely be seen in superficial biopsies of patients with pneumatosis intestinalis when air tracks into the bowel wall, frequently as a result of infection with air-forming bacteria (e-Figs. 4.241–4.244).

MISCELLANEOUS CONDITIONS

Diverticular Disease–Associated Colitis

In the early 1990s, clinicians became aware of a subset of patients with diverticular disease (usually involving the sigmoid colon) who developed segmental colitis in the area of diverticular disease (206,207). The pathologic findings were subsequently described in detail and it was noted

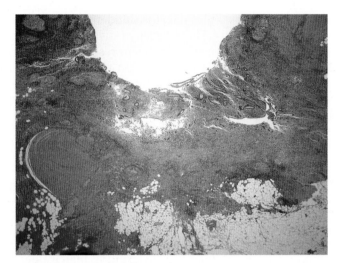

FIGURE 4.56 **Diverticular disease–associated colitis.** These cases may mimic IBD. This particular case shows ulceration with transmural inflammation and lymphoid aggregates similar to Crohn disease.

that, sometimes, cases perfectly mimicked ulcerative colitis (208) or Crohn disease (209). It was also noted that there is a minority of patients who later manifest ulcerative colitis or Crohn disease, following their episode of diverticular disease–associated colitis. The key principle is that these cases may mimic either Crohn disease or ulcerative colitis flawlessly, and the pathologist is cautioned against diagnosing idiopathic inflammatory disease affecting only the sigmoid colon, in patients with diverticular disease (Figs. 4.56 and 4.57, e-Figs. 4.245–4.250). Cases may display features

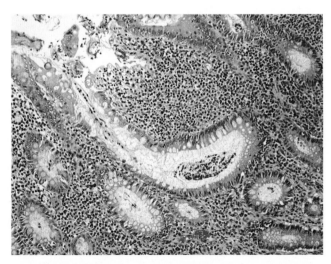

FIGURE 4.57 **Diverticular disease–associated colitis.** These cases may mimic IBD. This particular case shows lymphoplasmacytic expansion of the lamina propria with mild crypt distortion and abscess formation.

of chronicity, including basal plasmacytosis and crypt distortion, although most show mild active colitis. Those cases of diverticular disease displaying granulomas may even have granulomas in resected lymph nodes (209) (e-Fig. 4.251). In general, most patients with diverticular disease simply have "floppy" mucosa that is quite prone to prolapse changes, but one should always exercise caution in reviewing specimens showing colitis confined to the sigmoid colon. Patients with diverticular disease–associated colitis usually respond to antibiotics.

Occasionally, an endoscopist biopsies an inverted diverticulum, seeing it as a polyp. This can result in perforation if the inverted diverticulum is associated with muscularis propria.

Handling Aganglionosis Cases

Hirschsprung disease (HD, aganglionosis) is difficult to spell and can be similarly tricky to diagnose on small biopsies. It is an exciting research area, and new genetic discoveries may lead to exciting management decisions (210), but presently, the pathologist is faced with major decisions on tiny biopsies that can result in major surgery for tiny infants. There is much in the literature on so-called "neuronal dysplasia," an entity that has not been diagnosed at our hospital, as we remain unconvinced that it exists (211). In evaluating aganglionosis, we rely on H&E, acetylcholinesterase, and calretinin stains (Figs. 4.58–4.61, e-Figs. 4.252–4.255). Acetylcholinesterase is a histochemical test used on fresh frozen tissue (the enzyme is destroyed on fixation) (212). The test was first described in 1964 (213). Essentially, thiocholine reduces ferricyanide to ferrocyanide; the latter combines with Cu^{++} ions to form an insoluble copper-ferrocyanide complex. The Cu^{++} ions in the medium are combined with citrate to prevent formation of copper ferricyanide. With this method, the color is produced directly at

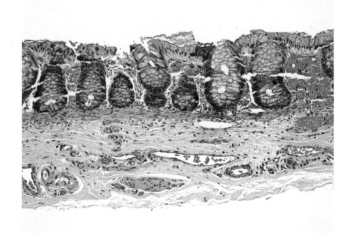

FIGURE 4.58 **Hirschsprung disease (aganglionosis).** There are no submucosal ganglion cells.

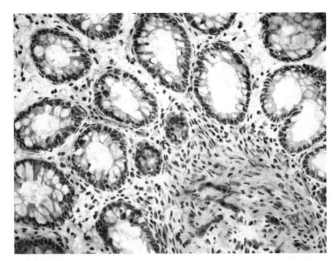

FIGURE 4.59 Hirschsprung disease (aganglionosis). Acetylcholinesterase identifies abnormal twigs of nerves, which aberrantly proliferate into the mucosa in the absence of submucosal ganglion cells.

the site of enzymatic activity, facilitating the estimation of optimal incubation time. This test remains "tried and true." Calretinin is an intracellular calcium-binding protein that can be identified immunohistochemically in nerve cell bodies within the submucosa, myenteric ganglia, and lamina propria of the ganglionated colon (Fig. 4.59). Staining is absent in cases of HD (Fig. 4.60). Based on calretinin evaluation, Guinard-Samuel and others were able to classify 12 cases of HD initially considered "suspicious for HD" using H&E and acetylcholinesterase stains. Calretinin is becoming

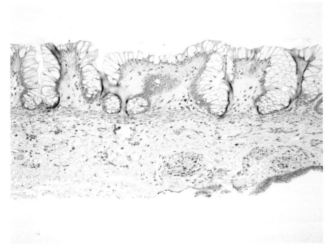

FIGURE 4.60 Hirschsprung disease (aganglionosis), calretinin immunostain. Note nearly absent staining (compare to Fig. 4.61). A few inflammatory cells show nonspecific labeling.

increasingly popular and is gaining preference over acetylcholinesterase histochemistry due to ease of interpretation and superior interobserver agreement (214,215). More recently, peripherin has been reported as a ganglion cell stain (216), but as of this writing, there is little experience with this marker.

HD is the most common cause of neonatal constipation, affecting 1 in 5,000 to 1 in 8,000 children. It can manifest in neonates, toddlers, and even school children. It results from abnormal migration of neural crest cells to the hindgut and is associated with germline mutations in *RET*, *EDNRB*, and other genes (217). It is found in association with other genetic disorders (e.g., Down syndrome). It has been classified as short segment (affecting rectum and rectosigmoid), which has a male predilection; long segment (subtotal colon), which also affects more boys than girls; total colonic aganglionosis (colon and part of small intestine), which affects the sexes equally; and ultrashort (<3 cm of rectum). The most common variant is short segment HD.

Of course, using mucosal biopsies for diagnosis has pitfalls. The findings sought are the absence of submucosal ganglion cells and an increase in presynaptic, parasympathetic fibers with abnormal extension into the mucosa (Figs. 4.58–4.61, e-Figs. 4.252–4.255). Identifying the abnormal twigs of nerves in the mucosa is the role of the acetylcholinesterase. Essentially, in the developing infant, the small nerve fibrils seek synapsis with ganglion cells. Finding none, they aberrantly proliferate into the mucosa (Fig. 4.61).

The ideal biopsy is a rectal suction biopsy (0.2 cm, two or three fragments). Ideally, there is one biopsy in formalin and one is frozen for acetylcholinesterase staining. A minimum of 75 cuts should be seen. At our

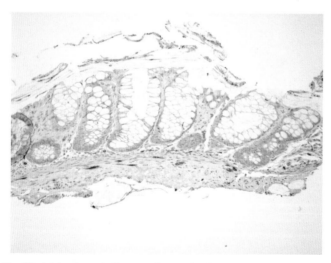

FIGURE 4.61 **Normal colon.** In the ganglionated colon, calretinin can be identified immunohistochemically in nerves within the submucosa, myenteric ganglia, and muscularis mucosae with wispy lamina propria staining (compare to Fig. 4.60).

hospital, we prepare 10 slides, each with 7 to 8 sections per ribbon for H&E staining. Then, we search for ganglion cells. Although some experts have suggested cutting the entire block, we do not follow this suggestion. The material for acetylcholinesterase is stable at 4°C for nearly 2 weeks, so a specimen accidentally left in a refrigerator all weekend can still be used for staining. This stain allows the pathologist to suspect the diagnosis on biopsies that lack submucosa. Of many standard immunohistochemical stains studied (NSE, S100, NCAM, PGP9.5, calretinin), only calretinin appears as or even more useful than acetylcholinesterase. The acetylcholinesterase stain highlights thick, coarse fibrils in the muscularis mucosae and lamina propria. These fibrils can be found in the muscularis mucosae at as early as 30 weeks gestation. When a good quality biopsy lacks ganglion cells and has the characteristic fibrils in the correct clinical setting, a diagnosis can be made.

There are essentially four pitfall areas when trying to diagnose HD (Table 4.7). The first is the physiologic zone of hypoganglionosis at the lower 1.5 to 2 cm of the rectum (218). This zone can also have prominent nerve trunks. Therefore, if anal squamous mucosa is seen on the slide, do *not* make a diagnosis of aganglionosis. Send the endoscopist back for a proper biopsy from at least 2 cm above the pectinate line.

The second pitfall is making a *de novo* diagnosis of HD on a frozen mucosal biopsy, which the surgeon plans to act upon without awaiting the permanent sections cut at multiple levels. Do *not* do it. Nonneural

TABLE 4.7 Evaluation of HD: Suction Biopsies	
Ganglion Cells present, Normal Acetylcholinesterase Pattern	Normal
Ganglion cells absent, abnormal acetylcholinesterase pattern	HD
Ganglion cells absent, normal acetylcholinesterase pattern	Probably not HD
	Biopsy too low Total colonic HD Assure adequate submucosa to evaluate
Ganglion cells absent, normal acetylcholinesterase pattern, immunoreactive nerves with calretinin	Not HD
Ganglion cells absent, normal acetylcholinesterase pattern, absent immunoreactivity for calretinin	HD
Ganglion cells present, abnormal acetylcholinesterase pattern	Consider transitional zone biopsy Consider ultrashort segment HD

tissue can be mistaken for nerves on frozen sections; tangential cuts of endothelial cells can mimic nerves extremely well on frozen sections. Also, very immature ganglion cells lack well-developed cytoplasm and are easily mistaken for lymphocytes. On the other hand, it is perfectly acceptable for surgeons to request frozen sections for positive identification of ganglion cells on full-thickness sections in order to perform an anastomosis to healthy tissue at the time of the definitive operation.

The third pitfall involves making a diagnosis of *no* aganglionosis, based on the acetylcholinesterase stain alone, when the biopsy contains little submucosal tissue. This could have serious consequences. Neonatal disease may display neural fibrils *only* in the muscularis mucosae and not yet into the lamina propria. As mentioned above, we regard calretinin immunostain a helpful adjunct in these problematic cases.

The final pitfall is that the acetylcholinesterase-positive pattern is not seen in total colonic aganglionosis.

It is important to note that some biopsies might have obvious ganglion cells and still show aberrant nerve fibrils on acetylcholinesterase staining. This finding is evident at the transitional area between ganglionic and aganglionic zones. It is of clinical significance if the surgeon performs a pullthrough, at the level of the transition zone, because the patient will continue to have postoperative dysmotility.

Changes in Cystic Fibrosis

Cystic fibrosis (CF) is the most common fatal autosomal recessive disease among whites with a U.S. incidence of 1 in 1,900 to 1 in 3,700 (219). Defective chloride ion transport across epithelial cell membranes results from mutations affecting the cystic fibrosis transmembrane conductance regulator (CFTR) gene located in the long arm of chromosome 7. As of the time of this writing, more than 1,800 mutations were listed in the CFTR mutation database (http://www.genet.sickkids.on.ca/cftr/StatisticsPage. html), the most common of which is the ΔF508 mutation, a 3 bp deletion occurring in the coding region of the gene (220). The CFTR gene encodes for a large transmembrane protein that serves as a chloride channel in a variety of epithelial cells. In respiratory and intestinal epithelium, the aberrant protein results in reduced luminal chloride secretion with increased sodium absorption. This in turn results in dehydrated luminal mucus due to passive water flow into the cell.

While pancreatic insufficiency and chronic respiratory tract infections are the most salient clinical manifestations, these may be preceded by luminal GI symptoms. For example, neonates may present with intestinal obstruction as a result of dessicated, impacted meconium within the terminal ileum. Known as meconium ileus, this manifestation may be the earliest manifestation of CF. Contrary to the initial belief that it is almost invariably associated with CF, it is now known to affect patients without the disease as well (221). Some patients develop fibrosing colonopathy, a stricturing disorder associated with the use of high-dose pancreatic enzyme replacement

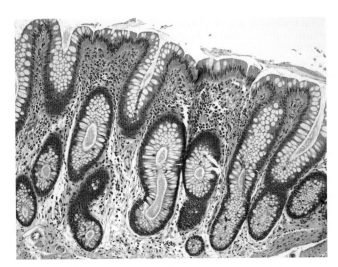

FIGURE 4.62 **Cystic fibrosis.** This colon biopsy from a patient with CF is near normal, save for inspissation of intraluminal mucus.

therapy (222,223). The most striking histologic changes are seen in resection specimens and include fibrosis and thickening of the muscularis propria (with preference for the inner circular layer), submucosal fibrosis, and prominent submucosal and muscularis propria mast cells (222,224). Superficial biopsies may be normal or may show disorganization or disintegration of the muscularis mucosae, intramucosal ganglion cells, prominent mucosal mast cells, eosinophilia, increased lamina propria cellularity and fibrosis, active inflammation, and goblet cell depletion (222,224) (Fig. 4.62, e-Fig. 4.256). Patients may require surgical resection of the affected colonic segment (223). Though believed to associate with high-dose pancreatic enzyme replacement, (a) cases of fibrosing colonopathy in patients who have never received such treatment are documented in the literature (225,226) and (b) many patients on high-dose replacement therapy do not develop this condition (223). The pathogenesis of this entity remains enigmatic.

Other miscellaneous conditions that may be encountered on rare occasion include bullous pemphigoid (e-Fig. 4.257–4.260) and histologic changes as a result of portal hypertension (e-Fig. 4.261–4.264).

REFERENCES

1. Tsang P, Rotterdam H. Biopsy diagnosis of colitis: possibilities and pitfalls. *Am J Surg Pathol*. 1999;23:423–430.
2. Drossman DA, Camilleri M, Mayer EA, et al. AGA technical review on irritable bowel syndrome. *Gastroenterology*. 2002;123:2108–2131.
3. Pascal RR, Gramlich TL, Parker KM, et al. Geographic variations in eosinophil concentration in normal colonic mucosa. *Mod Pathol*. 1997;10:363–365.
4. Leriche M, Devroede G, Sanchez G, et al. Changes in the rectal mucosa induced by hypertonic enemas. *Dis Colon Rectum*. 1978;21:227–236.

5. Driman DK, Preiksaitis HG. Colorectal inflammation and increased cell proliferation associated with oral sodium phosphate bowel preparation solution. *Hum Pathol* 1998;29;972–978.

6. Snover DC, Sandstad J, Hutton S. Mucosal pseudolipomatosis of the colon. *Am J Clin Pathol.* 1985;84:575–580.

7. Greenson JK, Stern RA, Carpenter SL, et al. The clinical significance of focal active colitis. *Hum Pathol.* 1997;28:729–733.

8. Volk EE, Shapiro BD, Easley KA, et al. The clinical significance of a biopsy-based diagnosis of focal active colitis: a clinicopathologic study of 31 cases. *Mod Pathol.* 1998;11:789–794.

9. Schneider EN, Havens JM, Scott MA, et al. Molecular diagnosis of Campylobacter jejuni infection in cases of focal active colitis. *Am J Surg Pathol.* 2006;30:782–785.

10. Xin W, Brown PI, Greenson JK. The clinical significance of focal active colitis in pediatric patients. *Am J Surg Pathol.* 2003;27:1134–1138.

11. Salto-Tellez M, Price AB. What is the significance of muciphages in colorectal biopsies? The significance of muciphages in otherwise normal colorectal biopsies. *Histopathology.* 2000;36:556–559.

12. Lou TY, Teplitz C, Thayer WR Jr. Ultrastructural morphogenesis of colonic PAS-positive macrophages ("colonic histiocytosis"). *Hum Pathol.* 1971;2:421–439.

13. Bejarano PA, Aranda-Michel J, Fenoglio-Preiser C. Histochemical and immunohistochemical characterization of foamy histiocytes (muciphages and xanthelasma) of the rectum. *Am J Surg Pathol.* 2000;24:1009–1015.

14. Koskela E, Kulju T, Collan Y. Melanosis coli. Prevalence, distribution, and histologic features in 200 consecutive autopsies at Kuopio University Central Hospital. *Dis Colon Rectum.* 1989;32:235–239.

15. Byers RJ, Marsh P, Parkinson D, et al. Melanosis coli is associated with an increase in colonic epithelial apoptosis and not with laxative use. *Histopathology.* 1997;30:160–164.

16. Ghadially FN, Parry EW. An electron-microscope and histochemical study of melanosis coli. *J Pathol Bacteriol.* 1966;92:313–317.

17. Walker NI, Smith MM, Smithers BM. Ultrastructure of human melanosis coli with reference to its pathogenesis. *Pathology.* 1993;25:120–123.

18. Ewing CA, Kalan M, Chucker F, et al. Melanosis coli involving pericolonic lymph nodes associated with the herbal laxative Swiss Kriss: a rare and incidental finding in a patient with colonic adenocarcinoma. *Arch Pathol Lab Med.* 2004;128:565–567.

19. Nascimbeni R, Donato F, Ghirardi M, et al. Constipation, anthranoid laxatives, melanosis coli, and colon cancer: a risk assessment using aberrant crypt foci. *Cancer Epidemiol Biomarkers Prev.* 2002;11:753–757.

20. Willems M, van Buuren HR, de Krijger R. Anthranoid self-medication causing rapid development of melanosis coli. *Neth J Med.* 2003;61:22–24.

21. Kunkel J, Schmidt S, Loddenkemper C, et al. Chronic diarrhea and melanosis coli caused by wellness drink. *Int J Colorectal Dis.* 2009;24:595–596.

22. Pardi DS, Tremaine WJ, Rothenberg HJ, et al. Melanosis coli in inflammatory bowel disease. *J Clin Gastroenterol.* 1998;26:167–170.

23. Nowicki MJ, Bishop PR, Subramony C, et al. Colonic chicken-skin mucosa in children with polyps is not a preneoplastic lesion. *J Pediatr Gastroenterol Nutr.* 2005;41:600–606.

24. Nowicki MJ, Subramony C, Bishop PR, et al. Colonic chicken skin mucosa: association with juvenile polyps in children. *Am J Gastroenterol.* 2001;96:788–792.

25. Shatz BA, Weinstock LB, Thyssen EP, et al. Colonic chicken skin mucosa: an endoscopic and histological abnormality adjacent to colonic neoplasms. *Am J Gastroenterol.* 1998;93:623–627.

26. Dimet S, Lazure T, Bedossa P. Signet-ring cell change in acute erosive gastropathy. *Am J Surg Pathol.* 2004;28:1111–1112.

27. Cameselle-Teijeiro J, Abdulkader I, Forteza J. Signet-ring cell change in pseudomembranous colitis versus signet-ring cell carcinoma. *Am J Surg Pathol*. 2004;28:1111.

28. Suri VS, Sakhuja P, Malhotra V, et al. Benign signet ring cell change with multilayering in the gallbladder mucosa–a case report. *Pathol Res Pract*. 2001;197:785–788.

29. Wang K, Weinrach D, Lal A, et al. Signet-ring cell change versus signet-ring cell carcinoma: a comparative analysis. *Am J Surg Pathol*. 2003;27:1429–1433.

30. Jessurun J, Paplanus SH, Nagle RB, et al. Pseudosarcomatous changes in inflammatory pseudopolyps of the colon. *Arch Pathol Lab Med*. 1986;110:833–836.

31. Shekitka KM, Helwig EB. Deceptive bizarre stromal cells in polyps and ulcers of the gastrointestinal tract. *Cancer*. 1991;67:2111–2117.

32. Odze R. Diagnostic problems and advances in inflammatory bowel disease. *Mod Pathol*. 2003;16:347–358.

33. Odze RD. Pathology of indeterminate colitis. *J Clin Gastroenterol*. 2004;38:S36–S40.

34. Glickman JN, Bousvaros A, Farraye FA, et al. Pediatric patients with untreated ulcerative colitis may present initially with unusual morphologic findings. *Am J Surg Pathol*. 2004;28:190–197.

35. Washington K, Greenson JK, Montgomery E, et al. Histopathology of ulcerative colitis in initial rectal biopsy in children. *Am J Surg Pathol*. 2002;26:1441–1449.

36. Emory T, Carpenter H, Gostout C, et al. Large intestine–Active chronic destructive colitis. *Atlas of gastrointestinal endoscopy and endoscopic biopsies*. Armed Forces Institute of Pathology/ American Registry of Pathology, 2000:312–327.

37. Rubenstein J, Sherif A, Appelman H, *et al*. Ulcerative colitis associated enteritis: is ulcerative colitis always confined to the colon? *J Clin Gastroenterol*. 2004;38:46–51.

38. Valdez R, Appelman HD, Bronner MP, et al. Diffuse duodenitis associated with ulcerative colitis. *Am J Surg Pathol*. 2000;24:1407–1413.

39. Lin J, McKenna BJ, Appelman HD. Morphologic findings in upper gastrointestinal biopsies of patients with ulcerative colitis: a controlled study. *Am J Surg Pathol*. 2010;34:1672–1677.

40. Bonen DK, Cho JH. The genetics of inflammatory bowel disease. *Gastroenterology*. 2003;124:521–536.

41. Benor S, Russell GH, Silver M, et al. Shortcomings of the inflammatory bowel disease Serology 7 panel. *Pediatrics*. 2010;125:1230–1236.

42. Gupta A, Derbes C, Sellin J. Clinical indications of the use of antineutrophil cytoplasmic antibodies and anti-Saccharomyces cerevisiae antibodies in the evaluation of inflammatory bowel disease at an Academic Medical Center. *Inflamm Bowel Dis*. 2005;11:898–902.

43. Sandborn WJ. Serologic markers in inflammatory bowel disease: state of the art. *Rev Gastroenterol Disord*. 2004;4:167–174.

44. Kim B, Barnett JL, Kleer CG, et al. Endoscopic and histological patchiness in treated ulcerative colitis. *Am J Gastroenterol*. 1999;94:3258–3262.

45. Kleer CG, Appelman HD. Ulcerative colitis: patterns of involvement in colorectal biopsies and changes with time. *Am J Surg Pathol*. 1998;22:983–989.

46. Assasi N, Blackhouse G, Xie F, et al. Patient outcomes after anti TNF-alpha drugs for Crohn's disease. *Expert Rev Pharmacoecon Outcomes Res*. 2010;10:163–175.

47. Seow CH, Benchimol EI, Steinhart AH, et al. Budesonide for Crohn's disease. *Expert Opin Drug Metab Toxicol*. 2009;5:971–979.

48. Kock NG. Intra-abdominal "reservoir" in patients with permanent ileostomy. Preliminary observations on a procedure resulting in fecal "continence" in five ileostomy patients. *Arch Surg*. 1969;99:223–231.

49. Kock NG. Construction of a continent ileostomy. *Schweiz Med Wochenschr*. 1971;101:729–734.

50. Kock NG, Myrvold HE, Nilsson LO, et al. Continent ileostomy. An account of 314 patients. *Acta Chir Scand*. 1981;147:67–72.

51. Yantiss RK, Sapp HL, Farraye FA, et al. Histologic predictors of pouchitis in patients with chronic ulcerative colitis. *Am J Surg Pathol*. 2004;28:999–1006.

52. Schmidt CM, Lazenby AJ, Hendrickson RJ, et al. Preoperative terminal ileal and colonic resection histopathology predicts risk of pouchitis in patients after ileoanal pull-through procedure. *Ann Surg*. 1998;227:654–662; discussion 663–655.

53. Stocchi L, Pemberton JH. Pouch and pouchitis. *Gastroenterol Clin North Am*. 2001;30:223–241.

54. Kmiot WA, Hesslewood SR, Smith N, et al. Evaluation of the inflammatory infiltrate in pouchitis with 111In-labeled granulocytes. *Gastroenterology*. 1993;104:981–988.

55. Kmiot WA, Youngs D, Tudor R, et al. Mucosal morphology, cell proliferation and faecal bacteriology in acute pouchitis. *Br J Surg*. 1993;80:1445–1449.

56. Shepherd NA. The pelvic ileal reservoir: pathology and pouchitis. *Neth J Med*. 1990;37(Suppl 1):S57–S64.

57. Moskowitz RL, Shepherd NA, Nicholls RJ. An assessment of inflammation in the reservoir after restorative proctocolectomy with ileoanal ileal reservoir. *Int J Colorectal Dis*. 1986;1:167–174.

58. Veress B, Reinholt FP, Lindquist K, et al. Different types of mucosal adaptation in the ileal reservoir after restorative proctocolectomy. A two-year follow-up study. *Apmis*. 1990;98:786–796.

59. Veress B, Reinholt FP, Lindquist K, et al. Prospective studies of the mucosa of the ileo-anal pouch. *Gastroenterology*. 1995;108:953–954.

60. Veress B, Reinholt FP, Lindquist K, et al. Long-term histomorphological surveillance of the pelvic ileal pouch: dysplasia develops in a subgroup of patients. *Gastroenterology*. 1995;109:1090–1097.

61. Sandborn WJ, Tremaine WJ, Batts KP, et al. Pouchitis after ileal pouch-anal anastomosis: a Pouchitis Disease Activity Index. *Mayo Clin Proc*. 1994;69:409–415.

62. Goldstein NS, Sanford WW, Bodzin JH. Crohn's-like complications in patients with ulcerative colitis after total proctocolectomy and ileal pouch-anal anastomosis. *Am J Surg Pathol*. 1997;21:1343–1353.

63. Scarpa M, van Koperen PJ, Ubbink DT, et al. Systematic review of dysplasia after restorative proctocolectomy for ulcerative colitis. *Br J Surg*. 2007;94:534–545.

64. Chambers WM, Mc CMNJ. Should ileal pouch-anal anastomosis include mucosectomy? *Colorectal Dis*. 2007;9:384–392.

65. Lowichik A, Weinberg AG. A quantitative evaluation of mucosal eosinophils in the pediatric gastrointestinal tract. *Mod Pathol*. 1996;9:110–114.

66. Polydorides AD, Banner BF, Hannaway PJ, et al. Evaluation of site-specific and seasonal variation in colonic mucosal eosinophils. *Hum Pathol*. 2008;39:832–836.

67. Bischoff SC. Food allergy and eosinophilic gastroenteritis and colitis. *Curr Opin Allergy Clin Immunol*. 2010;10:238–245.

68. Behjati S, Zilbauer M, Heuschkel R, et al. Defining eosinophilic colitis in children: insights from a retrospective case series. *J Pediatr Gastroenterol Nutr*. 2009;49:208–215.

69. Kumar NB, Nostrant TT, Appelman HD. The histopathologic spectrum of acute self-limited colitis (acute infectious-type colitis). *Am J Surg Pathol*. 1982;6:523–529.

70. Surawicz CM, Haggitt RC, Husseman M, et al. Mucosal biopsy diagnosis of colitis: acute self-limited colitis and idiopathic inflammatory bowel disease. *Gastroenterology*. 1994;107:755–763.

71. Lewin-Smith M, Wahl SM, Orenstein JM. Human immunodeficiency virus-rich multi-nucleated giant cells in the colon: a case report with transmission electron microscopy, immunohistochemistry, and in situ hybridization. *Mod Pathol*. 1999;12:75–81.

72. Khashab M, Wilson S, Cho WK. Image of the month. Intestinal spirochetosis: an unusual cause of asymptomatic colonic ulceration. *Clin Gastroenterol Hepatol.* 2010;8:A22.

73. Tsuzawa K, Fujisawa N, Sekino Y, et al. Education and Imaging. Gastrointestinal: colonic spirochetosis. *J Gastroenterol Hepatol.* 2008;23:1160.

74. Umeno J, Matsumoto T, Nakamura S, et al. Intestinal spirochetosis due to Brachyspira pilosicoli: endoscopic and radiographic features. *J Gastroenterol.* 2007;42:253–256.

75. Koteish A, Kannangai R, Abraham SC, et al. Colonic spirochetosis in children and adults. *Am J Clin Pathol.* 2003;120:828–832.

76. Esteve M, Salas A, Fernandez-Banares F, et al. Intestinal spirochetosis and chronic watery diarrhea: clinical and histological response to treatment and long-term follow up. *J Gastroenterol Hepatol.* 2006;21:1326–1333.

77. Lamps LW, Molina CP, West AB, et al. The pathologic spectrum of gastrointestinal and hepatic histoplasmosis. *Am J Clin Pathol.* 2000;113:64–72.

78. Orenstein JM, Dieterich DT. The histopathology of 103 consecutive colonoscopy biopsies from 82 symptomatic patients with acquired immunodeficiency syndrome: original and look-back diagnoses. *Arch Pathol Lab Med.* 2001;125:1042–1046.

79. Klausner JD, Kohn R, Kent C. Etiology of clinical proctitis among men who have sex with men. *Clin Infect Dis.* 2004;38:300–302.

80. de la Monte SM, Hutchins GM. Follicular proctocolitis and neuromatous hyperplasia with lymphogranuloma venereum. *Hum Pathol.* 1985;16:1025–1032.

81. Furman DL, Patel SK, Arluk GM. Endoscopic and histologic appearance of rectal syphilis. *Gastrointest Endosc.* 2008;67:161; commentary 161–162.

82. Nazemi MM, Musher DM, Schell RF, et al. Syphilitic proctitis in a homosexual. *JAMA.* 1975;231:389.

83. Teitelman M, Wilson JA, Guy CD. Image of the month. Syphilitic proctitis. *Clin Gastroenterol Hepatol.* 2008;6:xxvi.

84. Nisheena R, Ananthamurthy A, Inchara YK. Fulminant amebic colitis: a study of six cases. *Indian J Pathol Microbiol.* 2009;52:370–373.

85. Koo JS, Choi WS, Park DW. Fulminant amebic colitis mimicking pseudomembranous colitis. *Gastrointest Endosc.* 2010;71:400–401; discussion 401.

86. Bethony J, Brooker S, Albonico M, et al. Soil-transmitted helminth infections: ascariasis, trichuriasis, and hookworm. *Lancet.* 2006;367:1521–1532.

87. Khuroo MS, Khuroo NS. Trichuris dysentery syndrome: a common cause of chronic iron deficiency anemia in adults in an endemic area (with videos). *Gastrointest Endosc.* 2010;71:200–204.

88. Diniz-Santos DR, Jambeiro J, Mascarenhas RR, et al. Massive Trichuris trichiura infection as a cause of chronic bloody diarrhea in a child. *J Trop Pediatr.* 2006;52:66–68.

89. Do KR, Cho YS, Kim HK, et al. Intestinal helminthic infections diagnosed by colonoscopy in a regional hospital during 2001–2008. *Korean J Parasitol.* 2010;48:75–78.

90. Wiebe BM. Appendicitis and Enterobius vermicularis. *Scand J Gastroenterol.* 1991;26:336–338.

91. da Silva DF, da Silva RJ, da Silva MG, et al. Parasitic infection of the appendix as a cause of acute appendicitis. *Parasitol Res.* 2007;102:99–102.

92. Cao J, Liu WJ, Xu XY, et al. Endoscopic findings and clinicopathologic characteristics of colonic schistosomiasis: a report of 46 cases. *World J Gastroenterol.* 2010;16:723–727.

93. Mohamed AR, al Karawi M, Yasawy MI. Schistosomal colonic disease. *Gut.* 1990;31:439–442.

94. Atik FA, Lopes Filho GJ, Linhares Mde M, et al. Large intestine obstruction complicated with perforation: a rare manifestation of Schistosoma mansoni infection. *Sao Paulo Med J.* 1998;116:1781–1783.

95. Ming-Chai C, Chi-Yuan C, Pei-Yu C, et al. Evolution of colorectal cancer in schistso-somiasis: transitional mucosal changes adjacent to large intestinal carcinoma in colec-tomy specimens. *Cancer.* 1980;46:1661–1675.

96. Wu TS, Chen TC, Chen RJ, et al. Schistosoma japonicum infection presenting with colon perforation: case report. *Changgeng Yi Xue Za Zhi.* 1999;22:676–681.

97. Li WC, Pan ZG, Sun YH. Sigmoid colonic carcinoma associated with deposited ova of Schistosoma japonicum: a case report. *World J Gastroenterol.* 2006;12:6077–6079.

98. Dignan CR, Greenson JK. Can ischemic colitis be differentiated from C difficile colitis in biopsy specimens? *Am J Surg Pathol.* 1997;21:706–710.

99. Yamazaki T, Shirai Y, Tada T, et al. Ischemic colitis arising in watershed areas of the colonic blood supply: a report of two cases. *Surg Today.* 1997;27:460–462.

100. Longstreth GF, Yao JF. Diseases and drugs that increase risk of acute large bowel isch-emia. *Clin Gastroenterol Hepatol.* 2010;8:49–54.

101. Magee CD, Moawad FJ, Moses F. NO-Xplode: a case of supplement-associated isch-emic colitis. *Mil Med.* 2010;175:202–205.

102. Zou X, Cao J, Yao Y, et al. Endoscopic findings and clinicopathologic characteristics of ischemic colitis: a report of 85 cases. *Dig Dis Sci.* 2009;54:2009–2015.

103. McCabe ME, 3rd, Peura DA, Kadakia SC, et al. Gastrointestinal blood loss associated with running a marathon. *Dig Dis Sci.* 1986;31:1229–1232.

104. Heer M, Repond F, Hany A, et al. Acute ischaemic colitis in a female long distance run-ner. *Gut.* 1987;28:896–899.

105. Lucas W, Schroy PC, 3rd. Reversible ischemic colitis in a high endurance athlete. *Am J Gastroenterol.* 1998;93:2231–2234.

106. Moses FM, Brewer TG, Peura DA. Running-associated proximal hemorrhagic colitis. *Ann Intern Med.* 1988;108:385–386.

107. Zeitz M. Shock-associated nonocclusive ischemic colitis: a very rare event in young patients after trauma. *Int J Colorectal Dis.* 2001;16:58–59.

108. Johnson WM, Lior H, Bezanson GS. Cytotoxic Escherichia coli O157:H7 associated with haemorrhagic colitis in Canada. *Lancet.* 1983;1:76.

109. Riley LW, Remis RS, Helgerson SD, et al. Hemorrhagic colitis associated with a rare Escherichia coli serotype. *N Engl J Med.* 1983;308:681–685.

110. Bopp DJ, Sauders BD, Waring AL, et al. Detection, isolation, and molecular subtyping of Escherichia coli O157:H7 and Campylobacter jejuni associated with a large water-borne outbreak. *J Clin Microbiol.* 2003;41:174–180.

111. Carroll KC, Adamson K, Korgenski K, et al. Comparison of a commercial reversed passive latex agglutination assay to an enzyme immunoassay for the detection of Shiga toxin-producing Escherichia coli. *Eur J Clin Microbiol Infect Dis.* 2003;22:689–692.

112. Karch H, Bielaszewska M. Sorbitol-fermenting Shiga toxin-producing Escherichia coli O157:H(-) strains: epidemiology, phenotypic and molecular characteristics, and micro-biological diagnosis. *J Clin Microbiol.* 2001;39:2043–2049.

113. Richardson SE, Karmali MA, Becker LE, et al. The histopathology of the hemolytic uremic syndrome associated with verocytotoxin-producing Escherichia coli infections. *Hum Pathol.* 1988;19:1102–1108.

114. Kelly J, Oryshak A, Wenetsek M, et al. The colonic pathology of Escherichia coli O157:H7 infection. *Am J Surg Pathol.* 1990;14:87–92.

115. Su C, Brandt LJ, Sigal SH, et al. The immunohistological diagnosis of E. coli O157:H7 colitis: possible association with colonic ischemia. *Am J Gastroenterol.* 1998;93:1055–1059.

116. Boutros HH, Pautler S, Chakrabarti S. Cocaine-induced ischemic colitis with small-vessel thrombosis of colon and gallbladder. *J Clin Gastroenterol.* 1997;24:49–53.

117. Brown DN, Rosenholtz MJ, Marshall JB. Ischemic colitis related to cocaine abuse. *Am J Gastroenterol.* 1994;89:1558–1561.

118. Linder JD, Monkemuller KE, Raijman I, et al. Cocaine-associated ischemic colitis. *South Med J.* 2000;93:909–913.

119. Niazi M, Kondru A, Levy J, et al. Spectrum of ischemic colitis in cocaine users. *Dig Dis Sci.* 1997;42:1537–1541.

120. Papi C, Candia S, Masci P, et al. Acute ischaemic colitis following intravenous cocaine use. *Ital J Gastroenterol Hepatol.* 1999;31:305–307.

121. Simmers TA, Vidakovic-Vukic M, Van Meyel JJ. Cocaine-induced ischemic colitis. *Endoscopy.* 1998;30:S8–S9.

122. Dowd J, Bailey D, Moussa K, et al. Ischemic colitis associated with pseudoephedrine: four cases. *Am J Gastroenterol.* 1999;94:2430–2434.

123. Klestov A, Kubler P, Meulet J. Recurrent ischaemic colitis associated with pseudo-ephedrine use. *Intern Med J.* 2001;31:195–196.

124. Lichtenstein GR, Yee NS. Ischemic colitis associated with decongestant use. *Ann Intern Med.* 2000;132:682.

125. Deana DG, Dean PJ. Reversible ischemic colitis in young women. Association with oral contraceptive use. *Am J Surg Pathol.* 1995;19:454–462.

126. Frossard JL, Spahr L, Queneau PE, et al. Ischemic colitis during pregnancy and contraceptive medication. *Digestion.* 2001;64:125–127.

127. Garcia B, Ramaholimihaso F, Diebold MD, et al. Ischaemic colitis in a patient taking meloxicam. *Lancet.* 2001;357:690.

128. Yarze JC. Ischaemic colitis and meloxicam. *Lancet.* 2001;357:1619.

129. Rashid A, Hamilton SR. Necrosis of the gastrointestinal tract in uremic patients as a result of sodium polystyrene sulfonate (Kayexalate) in sorbitol: an underrecognized condition. *Am J Surg Pathol.* 1997;21:60–69.

130. Knudsen JF, Friedman B, Chen M, et al. Ischemic colitis and sumatriptan use. *Arch Intern Med.* 1998;158:1946–1948.

131. Naik M, Potluri R, Almasri E, et al. Sumatriptan-associated ischemic colitis. *Dig Dis Sci.* 2002;47:2015–2016.

132. Horton R. Lotronex and the FDA: a fatal erosion of integrity. *Lancet.* 2001;357:1544–1545.

133. Lisi DM. Lotronex withdrawal. *Arch Intern Med.* 2002;162:101.

134. Miller DP, Alfredson T, Cook SF, et al. Incidence of colonic ischemia, hospitalized complications of constipation, and bowel surgery in relation to use of alosetron hydrochloride. *Am J Gastroenterol.* 2003;98:1117–1122.

135. Shen B, Soffer EE. Alosetron (Lotronex) is back: should I use it to treat my patients with irritable bowel syndrome? *Cleve Clin J Med.* 2003;70:64–65.

136. Chang L, Tong K, Ameen V. Ischemic colitis and complications of constipation associated with the use of alosetron under a risk management plan: clinical characteristics, outcomes, and incidences. *Am J Gastroenterol.* 2010;105:866–875.

137. Rahimi R, Nikfar S, Abdollahi M. Efficacy and tolerability of alosetron for the treatment of irritable bowel syndrome in women and men: a meta-analysis of eight randomized, placebo-controlled, 12-week trials. *Clin Ther.* 2008;30:884–901.

138. Tuppy H, Haidenthaler A, Schandalik R, et al. Idiopathic enterocolic lymphocytic phlebitis: a rare cause of ischemic colitis. *Mod Pathol.* 2000;13:897–899.

139. Trimble MA, Weisz MA. Infarction of the sigmoid colon secondary to giant cell arteritis. *Rheumatology (Oxford).* 2002;41:108–110.

140. Preventza OA, Lazarides K, Sawyer MD. Ischemic colitis in young adults: a single-institution experience. *J Gastrointest Surg.* 2001;5:388–392.

141. Theodoropoulou A, Sfiridaki A, Oustamanolakis P, et al. Genetic risk factors in young patients with ischemic colitis. *Clin Gastroenterol Hepatol.* 2008;6:907–911.

142. Wielosz E, Borys O, Zychowska I, et al. Gastrointestinal involvement in patients with systemic sclerosis. *Pol Arch Med Wewn*. 2010;120:132–136.

143. Jaovisidha K, Csuka ME, Almagro UA, et al. Severe gastrointestinal involvement in systemic sclerosis: report of five cases and review of the literature. *Semin Arthritis Rheum*. 2005;34:689–702.

144. Krishnamurthy S, Schuffler MD. Pathology of neuromuscular disorders of the small intestine and colon. *Gastroenterology*. 1987;93:610–639.

145. Geboes K, Dalle I. Vasculitis and the gastrointestinal tract. *Acta Gastroenterol Belg*. 2002;65:204–212.

146. Iwashita A, Yao T, Schlemper RJ, et al. Mesenteric phlebosclerosis: a new disease entity causing ischemic colitis. *Dis Colon Rectum*. 2003;46:209–220.

147. Passam FH, Diamantis ID, Perisinaki G, et al. Intestinal ischemia as the first manifestation of vasculitis. *Semin Arthritis Rheum*. 2004;34:431–441.

148. Saraga E, Bouzourenne H. Enterocolic (lymphocytic) phlebitis: a rare cause of intestinal ischemic necrosis: a series of six patients and review of the literature. *Am J Surg Pathol*. 2000;24:824–829.

149. Schuler JG, Hudlin MM. Cecal necrosis: infrequent variant of ischemic colitis. Report of five cases. *Dis Colon Rectum*. 2000;43:708–712.

150. Storesund B, Gran JT, Koldingsnes W. Severe intestinal involvement in Wegener's granulomatosis: report of two cases and review of the literature. *Br J Rheumatol*. 1998;37:387–390.

151. Flaherty MJ, Lie JT, Haggitt RC. Mesenteric inflammatory veno-occlusive disease. A seldom recognized cause of intestinal ischemia. *Am J Surg Pathol*. 1994;18:779–784.

152. Turan M, Sen M, Koyuncu A, et al. Sigmoid colon perforation as an unusual complication of Behcet's syndrome: report of a case. *Surg Today*. 2003;33:383–386.

153. Dowling CM, Hill AD, Malone C, et al. Colonic perforation in Behcet's syndrome. *World J Gastroenterol*. 2008;14:6578–6580.

154. Chou SJ, Chen VT, Jan HC, et al. Intestinal perforations in Behcet's disease. *J Gastrointest Surg*. 2007;11:508–514.

155. Kim JH, Choi BI, Han JK, et al. Colitis in Behcet's disease: characteristics on double-contrast barium enema examination in 20 patients. *Abdom Imaging*. 1994;19:132–136.

156. Koklu S, Yuksel O, Onur I, et al. Ileocolonic involvement in Behcet's disease: endoscopic and histological evaluation. *Digestion*. 2010;81:214–217.

157. Fujita H, Kiriyama M, Kawamura T, et al. Massive hemorrhage in a patient with intestinal Behcet's disease: report of a case. *Surg Today*. 2002;32:378–382.

158. Pagnoux C, Mahr A, Cohen P, et al. Presentation and outcome of gastrointestinal involvement in systemic necrotizing vasculitides: analysis of 62 patients with polyarteritis nodosa, microscopic polyangiitis, Wegener granulomatosis, Churg-Strauss syndrome, or rheumatoid arthritis-associated vasculitis. *Medicine (Baltimore)*. 2005;84:115–128.

159. Hill SM, Milla PJ, Bottazzo GF, et al. Autoimmune enteropathy and colitis: is there a generalised autoimmune gut disorder? *Gut*. 1991;32:36–42.

160. Carroccio A, Volta U, Di Prima L, et al. Autoimmune enteropathy and colitis in an adult patient. *Dig Dis Sci*. 2003;48:1600–1606.

161. Kyle RA, Gertz MA, Lacy MQ, et al. Localized AL amyloidosis of the colon: an unrecognized entity. *Amyloid*. 2003;10:36–41.

162. Parks RW, O'Rourke D, Bharucha H, et al. Perforation of the sigmoid colon secondary to localised amyloidosis. *Ulster Med J*. 2002;71:144–146.

163. Thaler W, Schatzer G, Eder P, et al. Amyloidosis–an unusual case of recurrent intestinal bleeding and sigmoid perforation: case report with review of the literature. *Int J Colorectal Dis*. 1999;14:297–299.

164. Akin C, Metcalfe DD. Systemic mastocytosis. *Ann Rev Med*. 2004;55:419–432.

165. Alto WA, Clarcq L. Cutaneous and systemic manifestations of mastocytosis. *Am Fam Physician*. 1999;59:3047–3054, 3059–3060.

166. Hahn HP, Hornick JL. Immunoreactivity for CD25 in gastrointestinal mucosal mast cells is specific for systemic mastocytosis. *Am J Surg Pathol*. 2007;31:1669–1676.

167. Jensen RT. Gastrointestinal abnormalities and involvement in systemic mastocytosis. *Hematol Oncol Clin North Am*. 2000;14:579–623.

168. Kirsch R, Geboes K, Shepherd NA, et al. Systemic mastocytosis involving the gastrointestinal tract: clinicopathologic and molecular study of five cases. *Mod Pathol*. 2008;21:1508–1516.

169. Ma Y, Zeng S, Metcalfe DD, et al. The c-KIT mutation causing human mastocytosis is resistant to STI571 and other KIT kinase inhibitors; kinases with enzymatic site mutations show different inhibitor sensitivity profiles than wild-type kinases and those with regulatory-type mutations. *Blood*. 2002;99:1741–1744.

170. Bedeir A, Jukic DM, Wang L, et al. Systemic mastocytosis mimicking inflammatory bowel disease: a case report and discussion of gastrointestinal pathology in systemic mastocytosis. *Am J Surg Pathol*. 2006;30:1478–1482.

171. Jakate S, Demeo M, John R, et al. Mastocytic enterocolitis: increased mucosal mast cells in chronic intractable diarrhea. *Arch Pathol Lab Med*. 2006;130:362–367.

172. Nanduri VR, Kelly K, Malone M, et al. Colon involvement in Langerhans' cell histiocytosis. *J Pediatr Gastroenterol Nutr*. 1999;29:462–466.

173. Kibria R, Gibbs PM, Novick DM. Adult Langerhans cell histiocytosis: a rare cause of colon polyp. *Endoscopy*. 2009;41(Suppl 2);E160–E161.

174. Hyams JS, Haswell JE, Gerber MA, et al. Colonic ulceration in histiocytosis X. *J Pediatr Gastroenterol Nutr*. 1985;4:286–290.

175. Gilmore BS, Cohen M. Barium enema findings in a case of Langerhans cell histiocytosis involving the colon. *Pediatr Radiol*. 1993;23:589–590.

176. Singhi A, Montgomery E. Langerhans' cell histiocytosis of the gastrointestinal tract. *Am J Surg Pathol*. 2011;35(2):305–10.

177. Daniels JA, Lederman HM, Maitra A, et al. Gastrointestinal tract pathology in patients with common variable immunodeficiency (CVID): a clinicopathologic study and review. *Am J Surg Pathol*. 2007;31:1800–1812.

178. Levine S, Smith VV, Malone M, et al. Histopathological features of chronic granulomatous disease (CGD) in childhood. *Histopathology*. 2005;47:508–516.

179. Washington K, Stenzel TT, Buckley RH, et al. Gastrointestinal pathology in patients with common variable immunodeficiency and X-linked agammaglobulinemia. *Am J Surg Pathol*. 1996;20:1240–1252.

180. Weidner N, Askin FB, Berthrong M, et al. Bizarre (pseudomalignant) granulation-tissue reactions following ionizing-radiation exposure. A microscopic, immunohistochemical, and flow-cytometric study. *Cancer*. 1987;59:1509–1514.

181. Papadimitriou JC, Cangro CB, Lustberg A, et al. Histologic features of mycophenolate mofetil-related colitis: a graft-versus-host disease-like pattern. *Int J Surg Pathol*. 2003;11:295–302.

182. Oble DA, Mino-Kenudson M, Goldsmith J, et al. Alpha-CTLA-4 mAb-associated panenteritis: a histologic and immunohistochemical analysis. *Am J Surg Pathol*. 2008;32:1130–1137.

183. Villanacci V, Talbot IC, Rossi E, et al. Ischaemia: a pathogenetic clue in diversion colitis? *Colorectal Dis*. 2007;9:601–605.

184. Abbasakoor F, Mahon C, Boulos PB. Diversion colitis in sigmoid neovagina. *Colorectal Dis*. 2004;6:290–291.

185. Syed HA, Malone PS, Hitchcock RJ. Diversion colitis in children with colovaginoplasty. *BJU Int.* 2001;87:857–860.

186. Toolenaar TA, Freundt I, Huikeshoven FJ, et al. The occurrence of diversion colitis in patients with a sigmoid neovagina. *Hum Pathol.* 1993;24:846–849.

187. Harig JM, Soergel KH, Komorowski RA, et al. Treatment of diversion colitis with short-chain-fatty acid irrigation. *N Engl J Med.* 1989;320:23–28.

188. Read NW, Krejs GJ, Read MG, et al. Chronic diarrhea of unknown origin. Gastroenterology 1980;78:264–271.

189. Kao KT, Pedraza BA, McClune AC, et al. Microscopic colitis: a large retrospective analysis from a health maintenance organization experience. *World J Gastroenterol.* 2009;15:3122–3127.

190. Lindstrom CG. 'Collagenous colitis' with watery diarrhoea–a new entity? *Pathol Eur.* 1976;11:87–89.

191. Nomura E, Kagaya H, Uchimi K, et al. Linear mucosal defects: a characteristic endoscopic finding of lansoprazole-associated collagenous colitis. *Endoscopy.* 2010;42(Suppl 2);E9–E10.

192. Umeno J, Matsumoto T, Nakamura S, et al. Linear mucosal defect may be characteristic of lansoprazole-associated collagenous colitis. *Gastrointest Endosc.* 2008;67:1185–1191.

193. Yusuke H, Jun T, Naotaka M, *et al.* Lansoprazole-associated collagenous colitis: unique presentation, similar to ischemic colitis. *Endoscopy.* 2009;41(Suppl 2):E281–E282.

194. Bohr J, Tysk C, Eriksson S, et al. Collagenous colitis: a retrospective study of clinical presentation and treatment in 163 patients. *Gut.* 1996;39:846–851.

195. Lazenby AJ, Yardley JH, Giardiello FM, et al. Pitfalls in the diagnosis of collagenous colitis: experience with 75 cases from a registry of collagenous colitis at the Johns Hopkins Hospital. *Hum Pathol.* 1990;21:905–910.

196. Kakar S, Pardi DS, Burgart LJ. Colonic ulcers accompanying collagenous colitis: implication of nonsteroidal anti-inflammatory drugs. *Am J Gastroenterol.* 2003;98:1834–1837.

197. Allende DS, Taylor SL, Bronner MP. Colonic perforation as a complication of collagenous colitis in a series of 12 patients. *Am J Gastroenterol.* 2008;103:2598–2604.

198. Lazenby AJ, Yardley JH, Giardiello FM, et al. Lymphocytic ("microscopic") colitis: a comparative histopathologic study with particular reference to collagenous colitis. *Hum Pathol.* 1989;20:18–28.

199. Jessurun J, Yardley JH, Lee EL, et al. Microscopic and collagenous colitis: different names for the same condition? *Gastroenterology.* 1986;91:1583–1584.

200. Rubio CA, Orrego A, Hoog A, et al. Quantitative assessment of the subepithelial collagen band does not increase the accuracy of diagnosis of collagenous colitis. *Am J Clin Pathol.* 2008;130:375–381.

201. Wang HH, Owings DV, Antonioli DA, et al. Increased subepithelial collagen deposition is not specific for collagenous colitis. *Mod Pathol.* 1988;1:329–335.

202. Goldstein NS, Gyorfi T. Focal lymphocytic colitis and collagenous colitis: patterns of Crohn's colitis? *Am J Surg Pathol.* 1999;23:1075–1081.

203. Najarian RM, Hait EJ, Leichtner AM, et al. Clinical significance of colonic intraepithelial lymphocytosis in a pediatric population. *Mod Pathol.* 2009;22:13–20.

204. Ayata G, Ithamukkala S, Sapp H, et al. Prevalence and significance of inflammatory bowel disease-like morphologic features in collagenous and lymphocytic colitis. *Am J Surg Pathol.* 2002;26:1414–1423.

205. Brown IS, Lambie DL. Microscopic colitis with giant cells: a clinico-pathological review of 11 cases and comparison with microscopic colitis without giant cells. *Pathology.* 2008;40:671–675.

206. Gore S, Shepherd NA, Wilkinson SP. Endoscopic crescentic fold disease of the sigmoid colon: the clinical and histopathological spectrum of a distinctive endoscopic appearance. *Int J Colorectal Dis.* 1992;7:76–81.

207. Peppercorn MA. Drug-responsive chronic segmental colitis associated with diverticula: a clinical syndrome in the elderly. *Am J Gastroenterol.* 1992;87:609–612.

208. Makapugay LM, Dean PJ. Diverticular disease-associated chronic colitis. *Am J Surg Pathol.* 1996;20:94–102.

209. Goldstein NS, Leon-Armin C, Mani A. Crohn's colitis-like changes in sigmoid diverticulitis specimens is usually an idiosyncratic inflammatory response to the diverticulosis rather than Crohn's colitis. *Am J Surg Pathol.* 2000;24:668–675.

210. McCallion AS, Stames E, Conlon RA, et al. Phenotype variation in two-locus mouse models of Hirschsprung disease: tissue-specific interaction between Ret and Ednrb. *Proc Natl Acad Sci USA.* 2003;100:1826–1831.

211. Kapur RP. Neuronal dysplasia: a controversial pathological correlate of intestinal pseudo-obstruction. *Am J Med Genet.* 2003;122A:287–293.

212. Galvis DA, Yunis EJ. Comparison of neuropeptide Y, protein gene product 9.5, and acetylcholinesterase in the diagnosis of Hirschsprung's disease. *Pediatr Pathol Lab Med.* 1997;17:413–425.

213. Karnovsky MJ, Roots L. A "Direct-Coloring" Thiocholine Method for Cholinesterases. *J Histochem Cytochem.* 1964;12:219–221.

214. Guinard-Samuel V, Bonnard A, De Lagausie P, et al. Calretinin immunohistochemistry: a simple and efficient tool to diagnose Hirschsprung disease. *Mod Pathol.* 2009;22:1379–1384.

215. Kapur RP, Reed RC, Finn LS, et al. Calretinin immunohistochemistry versus acetylcholinesterase histochemistry in the evaluation of suction rectal biopsies for Hirschsprung Disease. *Pediatr Dev Pathol.* 2009;12:6–15.

216. Holland SK, Hessler RB, Reid-Nicholson MD, et al. Utilization of peripherin and S-100 immunohistochemistry in the diagnosis of Hirschsprung disease. *Mod Pathol.* 2010;23:1173–1179.

217. Parisi MA, Kapur RP. Genetics of Hirschsprung disease. *Curr Opin Pediatr.* 2000;12:610–617.

218. Aldridge RT, Campbell PE. Ganglion cell distribution in the normal rectum and anal canal. A basis for the diagnosis of Hirschsprung's disease by anorectal biopsy. *J Pediatr Surg.* 1968;3:475–490.

219. Gibson RL, Burns JL, Ramsey BW. Pathophysiology and management of pulmonary infections in cystic fibrosis. *Am J Respir Crit Care Med.* 2003;168:918–951.

220. Worldwide survey of the delta F508 mutation–report from the cystic fibrosis genetic analysis consortium. *Am J Hum Genet.* 1990;47:354–359.

221. Gorter RR, Karimi A, Sleeboom C, et al. Clinical and genetic characteristics of meconium ileus in newborns with and without cystic fibrosis. *J Pediatr Gastroenterol Nutr.* 2010;50:569–572.

222. Schwarzenberg SJ, Wielinski CL, Shamieh I, et al. Cystic fibrosis-associated colitis and fibrosing colonopathy. *J Pediatr.* 1995;127:565–570.

223. Stevens JC, Maguiness KM, Hollingsworth J, et al. Pancreatic enzyme supplementation in cystic fibrosis patients before and after fibrosing colonopathy. *J Pediatr Gastroenterol Nutr.* 1998;26:80–84.

224. Pawel BR, de Chadarevian JP, Franco ME. The pathology of fibrosing colonopathy of cystic fibrosis: a study of 12 cases and review of the literature. *Hum Pathol.* 1997;28:395–399.

225. Waters BL. Cystic fibrosis with fibrosing colonopathy in the absence of pancreatic enzymes. *Pediatr Dev Pathol.* 1998;1:74–78.

226. Serban DE, Florescu P, Miu N. Fibrosing colonopathy revealing cystic fibrosis in a neonate before any pancreatic enzyme supplementation. *J Pediatr Gastroenterol Nutr.* 2002;35:356–359.

5

ANUS

It is probably most important for pathologists to remember that a biopsy from the anatomic (clinical) anus can display glandular, transitional, or squamous mucosa, and a biopsy labeled "anus," showing colonic-type mucosa, is not necessarily labeled incorrectly or obtained ineptly (Fig. 5.1). The anal canal, by anatomic definition, begins as the rectum enters the puborectalis sling (palpated as the anorectal ring on a digital exam) and ends at the squamous mucocutaneous junction with the perianal skin (1). The anal canal forms during the fourth and seventh weeks of gestation; the upper two thirds are endoderm-derived, and the lower one third is ectodermally derived. The dentate, or pectinate line, is where these zones meet.

The anus can also be divided into the mucosa-lined anal canal and the more distal epidermis-covered anal margin. Where the skin meets the canal, apocrine glands may be prominent and, like in skin, melanocytes can be encountered (e-Figs. 5.1–5.4). Cancers arising in the anal margin are regarded as skin cancers and are treated with local excision. The anal canal extends proximally from the anal verge to the rectal mucosa. Most of the anal canal is lined with squamous mucosa, which is present between the anal verge and the dentate (or pectinate) line. The dentate line is a visually identifiable border between the more distal squamous mucosa and a transitional area of squamous and nonsquamous mucosa. The adjacent nonsquamous lining can consist of either transitional (urothelium-like) or rectal glandular mucosa (Fig. 5.1) (2,3). Anal ducts and glands are found at the transition zone and lymphatic spaces are often prominent in these areas (e-Figs. 5.5–5.9).

The anal canal has a variable number of anal glands, ranging from 3 to 10 with a median number of 6 (Fig. 5.2). Most are located within the submucosa but some may be found within the anal sphincters. These mucus-secreting glands are lined by stratified columnar epithelium, sometimes with goblet cells; are typically associated with a lymphocytic infiltrate; and are surrounded by one or two layers of myoepithelial cells (4). Their secretions empty within the anal sinuses. Like their salivary counterparts, these glands can undergo squamous metaplasia (Fig. 5.2, e-Figs. 5.10 and 5.11). Neoplasms arising in association with these glands are rare and are addressed in Volume 2.

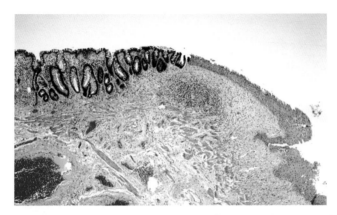

FIGURE 5.1 **Anal transitional zone.** This image shows an abrupt transitional zone between squamous and rectal-type mucosa.

Biopsies of the anal canal are less frequently encountered than those from the remainder of the gastrointestinal (GI) tract. Of course, the length of the anus accounts for the minority of the GI tract. For example, in our material, we receive colon biopsy accessions from about 5,000 patients each year, but only about 250 patients have anal biopsies. We would probably receive fewer anal biopsies if a clinic in our hospital were not directed at detecting human papillomavirus (HPV)-related intraepithelial lesions in high-risk individuals. Anal cancers are uncommon (estimated new cases for 2010 were about 5,260, in contrast to about 142,570 for the colon

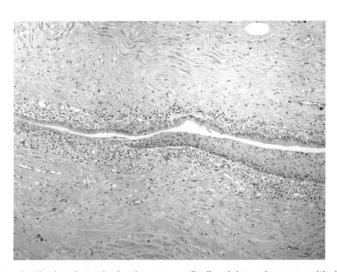

FIGURE 5.2 **Anal gland.** Anal glands are usually lined by columnar epithelium. Note the surrounding lymphocytic infiltrate. Like their salivary counterparts, these glands can undergo squamous metaplasia, as illustrated in the right side of the field.

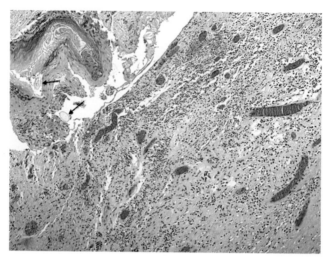

FIGURE 5.3 **Pilonidal disease.** Note fibrous tissue, chronic inflammatory cells, and associated hair shafts (*arrows*).

and rectum) (5); pilonidal disease, which is common, is seldom biopsied (Figs. 5.3 and 5.4).

Of course, the anus can be the site for a host of conditions affecting the skin, a topic beyond the scope of this slim manual, but, e.g., various keratoses can be found in the anal area. When typical seborrheic keratoses present in this area, they raise the possibility of condyloma based on their site, despite their lack of viral cytopathic changes (Fig. 5.5, e-Figs. 5.12 and 5.13). In patients who have been irradiated (typically for prostate or

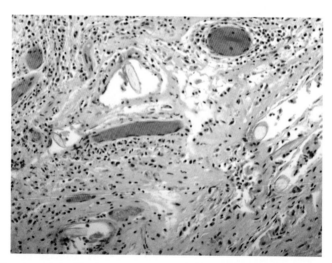

FIGURE 5.4 **Pilonidal disease.** This is a higher power image of Figure 5.3, showing portions of hair shafts and associated fibroinflammatory reaction.

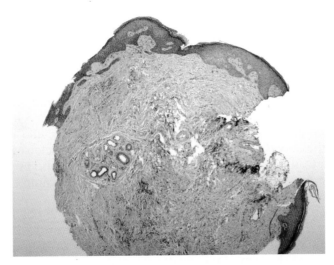

FIGURE 5.5 **Radiation injury affecting the epidermis-covered anal margin.** The most striking finding at this power is the dense fibrous scarring. Note apocrine glands to the left-hand side of the field.

cervical cancer), the usual radiation-associated changes are seen (6) including hyalinized vessels and collagen (Figs. 5.5 and 5.6, e-Figs. 5.14–5.18).

HEMORRHOIDS

Hemorrhoids are common and were the subject of both a review and a position statement by the American Gastroenterologic Association in 2004 (7,8). They were traditionally viewed as varicosities of submucosal veins

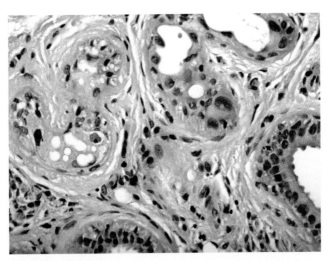

FIGURE 5.6 **Radiation injury.** This higher magnification image of Figure 5.5 shows effects of radiation on the apocrine glands. Note nuclear atypia and cytoplasmic vacuolation with a low nuclear-to-cytoplasmic ratio.

but are now believed to reflect sagging or slippage of normal structures, probably exacerbated by straining at defecation. Hemorrhoids are normal anatomic structures found in the subepithelial space of the anal canal (7–9). They consist of connective tissue cushions surrounding the direct arteriovenous communications between the terminal branches of the superior rectal arteries and the superior, inferior, and middle rectal veins. Anal subepithelial smooth muscle arises from the conjoined longitudinal muscle layer, passes through the internal anal sphincter, and inserts into the subepithelial vascular space. There, the smooth muscle suspends and contributes to the bulk of the hemorrhoidal cushions. The hemorrhoidal cushions serve as a conformable "stopper" to ensure complete closure of the anal canal.

Hemorrhoidal vessels are usually located above the dentate line on the left lateral, right anterior, and right posterior aspects of the anal canal. Symptomatic hemorrhoids may be above (internal) or below (external) the dentate line. In some individuals, external hemorrhoids are actually prolapsed internal hemorrhoids.

Symptoms attributed to hemorrhoids include bleeding, protrusion, itching, and pain. For the most part, external hemorrhoids are asymptomatic unless they become thrombosed, in which case they present as an acutely painful, perianal lump. Persisting skin tags after resolution of the thrombosis can lead to problems with hygiene and secondary irritation.

Most hemorrhoidal symptoms arise from enlarged internal hemorrhoids. Abnormal swelling of the anal cushions, stretching of the suspensory muscles, and dilation of the submucosal arteriovenous plexus result in the prolapse of upper anal and lower rectal tissue through the anal canal. This tissue is easily traumatized and leads to bleeding.

The pathogenesis of the enlarged, prolapsing cushions is unknown. Many clinicians believe that inadequate fiber intake, prolonged sitting on the toilet, and chronic straining at stool are all factors, but there are few evidence-based studies to support these assertions. On the other hand, there is evidence that ingestion of fiber can improve symptomatic hemorrhoids (10).

The community-wide prevalence of hemorrhoids in the United States is reported to be 4.4%, with a peak prevalence occurring between 45 and 65 years of age. There is no gender predilection, but they are frequent during pregnancy. Increased prevalence rates are associated with higher socioeconomic status, but this association may reflect differences in health-seeking behavior. Population-based surveys suggest that the prevalence of hemorrhoids decreased in both the United States and the United Kingdom during the second half of the 20th century. Hemorrhoids are frequent in patients with spinal cord injury. Prominent hemorrhoids had been touted in patients with the so-called "gay bowel" syndrome in early literature (11) but a 2004 study of anal disease in human immunodeficiency virus (HIV) patients (presumably an overlapping patient group) listed an incidence of hemorrhoids from 4% to 5% (12), a figure identical to that in the community at large. Patients with portal hypertension have been reported to have hemorrhoids more frequently than controls (in one study, about half of the control group had hemorrhoids vs. 70% of those with cirrhosis and portal hypertension) (13), but, in fact, portal hypertension causes varices of the anal canal. These varices are distinct from hemorrhoids. Rectal variceal bleeding is best treated by correction of the underlying portal hypertension. Because symptoms caused by other conditions are frequently attributed to hemorrhoids, a careful clinical examination is warranted to exclude other diseases (14).

As above, hemorrhoids are defined as internal or external, according to their position relative to the dentate line. External hemorrhoids become symptomatic only when thrombosed, or when skin tags are so large that hygiene is impossible. Thrombosed external hemorrhoids are common. Such patients present with acute-onset anal pain and a palpable perianal lump. Thrombosed external hemorrhoids occasionally bleed when local pressure causes erosion through the overlying skin. Thrombosed internal hemorrhoids are far less common; typical symptoms include pain, pressure, bleeding, mucus production, and an inability to reduce spontaneously prolapsing tissue.

Symptoms of internal hemorrhoids include bleeding and protrusion. Prolapsed hemorrhoids are a cause of soiling and mucus discharge, and both lead to secondary *pruritus ani*. Advanced prolapsed hemorrhoids may become incarcerated and strangulated.

Most colorectal surgeons use the grading system published in 1985 by Banov et al. (15). Internal hemorrhoids that bleed, but do not prolapse, are designated as first-degree hemorrhoids. Those that prolapse and reduce spontaneously (with or without bleeding) are second-degree hemorrhoids. Prolapsed hemorrhoids that require reduction are third-degree hemorrhoids. Prolapsed internal hemorrhoids that cannot be reduced are fourth-degree hemorrhoids; they usually include both internal and external components and are confluent from skin tag to inner anal canal. Acutely thrombosed, incarcerated internal hemorrhoids and incarcerated, thrombosed hemorrhoids involving circumferential rectal mucosal prolapse are also fourth-degree hemorrhoids.

Surgical treatment of hemorrhoids is suggested in only a minority of cases. The indications for surgery are (a) failure of medical and nonoperative therapy; (b) symptomatic third-degree, fourth-degree, or mixed internal and external hemorrhoids; (c) symptomatic hemorrhoids in the presence of a concomitant anorectal condition that requires surgery; and (d) patient preference (7).

When hemorrhoids are seen in excised material, they feature large ectatic vessels, and the associated mucosa typically displays prolapse changes (16) (Fig. 5.7, e-Figs. 5.19 and 5.20). "Pagetoid dyskeratosis" in overlying squamous mucosa, similar to that seen in prolapsed uterine cervices, is also observed (17) (e-Fig. 5.20). We would not suggest reporting this peculiar pattern of dyskeratosis using such terminology (which might

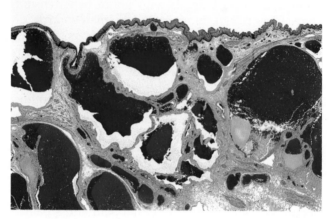

FIGURE 5.7 **Low magnification image of hemorrhoids.** Note the ectatic vessels.

prompt excessive concern on the part of the surgeon), but we would suggest that it is not to be mistaken for HPV cytopathic changes. The mucosa overlying hemorrhoids should always be examined for the possibility of squamous neoplasia (further discussed in Volume 2).

PAPILLARY ENDOTHELIAL HYPERPLASIA (VEGETANT INTRAVASCULAR HEMANGIOENDOTHELIOMA)

Papillary endothelial hyperplasia (PEH) has been reported all over the body (18–25), but the very first report was in hemorrhoidal vessels, imparting a gross appearance that Masson likened to a cherry (26) (and first year pathology residents have been hearing about this with glazed eyes ever since).

This benign reactive process is an unusually exuberant form of organizing vascular thrombus. PEH may occur at any age and involve virtually any vessel, including those of neoplastic processes and vascular malformations. However, in its "pure" form, it typically presents as a solitary, superficial, firm, bluish or erythematous mass, involving the fingers, head, neck, or anorectal region.

Histologically, the lesion shows papillary fronds with a core of fibrin or hyalinized collagen, lined by a single layer of endothelial cells, which may be plump or swollen but lack significant atypia or mitotic activity (Fig. 5.8, e-Figs. 5.21–5.28). Occasionally, the fronds appear to be "free-floating" within the vessel lumen. Extravascular extension may occasionally be seen, although it is usually not extensive.

The following features differentiate PEH from angiosarcoma, a tumor with which it has occasionally been confused: (a) the frequent confinement of the process to a vascular lumen; (b) lack of cellular pleomorphism; (c) the typical arrangement of the endothelium in a monolayer; (d) low mitotic rate; and (e) lack of cellular necrosis (e-Figs. 5.27 and 5.28).

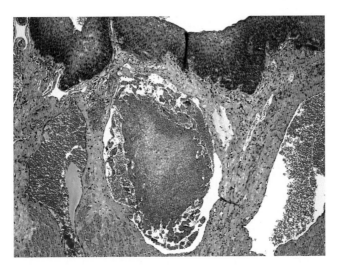

FIGURE 5.8 **Papillary endothelial hyperplasia (PEH).** PEH is characterized by papillary fronds with a core of fibrin or hyalinized collagen, lined by a single layer of endothelial cells. Note the lack of atypia.

INFECTIOUS PROCTITIS

Herpes Simplex Virus Proctitis

Herpes simplex virus (HSV) proctitis has the same viral cytopathic features as HSV elsewhere in the body. It is associated with the presence of genital lesions, as well as with penoanal intercourse (27–30). Biopsies usually show characteristic multinucleated cells, with smudged intranuclear inclusions in squamous epithelial cells at the edge of ulcers (Fig. 5.9,

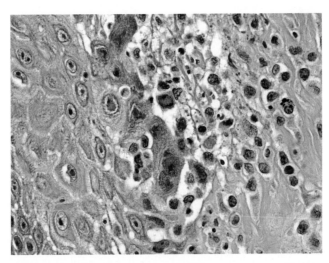

FIGURE 5.9 **Herpes simplex virus (HSV) proctitis.** Squamous epithelial cells infected with HSV show smudged intranuclear inclusions with chromatin margination of squamous epithelial cells.

e-Figs. 5.29 and 5.30). Immunohistochemistry can be helpful in confirming an impression of HSV proctitis (e-Fig. 5.30).

Cytomegalovirus Proctitis

Cytomegalovirus (CMV) proctitis is typically encountered in HIV/AIDS patients but can also arise in individuals with inflammatory bowel disease taking immunomodulation therapy and diabetics occasionally in immuno-competent persons (31). Patients can present with hematochezia second-ary to the ischemia that results from infected endothelial cells. The viral cytopathic effect in CMV proctitis is the same as that in other sites with both nuclear and cytoplasmic inclusions that enlarge the infected cells—typically endothelial cells or fibroblasts. The neighboring epithelium often displays prominent apoptosis. Most examples can be readily diagnosed on H&E stains but immunolabeling can be helpful in some examples (Fig. 5.10, e-Figs. 5.31 and 5.32). As in other anatomic locations, viral proctitis is often accompanied by a mononuclear infiltrate (e-Fig. 5.31).

Syphilis Proctitis

Treponema pallidum is the causative agent of syphilis, a sexually transmitted disease characterized by primary, secondary, and tertiary stages. As noted in Chapter 4, the primary stage presents with a chancre, a painless firm, red lesion at the site of inoculation, which heals after 3 to 6 weeks. The second-ary stage, characterized by a maculopapular rash, is the result of spirochete multiplication within the skin and mucous membranes and occurs 2 to 10 weeks after the initial stage. Condyloma lata (raised, broad-based plaques) may be seen during this stage and may provoke concern for HPV infection,

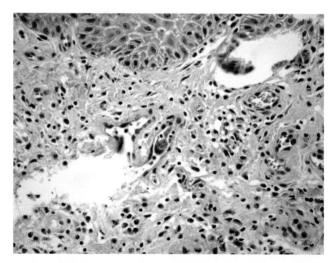

FIGURE 5.10 **Cytomegalovirus (CMV) proctitis.** The classic viral cytopathic changes with large intranuclear and smaller intracytoplasmic inclusions are seen here within an endothe-lial cell. Note the associated mononuclear response.

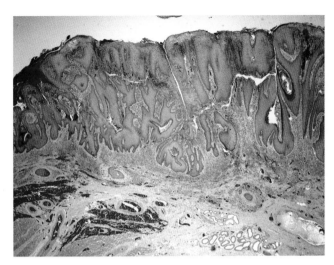

FIGURE 5.11 **Condyloma lata**. Note the striking acanthosis, broadening, and elongation of rete ridges associated with a massive mononuclear response.

especially in the anal area. Condyloma lata displays acanthosis that can be striking, surface erosion, broadening and elongation of rete ridges, exocytosis and neutrophils in the most superficial layers, and spongiosis (32). Vessels may show endothelial swelling and proliferation and may be encircled by a cuff of plasma cells (32) (Fig. 5.11, e-Figs. 5.33–5.38). Although it is not widely available, there is an antibody to *T. pallidum* that can be used to confirm the diagnosis (33–35) (Fig. 5.12, e-Fig. 5.39). The antibody cross reacts with the agent of "intestinal spirochetosis" (e-Figs. 5.40 and 5.41).

The tertiary stage of syphilis is now rare since antibiotics are readily available but is characterized by aortitis, tabes dorsalis, and gummas

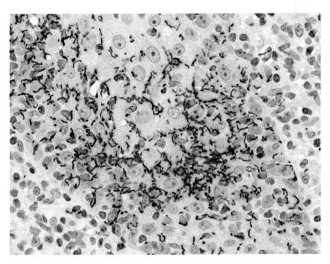

FIGURE 5.12 **Syphilis proctitis**. Though not widely available, an immunohistochemical stain for *T. pallidum* may be used to confirm the diagnosis.

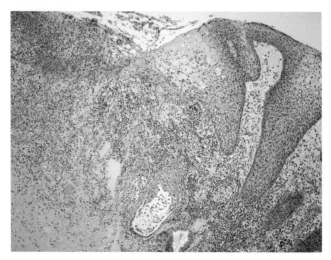

FIGURE 5.13 **Syphilis proctitis.** This ulcerated lesion is at the junction between squamous and colorectal mucosa. The process is rich in plasma cells.

(rubbery nodules composed of a necrotic center with surrounding macrophages, fibroblasts, lymphocytes, and plasma cells).

Endoscopically, syphilitic proctitis may present granular, friable, erythematous, thick, or ulcerated mucosa (36–38). On histologic exam of anal mucosa, one sees ulceration, granulation tissue, and massive associated mucosal and submucosal lymphoplasmacytic infiltration that tends to be angiocentric (Figs. 5.13 and 5.14, e-Figs. 5.42–5.46). Poorly formed

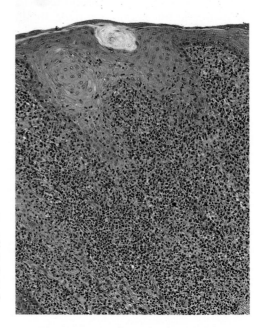

FIGURE 5.14 **Anal syphilis.** Though the findings are not wholly specific, one should consider this diagnostic possibility when one sees a massive mononuclear inflammatory response rich in plasma cells (photomicrograph provided as a kind courtesy of Dr. Fabio Facchetti).

granulomas may be present (e-Fig. 5.46). Although silver stains can highlight the spirochetes, these are frequently not identified. Definitive diagnosis requires serologic confirmation with rapid plasma reagin (RPR), fluorescent treponemal antibody-absorption test (FTA), or immunolabeling.

Lymphogranuloma Venereum Proctitis

Chlamydia trachomatis, serotypes L1, L2, and L3, is the causative agent of lymphogranuloma venereum (LGV), although other subtypes of this organism can cause cervicitis, endometritis, urethritis, and trachoma (39). Recently, outbreaks have been reported in men who have sex with men (MSM) (39). Traditionally, LGV initially presented with a penile papule followed by a secondary stage featuring tender inguinal lymphadenitis (Bubos). However, in the MSM population, the presentation at all stages may include rectal discharge and proctitis with a tertiary stage of anorectal strictures, perirectal abscesses, genital elephantiasis, penile deformities, and esthiomene (a chronic ulcer) (39). The diagnosis can be established by serology or PCR and the infection is treated with doxycycline.

The reported histologic findings in LGV are relatively nonspecific and overlap with those of syphilis proctitis and thus the diagnosis must be confirmed by laboratory testing. Depending on the stage of the disease, biopsies may demonstrate mucosal ulcers, prominent chronic inflammation, and fibrosis. Biopsies showing rectal mucosa may display distorted crypt architecture and lamina propria fibrosis (40) (e-Figs. 5.47–5.50).

CONDYLOMA AND HUMAN PAPILLOMA VIRUS–ASSOCIATED LESIONS

Condylomas and anal intraepithelial neoplasia are considered in Volume 2.

CROHN DISEASE

In patients with Crohn disease, a variety of perianal manifestations may occur, including anogenital skin lesions (anal skin tags, hemorrhoids, tumor-like lesions (41) [rare]), anal canal lesions (anal fissures, anal ulcers, and anorectal strictures), perianal fistulas and abscesses, rectovaginal fistulas, and cancer (42). However, some observers contest whether the risk of anal cancer is truly elevated (3). The etiology of Crohn perianal fistulas may be a *fistula-in-ano*, arising from dilated and inflamed, or infected anal glands and/or the penetration of fissures or ulcers in the rectum or anal canal. Most patients with Crohn disease who have anorectal or rectovaginal fistulas also have inflammatory involvement of the colon/rectum, while those with disease limited to the small bowel uncommonly develop anorectal/rectovaginal complications (43). In 1978, Hughes proposed an anatomic and pathologic classification for perianal Crohn disease (the Cardiff classification), in which each major manifestation of perianal Crohn disease (ulceration, fistula, and stricture) is graded on a scale of

0 to 2 (0, absent; 2, severe). Fistulas are also classified as low (not extending above the dentate line) or high (extending above the dentate line, sometimes to the levator muscles). Also noted in Hughes work are other associated anal conditions, the intestinal location of other sites of Crohn disease, and a global assessment of the activity of the perianal disease (44). Despite its descriptive accuracy and comprehensiveness, the Cardiff classification system has never gained widespread acceptance because of the perception by clinicians that it is of limited clinical relevance (45,46).

In ulcerative colitis, involvement of the anal canal is typically nonspecific and unrelated to the inflammatory disease. In contrast, in Crohn disease, the anal canal itself is affected in about 25% of patients with classic small intestinal disease and in up to 80% of those with colonic involvement. Anal disease may be the initial manifestation in about one-third of patients with Crohn disease. Biopsies may display a patchy, active chronic inflammatory process, but fissures, fistulas, and striking chronic inflammatory infiltrates are the hallmark (Figs. 5.15–5.16, e-Figs. 5.51–5.57). However, unless granulomas are detected, biopsy features are not specific and must be correlated with clinical ones. Anal biopsies are not commonly encountered in Crohn disease simply because they cause a certain amount of morbidity, themselves, so clinicians are reluctant to perform them. With anal Crohn disease, the issue of treatment is far more compelling than that of biopsy interpretation (42).

There are no controlled trials showing that antibiotics are effective in the treatment of Crohn perianal fistulas. However, metronidazole, as well as antimetabolites (such as azathioprine, 6-mercaptopurine, tacrolimus, and cyclosporine), has been used with some reported success. In addition, infliximab (Remicade, a mouse/human chimeric monoclonal antibody to tumor necrosis factor) is effective in the treatment of Crohn

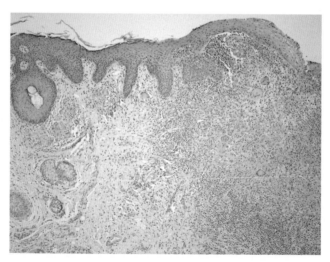

FIGURE 5.15 **Anal Crohn disease.** Note the prominent granulomatous inflammation.

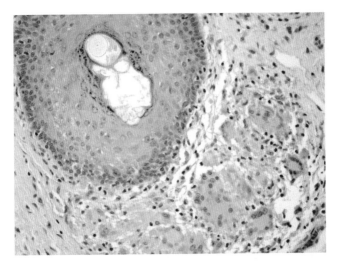

FIGURE 5.16 **Anal Crohn disease.** Higher magnification image of Figure 5.15 highlighting giant cells.

perianal fistulas. Adverse events observed in patients treated with infliximab include infusion reactions, delayed hypersensitivity reactions, formation of human antichimeric antibodies, formation of antinuclear antibodies, and anti–double-stranded DNA antibodies, and drug-induced lupus. Concomitant immunosuppressive therapy with azathioprine, 6-mercaptopurine, or methotrexate has been recommended to reduce the frequency of these reactions, which are largely due to an immunogenic response to the murine component of the chimeric antibody. There is also an increased overall rate of infection and, rarely, serious infections including pneumonia, sepsis, tuberculosis, histoplasmosis, coccidioidomycosis, listeriosis, *Pneumocystis carinii* pneumonia, and aspergillosis occur.

Surgical intervention for minor anal conditions is not without difficulties in these patients. Individuals with Crohn disease may have typical Crohn disease skin tags, which are large, edematous, hard, cyanotic, and often tender or painful, and a variety of other skin tags including long (up to 2 cm), narrow polypoid lesions (fibroepithelial polyp, see below) and large, flat "elephant ear" tags, which are soft and painless. Although some investigators have advocated excisional biopsy of typical Crohn disease skin tags to aid in the diagnosis, the typical appearance and risk of postoperative complications, poor wound healing, and rare requisite for proctectomy preclude routine biopsy or excision. On the other hand, the fibroepithelial polypoid tags and elephant ear tags can be locally excised if clinically indicated in patients experiencing difficulty with perianal hygiene or toileting, without concerns about wound healing (however, excision of these innocuous tags is rarely required). When symptomatic prolapsing or bleeding hemorrhoids fail to respond to conservative measures, in the absence of active anorectal Crohn disease, elastic band ligation may be used with great effect. It should also be noted that in patients without a preceding history or diagnosis of Crohn disease, who have a nonhealed hemorrhoidectomy wound from 2 to 3 months postoperatively, investigation (including colonoscopy) is warranted to rule out occult Crohn disease.

Anal fissures in patients with Crohn disease are usually painless and heal spontaneously. Surgical intervention in unselected patients does not improve the outcome and should generally be avoided.

Anal or rectal strictures may arise as complications of ulceration of the anal canal or rectum, perianal abscesses, and perianal fistulas and are often associated with ongoing rectal inflammation, complex perianal fistulas, and rectovaginal fistulas. Anal strictures may be short (< 2 cm in length) and annular (which result in a diaphragm-like deformity) or long and tubular. Symptoms related to toileting are typically those of urgency, incontinence, tenesmus, frequency, and difficulty with defecation. Many patients are asymptomatic and do not require treatment. For symptomatic patients, treatment consists of dilation; often, multiple dilations are required.

Deep perianal abscesses may be associated with a high perianal fistula and should be treated with incision and drainage.

The surgical treatment of perianal fistulas in patients with Crohn disease is determined by the presence or absence of macroscopic evidence of inflammation in the rectum, and the type and location of the fistula. Patients who have low fistulas (superficial, low intersphincteric, or low transsphincteric) may be treated by laying open the fistula tract through 1- or 2-stage fistulotomy. Fistulotomy is widely used by surgeons to treat simple fistulas, and this procedure results in a high rate of healing that is often sustained. The prevailing view among surgeons is that patients with a simple fistula, but who do not respond to a short course of antibiotics, are best treated with fistulotomy. More recently, fibrin glue and bioprosthetic fistula plugs have been tested with some success in patients with Crohn disease (47,48). The immunosuppressive medications azathioprine and 6-mercaptopurine can be used to treat simple fistulas and are recommended in practice guidelines. However, they have not been evaluated in placebo-controlled trials.

Infliximab has been proven effective in placebo-controlled trials for the indications of both reduction in the number of draining fistulas and maintenance of that reduction.

REFERENCES

1. Edge S, Byrd D, Compton C, et al. eds. *AJCC cancer staging manual.* New York: Springer; 2010.
2. Rickert RR, Compton CC. Protocol for the examination of specimens from patients with carcinomas of the anus and anal canal: a basis for checklists. Cancer Committee of the College of American Pathologists. *Arch Pathol Lab Med.* 2000;124:21–25.
3. Ryan DP, Compton CC, Mayer RJ. Carcinoma of the anal canal. *N Engl J Med.* 2000;342:792–800.

4. Seow-Choen F, Ho JM. Histoanatomy of anal glands. *Dis Colon Rectum*. 1994; 37:1215–1218.

5. Jemal A, Siegel R, Xu J, et al. Cancer statistics, 2010. *CA Cancer J Clin*. 2010;60:277–300.

6. Da Silva GM, Berho M, Wexner SD, et al. Histologic analysis of the irradiated anal sphincter. *Dis Colon Rectum*. 2003;46:1492–1497.

7. American Gastroenterological Association medical position statement: diagnosis and treatment of hemorrhoids. *Gastroenterology*. 2004;126:1461–1462.

8. Madoff RD, Fleshman JW. American Gastroenterological Association technical review on the diagnosis and treatment of hemorrhoids. *Gastroenterology*. 2004;126:1463–1473.

9. Hulme-Moir M, Bartolo DC. Hemorrhoids. *Gastroenterol Clin North Am*. 2001;30: 183–197.

10. Gearhart S. Is fiber beneficial for the treatment of hemorrhoids? *Nat Clin Pract Gastroenterol Hepatol*. 2006;3:192–193.

11. Sohn N, Robilotti JG, Jr. The gay bowel syndrome. A review of colonic and rectal conditions in 200 male homosexuals. *Am J Gastroenterol*. 1977;67:478–484.

12. Gonzalez-Ruiz C, Heartfield W, Briggs B, et al. Anorectal pathology in HIV/AIDS-infected patients has not been impacted by highly active antiretroviral therapy. *Dis Colon Rectum*. 2004;47:1483–1486.

13. Bresci G, Gambardella L, Parisi G, et al. Colonic disease in cirrhotic patients with portal hypertension: an endoscopic and clinical evaluation. *J Clin Gastroenterol*. 1998; 26:222–227.

14. Gearhart SL. Symptomatic hemorrhoids. *Adv Surg*. 2004;38:167–182.

15. Banov L Jr, Knoepp LF Jr, Erdman LH, et al. Management of hemorrhoidal disease. *J S C Med Assoc*. 1985;81:398–401.

16. Kaftan SM, Haboubi NY. Histopathological changes in haemorrhoid associated mucosa and submucosa. *Int J Colorectal Dis*. 1995;10:15–18.

17. Val-Bernal JF, Pinto J. Pagetoid dyskeratosis is a frequent incidental finding in hemorrhoidal disease. *Arch Pathol Lab Med*. 2001;125:1058–1062.

18. Amerigo J, Berry CL. Intravascular papillary endothelial hyperplasia in the skin and subcutaneous tissue. *Virchows Arch A Pathol Anat Histol*. 1980;387:81–90.

19. Barr RJ, Graham JH, Sherwin LA. Intravascular papillary endothelial hyperplasia. A benign lesion mimicking angiosarcoma. *Arch Dermatol*. 1978;114:723–726.

20. Clearkin KP, Enzinger FM. Intravascular papillary endothelial hyperplasia. *Arch Pathol Lab Med*. 1976;100:441–444.

21. Dunphy CH, Sotelo-Avila C, Luisiri A, et al. Paroxysmal nocturnal hemoglobinuria associated with venous thrombosis and papillary endothelial hyperplasia presenting as ulcerated duodenal mass. *Arch Pathol Lab Med*. 1994;118:837–839.

22. Park JY, Chung-Park M, Snow M. Intravascular papillary endothelial hyperplasia of superior vena cava: a rare cause of the superior vena cava syndrome. *Thorax*. 1991;46:272–273.

23. Romani J, Puig L, Costa I, et al. Masson's intravascular papillary endothelial hyperplasia mimicking Stewart-Treves syndrome: report of a case. *Cutis*. 1997;59:148–150.

24. Schwartz IS, Parris A. Cutaneous intravascular papillary endothelial hyperplasia: a benign lesion that may simulate angiosarcoma. *Cutis*. 1982;29:66–69, 72–64.

25. Stewart M, Smoller BR. Multiple lesions of intravascular papillary endothelial hyperplasia (Masson's lesions). *Arch Pathol Lab Med*. 1994;118:315–316.

26. Masson P. Hemangioendotheliome vegetant intravasculaire. *Bull Soc Anat Paris*. 1923;93:517–523.

27. Evans BA, Kell PD, Bond RA, et al. Predictors of seropositivity to herpes simplex virus type 2 in women. *Int J STD AIDS*. 2003;14:30–36.

28. Jacobs E. Anal infections caused by herpes simplex virus. *Dis Colon Rectum*. 1976; 19:151–157.

29. Krone MR, Tabet SR, Paradise M, et al. Herpes simplex virus shedding among human immunodeficiency virus-negative men who have sex with men: site and frequency of shedding. *J Infect Dis*. 1998;178:978–982.

30. van de Laar MJ, Termorshuizen F, Slomka MJ, et al. Prevalence and correlates of herpes simplex virus type 2 infection: evaluation of behavioural risk factors. *Int J Epidemiol*. 1998;27:127–134.

31. Alam I, Shanoon D, Alhamdani A, et al. Severe proctitis, perforation, and fatal rectal bleeding secondary to cytomegalovirus in an immunocompetent patient: report of a case. *Surg Today*. 2007;37:66–69.

32. Pandhi RK, Singh N, Ramam M. Secondary syphilis: a clinicopathologic study. *Int J Dermatol*. 1995;34:240–243.

33. Buffet M, Grange PA, Gerhardt P, et al. Diagnosing *Treponema pallidum* in secondary syphilis by PCR and immunohistochemistry. *J Invest Dermatol*. 2007;127:2345–2350.

34. Facchetti F, Incardona P, Lonardi S, et al. Nodal inflammatory pseudotumor caused by luetic infection. *Am J Surg Pathol*. 2009;33:447–453.

35. Venturini M, Sala R, Semenza D, et al. Reflectance confocal microscopy for the in vivo detection of *Treponema pallidum* in skin lesions of secondary syphilis. *J Am Acad Dermatol*. 2009;60:639–642.

36. Furman DL, Patel SK, Arluk GM. Endoscopic and histologic appearance of rectal syphilis. *Gastrointest Endosc*. 2008;67:161; commentary 161–162.

37. Nazemi MM, Musher DM, Schell RF, et al. Syphilitic proctitis in a homosexual. *JAMA*. 1975;231:389.

38. Teitelman M, Wilson JA, Guy CD. Image of the month. Syphilitic proctitis. *Clin Gastroenterol Hepatol*. 2008;6:xxvi.

39. Kapoor S. Re-emergence of lymphogranuloma venereum. *J Eur Acad Dermatol Venereol*. 2008;22:409–416.

40. Martin IM, Alexander SA, Ison CA, et al. Diagnosis of lymphogranuloma venereum from biopsy samples. *Gut*. 2006;55:1522–1523.

41. Kim BS, Kim HS, Kim MB, et al. Perianal Crohn's disease with a clenched fist-like appearance. *J Eur Acad Dermatol Venereol*. 2009;23:1197–1198.

42. Sandborn WJ, Fazio VW, Feagan BG, et al. AGA technical review on perianal Crohn's disease. *Gastroenterology*. 2003;125:1508–1530.

43. Bell SJ, Williams AB, Wiesel P, et al. The clinical course of fistulating Crohn's disease. *Aliment Pharmacol Ther*. 2003;17:1145–1151.

44. Hughes LE. Surgical pathology and management of anorectal Crohn's disease. *J R Soc Med*. 1978;71:644–651.

45. Francois Y, Vignal J, Descos L. Outcome of perianal fistulae in Crohn's disease–value of Hughes' pathogenic classification. *Int J Colorectal Dis*. 1993;8:39–41.

46. Hughes LE. Clinical classification of perianal Crohn's disease. *Dis Colon Rectum*. 1992;35:928–932.

47. Grimaud JC, Munoz-Bongrand N, Siproudhis L, et al. Fibrin glue is effective healing perianal fistulas in patients with Crohn's disease. *Gastroenterology*. 2010;138:2275–2281, 2281 e2271.

48. Schwandner O, Fuerst A. Preliminary results on efficacy in closure of transsphincteric and rectovaginal fistulas associated with Crohn's disease using new biomaterials. *Surg Innov*. 2009;16:162–168.

INDEX